Educational Opportunities in

Integrative Medicine

A
know your source
GUIDE

Educational Opportunities in

Integrative Medicine

The A to Z Healing Arts Guide and Professional Resource Directory

Douglas "Las" Wengell, MBA

With Nathen Gabriel, ND

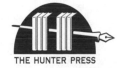

THE HUNTER PRESS

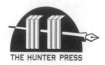

THE HUNTER PRESS

Cover design by Alison Scheel
Interior design by The Roberts Group

Manufactured in the United States of America

10 9 8 7 6 1 2 3 4 5

Publisher's Cataloging-in-Publication
(Provided by Quality Books, Inc.)

Wengell, Douglas A.
    Educational opportunities in integrative medicine :
the A to Z healing arts guide and professional resource
directory / Douglas "Las" Wengell ; with Nathen Gabriel.
    p. cm.
    Includes bibliographical references and index.
    LCCN 2008928503
    ISBN-13: 978-0-9776552-4-3
    ISBN-10: 0-9776552-4-5

    1. Integrative medicine--Vocational guidance.
2. Alternative medicine--Vocational guidance.
3. Integrative medicine--Study and teaching--Directories.
4. Alternative medicine--Study and teaching--
Directories. I. Gabriel, Nathen. II. Title.

R735.W46 2008   610.7
          QBI08-600179

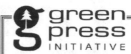

Know Your Source Inc. is committed to preserving ancient forests and natural resources. We elected to print this title on 30% post consumer recycled paper, processed chlorine free. As a result, for this printing, we have saved:

31 Trees (40' tall and 6-8" diameter)
11,255 Gallons of Wastewater
21 million BTU's of Total Energy
1,445 Pounds of Solid Waste
2,712 Pounds of Greenhouse Gases

Know Your Source Inc. made this paper choice because our printer, Thomson-Shore, Inc., is a member of Green Press Initiative, a nonprofit program dedicated to supporting authors, publishers, and suppliers in their efforts to reduce their use of fiber obtained from endangered forests.

For more information, visit www.greenpressinitiative.org

Environmental impact estimates were made using the Environmental Defense Paper Calculator. For more information visit: www.papercalculator.org.

Please send updates and new resources for future editions to updates@thehunterpress.com.

In Loving Memory of

David Wengell (1976–2008)
An iron-willed fighter with a heart of gold

TABLE OF CONTENTS

FOREWORD

Adam Perlman, MD, MPH, FACP

> **THERE IS** a yearning on the part of patients and many providers for a more patient-centered approach to care: an approach that values evidence, but respects patient's preferences; an approach that focuses on health and healing; and an approach that is inclusive and respectful of other healing traditions as well as individuals who practice those traditions. A term that has come to define that approach to care is integrative medicine.

That health care in the United States is in crisis is no surprise to patients or providers. Millions of people are under- or uninsured. Medicare is projected to run out of money in just a few years—and just at a time when seniors are the fastest growing segment of the population and dissatisfaction with the state of our health care system, by both health care providers and the public, is widespread. It is perhaps due to this state of crisis and concern that both the public and health professionals are looking for alternatives. One clear sign of this is the growing interest, utilization, and acceptance of methods and modalities currently categorized as complementary and alternative medicine (CAM). Although people have perhaps always used techniques for their health which were not considered part of the conventional or dominant health care system, never before in this country has the dominant system, allopathic medicine, been so accepting and willing to integrate therapies and practitioners from other systems.

Certainly, the entire conventional medical establishment is not embracing CAM with open arms. But the inclusion of CAM content in many medical, nursing, and allied health school curriculums; a National Institutes of Health Center dedicated to research on CAM; and the creation of the Consortium of Academic Health Centers for Integrative Medicine, made up of forty-one leading medical schools as of 2008, all with integrative medicine centers, are just a few examples of integration and acceptance that did not exist just a few years ago.

However, this trend is not driven by a desire to "substitute Saint John's Wort for Prozac," but rather a yearning on the part of patients and many providers for a more patient-centered approach to care: an approach that values evidence, but respects patient's preferences; an approach that focuses on health and healing; and an approach that is inclusive and respectful of other healing traditions as well as individuals who practice those traditions. A term that has come to define that approach to care is integrative medicine. Although initially coined by Dr Andrew Weil as a way to describe this practice by physicians, those using this term should not fail to recognize the significant number of nursing and allied health professionals with interest and expertise in this area, and the importance of the role of CAM providers.

As interest in integrative medicine has grown, so has the need for training and educational programs. At the University of Medicine and Dentistry of New Jersey, through our Institute for Complementary and Alternative Medicine, we have recently developed an integrative health and wellness track within the master's of health sciences program. In addition, we've incorporated significant content on integrative medicine into the medical and allied health schools curriculum and have partnered with a massage school to offer a certificate training program for massage therapists in orthopedic massage. These are just a few examples of the types of educational opportunities that exist across the country and are offered by both conventional and CAM institutions.

With the growth in the number and breadth of educational opportunities as well as interest in the CAM fields and integrative medicine, the need has developed for a reliable resource and education guide that can be used by health care providers, both conventional and CAM, as well as the general public. This book fulfills that need. My hope is that resources such as this will be used to facilitate the education of both conventional and CAM providers as well as the public, leading to an increase in the integrative approach to care and, ultimately, an improved health care system as well as improved health for all.

Yours in good health,
Adam Perlman, MD, MPH, FACP

INTRODUCTION

WE CAN improve our health care system dramatically by expanding our views of disease, prevention, and well-being beyond the relatively strict Western paradigm. This movement has already begun, and it's called integrative medicine.

The healing arts date back to the dawn of civilizations the world over. Nearly 2000 years before Hippocrates and the Greeks set in motion the Western scientific method, Asian and American cultures grappled with health and disease. It wasn't until the last two centuries that non-Western and folk traditions began to be widely noticed in the United States and only in the last two decades that they began to be tested and considered in the context of healing the whole person. This guidebook is designed to help students and practitioners discover where they fit along the wide spectrum between scientific, empirical, and soulful medicine, and what career track to pursue.

Whatever discipline you choose, whether just starting out or expanding your horizons, you should do so with a full understanding of the economic and social dimensions of our nation's health care system, and the opportunities and challenges it presents. Seven years ago, the World Health Organization made the first major effort to rank the health care systems of 191 nations. France and Italy took the top two spots; the United States was an embarrassing thirty-seventh. More recently, the highly regarded Commonwealth Fund, an American foundation advocating for a high performance health care system, ranked the U.S. last or next-to-last compared with five other advanced nations—Australia, Canada, Germany, New Zealand, and the United Kingdom—on most measures of objective performance, including quality of care and access to it.

We have long known that the United States has a high infant mortality rate, so it is no surprise that we rank last among twenty-three nations by that yardstick. But the problem is broader. We are also near the bottom in life expectancy at age sixty, and fifteenth among nineteen countries in deaths from a wide range of illnesses that would not have been fatal if treated with timely and effective care. We have done a better job than other industrialized nations in reducing smoking; however, our obesity epidemic is the worst in the world and it affects our nation's children in ways other first world nations think unconscionable.

All other major industrialized nations provide universal health coverage, and most of them have comprehensive benefit packages. The United States, the wealthiest and most powerful nation in the history of the world, has some 45 million people without health insurance and many more millions who have inadequate poor coverage. Studies have shown that people without insurance postpone treatment until a minor illness becomes worse, harming their own health and imposing greater costs to themselves, their community and all of society.

It is unfair to characterize allopathic medicine as the reason for our problems. For starters, consider the huge advances in public health such as fluorinated drinking water, infectious disease control, immunizations, lower infant mortality rates, fewer deaths from heart disease, and nutrition labeling. Much of the efficacy of allopathic medicine rests on the miraculous scientific advances seen in pharmacology, surgery, neurology, genetics, and technological tools such as MRIs and CT scans. These powerful techniques have dominated conventional health care during the last century—and for good reason. They work. If you require intrusive or emergency medicine in the event of a traumatic injury, there is nothing better than our world-class intensive care units. If you require the removal of a cancer or cataract, there is nothing better than a modern operating room under the steady hand of surgeons with a decade of arduous training. If you are one of the 20 or so million Americans who at any moment struggle with depression, SSRIs such as Prozac and Zoloft, while far from perfect and not a cure, mitigate suffering in ways previous generations could hardly imagine.

Whether or not our system of health care becomes socialized, we can improve it dramatically by expanding our views of disease, prevention, and well-being beyond the relatively strict Western paradigm. This movement has already begun, and it's called integrative medicine.

"Complementary and alternative medicine" describes any number of legitimate and unofficial non-allopathic modalities, many of which date back to the human potential movement of the 1960s, which in turn borrowed from Eastern and folk traditions. It was fed by Americans looking to heal chronic or difficult-to-diagnose diseases which allopathic medicine was unable to address, those seeking preventive care, or those wanting more authentic relationships with their health care provider.

With the launch in the 1990s of the National Center for Complementary and Alternative Medicine (part of the U.S. National Institutes of Health), many of these disciplines began to be researched and explored. By 1998, two seminal studies were published in the *Journal of the American Medical Association* and delivered surprising news: an astonishing 42 percent of Americans had sought some form of nontraditional medical care, most commonly chiropractic medicine, with this number surpassing the number of visits to traditional medical physicians. Patient encounters to CAM practitioners totaled an incredible 629 million visits in one year.

Only in the last decade has there been a concerted effort to merge the conventional and the alternative under the umbrella called integrative medicine. Astonishingly, in 2004, 18 percent of American hospitals offered complementary and alternative services, up from half that five years prior. During this time, the Consortium of Academic Health Centers for Integrative Medicine was inaugurated, dedicated to "transform medicine and health care through rigorous scientific studies, new models of clinical care, and innovative educational programs that integrate biomedicine, the complexity of human beings, the intrinsic nature of healing, and the rich diversity of therapeutic systems." Leading edge member institutions—the Program in Integrative Medicine at the University of Arizona School of Medicine, home of Dr. Andrew Weil; Georgetown School of Medicine; Harvard's Osher Institute; and the Centers for Integrative Medicine at Duke and University of California–San Francisco, among many others—represent the early signs of mainstream acceptance, with popular CAM offerings including acupuncture, massage therapy, mind-body therapies, nutritional counseling, physical Yoga, and mindfulness-based stress reduction (a secular form of meditation).

Integrative medicine lacks a clear definition because it is both interdisciplinary and includes dimensions of health that are not easily quantifiable. In general, integrative medicine:

- Recognizes that the mind affects the body, and the body the mind, and that there are modalities to influence one another in ways that foster comprehensive healing.

- Acknowledges the spiritual dimension of health and illness for the individual.

- Explores with an open mind global medical modalities not yet vetted by Western science.

- Fosters authentic empathic relationships between healer and patient.

- Promotes self-healing, prevention, tailored remedies, and personal responsibility.

- Advances evidence-based testing.

To be an integrative practitioner is not so much

to practice a predefined set of techniques, or to have a series of letters behind your name. At root, it's a perspective, an orientation, a worldview. Inherent to this view: inclusivity, tolerance, curiosity, pluralism, humility, personal experience, intellectual curiosity, empathy, and wonder. It's a belief that the human experience cannot be narrowly defined to merely one dimension; that we are physical beings governed by natural law but that we also have rich and complex inner lives. It's a deep and burning desire to realize our potential, find purpose in our life, and feel awe and reverence at being alive.

The next step is synthesis. In 2002, the White House Commission on Complementary and Alternative Medicine Policy report, written on behalf of the president, articulated the challenge of combining CAM and allopathic medicine: "The perception that conventional health care emphasizes high technology approaches to treating patients, while CAM health care emphasizes low technology approaches to promoting health and preventing disease, has led some to suggest that conventional and CAM health care may eventually converge to form a new health care system that integrates the best of each. However, there are not only scientific, but also educational, regulatory, and political obstacles to integration of the two systems."

In other words, integration is easier in theory than practice. One reality is that in order to categorize and make sense of knowledge, it's parceled into narrow sources of inquiry. In the tunnel vision of one discipline, it's easy to lose the big picture and difficult to teach a humanistic, patient-centered perspective if you haven't first mastered the basics. This is true in art as well as science. The body of medical knowledge is now so vast that it's impossible to know everything. Medical doctors become experts in sub-sub-subspecialties and refer clients to experts they sat next to in medical school. This has helped allopathic medicine explore the far reaches of disease and ailments in ways our ancestors would have a hard time believing. But in the process, with a paternal hubris and a denial of its limitations, mainstream medicine lost its soul.

The challenge is now to come full circle with a paradigm that is preventive, holistic, and integrative in orientation. In addition to the leadership of a new generation of practitioners, research centers, and foundations, there is a real possibility that a new administration will begin to address some of these hopes. During the 2008 primaries, for example, presidential candidates from both sides acknowledged that we should fund preventive medicine. Epidemiologists in general as well as other first world nations have long known that prevention is more economical in the long run, and this reasoning may be the most persuasive argument to Washington policy makers. Whatever the outcome of the election, however, transformation is inevitable. If you are a student looking at a career in health care, the upside is that, with the mainstream now on board and with the old school style of conventional medicine fading, you have the opportunity to be a powerful agent of change during your career.

The era of a mechanistic, reductionist, linear view of the world will not survive because it is an inadequate model when it comes to representing the complexities of our world. Advances in quantum physics already portend this revolution in thinking. As we move toward greater levels of connectivity, convergence, and integration—between old and new, East and West, ancient and modern—there is the hope that as the world gets smaller it also gets smarter. A medical pluralism is about taking the best of everything and moving forward. The transition will not be easy. But it is rich in possibility. Best of all, it's a future that can be embraced today.

I look forward to a medical establishment that puts as much focus on health and wellness as it does disease: a society in which a newborn comes into the world by a physician-midwife team; an adult is treated by holistic practitioners for everyday ailments and assisted by nurturing allopaths in all the many areas they excel; a frail elder is tended with compassion by a hospice counselor and a palliative care physician. I look forward to a health care system where engaged patients form healing partnerships with collaborative practitioners who offer a globalized range of both complementary and conventional modalities. Patients, practitioners, and planet—that's all we've got. Let's get to work.

Douglas "Las" Wengell
Burlington, Vermont

The Spectrum of Healing Modalities

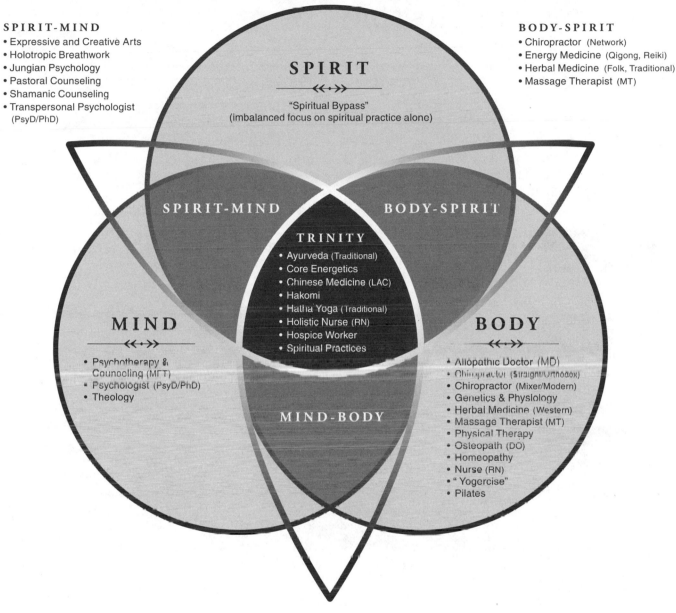

SPIRIT-MIND
- Expressive and Creative Arts
- Holotropic Breathwork
- Jungian Psychology
- Pastoral Counseling
- Shamanic Counseling
- Transpersonal Psychologist
  (PsyD/PhD)

BODY-SPIRIT
- Chiropractor (Network)
- Energy Medicine (Qigong, Reiki)
- Herbal Medicine (Folk, Traditional)
- Massage Therapist (MT)

SPIRIT
<<•>>
"Spiritual Bypass"
(imbalanced focus on spiritual practice alone)

SPIRIT-MIND

BODY-SPIRIT

TRINITY
- Ayurveda (Traditional)
- Core Energetics
- Chinese Medicine (LAC)
- Hakomi
- Hatha Yoga (Traditional)
- Holistic Nurse (RN)
- Hospice Worker
- Spiritual Practices

MIND
<<•>>
- Psychotherapy & Counseling (MFT)
- Psychologist (PsyD/PhD)
- Theology

BODY
<<•>>
- Allopathic Doctor (MD)
- Chiropractor (Straight/Orthodox)
- Chiropractor (Mixer/Modern)
- Genetics & Physiology
- Herbal Medicine (Western)
- Massage Therapist (MT)
- Physical Therapy
- Osteopath (DO)
- Homeopathy
- Nurse (RN)
- " Yogercise"
- Pilates

MIND-BODY

MIND-BODY
- Ayurvedic Medicine (modern)
- Aromatherapy
- Biofeedback
- Body-Centered Psychotherapy (MFT)
- Expressive & Creative Arts
- Holistic Allopathic Doctor (MD)
- Hypnotherapy
- Midwifery
- Naturopathic Doctor (ND)
- Psychiatrist (MD)
- Social Work (MSW)
- Somatic Therapies
- Hatha Yoga (Modern)

A BIRD'S EYE VIEW

ANCIENT PRE-HISTORY

30,000 BC   100 BC

← Age of Mysticism →

AFRICA

| Cave Paintings (30,000 BC) | Shamanism (8000 BC) | Goddess Worship (7000 BC) | Egyptian Civilization (3000 BC) First Medicine, Polytheism | Babylonian Civilization (2000 BC) Astrology, Polytheism | Zoroastrianism (1000 BC) mystical tradition |

SOUTHEAST ASIA INDIA

Vedas (1500 BC) **"KNOWLEDGE"** mystical philosophy

<u>Yoga</u> *Upanishads*   **Shankara** (788 BC)   **Patanjali** (300 BC)
      Bhagavad Gita Vedanta   (Raja)*Yoga Sutras*
Ayurvedic Healing (1200 BC)
<u>Hinduism</u>

NEPAL & HIMALAYAS

<u>Buddhism</u>   Siddhartha Gautama "Buddha" (483 BC)

CHINA

| I Ching (c 2800 BC) *Book of Changes* | Acupuncture (2500 BC) | <u>Confucianism</u> | Kung Fu Tzu Confucius (479 BC) | First Chinese Medical Text (100 BC) *The Yellow Emperor's Classic* |

Lao Tzu (c 550 BC) *Tao Te Ching*   <u>Taoism</u>   Chuang Tzu (c 300 BC)

JAPAN   <u>Shinto</u> "The Way of the Gods"

THE AMERICAS

<u>Polytheism, Shamanism, Animism</u>   Norte Chico (3000 BC) First America Civilization   Mayan Civilization (1800 BC)   Shaman "they who **KNOW**"

MIDDLE EAST PALISTINE

<u>Christianity</u>   *New Testament*
Gnosticism (100 BC) sacred **"KNOWLEDGE"** mystical tradition
Kabbalah   *Hebrew Bible*
Judaic mysticism

<u>Sufism</u>   <u>Islam</u>   Muhammad (632)
Mystical tradition   Whirling Dirvish Dance

GREECE

<u>Greek Mythology, Polytheism</u>   Socrates (399 BC) **"KNOW THYSELF"**   Hippocrates (370 BC) Father Western Medicine
Aristotle (322 BC) natural philosophy
Plato (347 BC) *apriori* principles

OF SCIENCE, SPIRITUALITY AND THE HEALING ARTS

LAST 2000 YEARS

TODAY

◄─────────── Age of Reason ───────────►

| SCIENCE: | Copernicus (1543) Astronomer | Newton (1727) Physicist, alchemist philosopher | Charles Darwin (1882) On the Origin of Species | Albert Einstein (1955) Relativity | Werner Heisenberg (1976) Quantum Physics Uncertainty Principle | Stephen Hawking (living) Grand Unification Theory | Science Physics |
| | | | Robert Oppenheimer (1967) Atomic Age / nuclear medicine | | | Human Genome (2000) | Genetics Nanotechnology |

| EAST-WEST PHILOSOPHY: | Ralph Emerson (1882) Transcendentalism | Rudolf Steiner (1925) Anthroposophy | Aldous Huxley (1963) Perennial Philosophy (living) Doors of Perception | Ken Wilber | |

| EXISTENTIALISM: | Soren Kierkegaard (1955) Self-Reflection | Martin Buber 1965) I and Thou | Martin Heidegger (1976) Being and Nothingness | Philosophy Psychology Meaning Existence |

| PSYCHOLOGY: | Sigmund Freud, MD (1939) Unconscious | Wilhelm Reich, MD (1957) Mind-Body Pioneer | Carl Jung, MD (1961) Archetypes & Mythology | Abraham Maslow (1970) Self Actualization | |

| Swami Swatmarama (1550) Father of Hatha Yoga | Swami Vivekananda (1902) Vedanta | Swami Aurobindo (1950) Integral Yoga | Paramhansa Yogananda (1952) and others Western introduction | Bikram Choudhury (living) Secularized Yoga | Ayurveda Yoga Therapy Meditation |

Mahayana Buddhism
East Asian and Tibetan Buddhism (700)

Tibetan Buddhism (650)

Early Bodywork

Theravada Buddhism

Gendun Drup (14/4)
First Dalai Lama

Mindfulness
Mandala
Tantra

Chinese Buddhism (650)

Zen Buddhism
D.T. Suzuki (1966)

Chinese Medicine
Acupuncture
Tai Chi
Qigong
Martial Arts

Zen (650)

| Native Americans "Medicine People," Nature Spirits | Inca civilization (1450) Polytheistic, Sun God | Naturopathy Herbal Medicine Aromatherapy Shamanism Entheogens |

| Jesus of Nazareth | Saint Augustine (430) Christian Philosopher | Thomas Aquinas (1274) Christian Theologian Natural Theology & Metaphysics | Martin Luther (1546) Protestant Reformation | Pastoral Counseling RN |

Talmud

Ibn al-Haytham (1039) Scientist Philosopher	Rationalism (deduction)	Descartes (1650) Spinoza (1677) Leibniz (1716)	William James, MD (1910) Varieties of Religious Experience	
Sunni (675)	Abd al-Rahman al-Khazini (1130) Scientist Philosopher			Scientist Allopathic Medicine
Shi'a (675)	Nasir al-Din Tusi (1274) Scientist Philosopher	"Science" Latin scire "TO KNOW"	Charles Peirce (1914) Pragmatism	Scientific Method	DO DC
Mystery Religions Eleusinian, Dionysus, Mithras	Empiricism (induction)	Hobbes (1679) Locke (1704)	John Dewey (1952) Art as Experience		ND RN
Druids		Hume (1776)			Homeopathy

HEALTH CARE DESIGNATIONS

Diplomat

Diplomat status occurs when a medical specialist's competence has been certified by a diploma granted by an appropriate professional group. Diplomas usually require credit hours from a particular academic program. These are not state-sanctioned degrees, but come strictly from private organizations.

Certification

Certification is a title received from a state-approved school after successfully completing the school's program. This is not to be confused with professional certification, which is a degree granted by a private organization. Certification is reserved for registered practitioners of a recognized and accredited field of healing.

Degree

Degrees are conferred by a college, university, or some other educational institution as official recognition for the successful completion of an academic or vocational program. This is not a license to practice any profession. Usually a degree is a necessary perquisite for applying to a graduate program. Degrees preclude licensure.

License

A license or permit usually refers to locally earned rights to practice a particular business or style of health care. They are granted by government agencies, which allow individuals to legally practice their modality in a particular city, state, or location. A license may be required in addition to certification in order to conduct practice. For instance, a massage therapist may be certified (CMT) after graduating from school, but she or he must also apply for and be granted a license or permit to practice in most states.

Degree Acronyms

AAMA: Member of the American Academy of Medical Acupuncturists

ACSW: Academy of Certified Social Worker

ACT: Acupuncture Therapist

ADTR: American Dance Therapy Registered

AHP: Advanced Hellerwork Practitioner

AMT: Advanced Massage Therapist by the California Bureau of Private Post-Secondary Vocational Education (BPPVE)

AP: Acupuncture Physician

APP: Associate Polarity Practitioner by the American Polarity Therapy Association (APTA)

ATI: Designates teaching members of Alexander Technique International (also MATI)

ATR: Art Therapist Registered by the Art Therapy Credentials Board (ATCB)

ATR-BC: Board Certified art therapists by the Art Therapy Credentials Board (ATCB)

BAMS:: Bachelor of Ayurvedic Medicine

BCIAC: Biofeedback certification by the Biofeedback Certification Institute of America

BCD: Board Certified Diplomat

BS: Bachelor of Science (Generic)

BSN: Bachelor of Science in Nursing

CA or CAc: Certified Acupuncturist

CAC: Certified Alcohol Counselor

CAMT: Certified Acupressure Massage Therapist

CAR: Certified Advanced Rolfer by the Rolf Institute

CAT: Certified Alexander Teacher

CBT: Certified Biofeedback Therapy

CBPM: Certified Bonnie Prudden Myotherapy

CCH: Certified in Classical Homeopathy by the Council for Homeopathic Certification

CHOM: Certified Homeopathic

CHT: Certified Hypnotherapist

CLMP: Certified Licensed Massage Practitioner

CLMT: Certified Licensed Massage Therapist

CMP: Certified Massage Practitioner

CMT: Certified Massage Therapist

CN: Clinical Nutritionist

CNC: Certified Nutritional Consultant

CNP: Certified Nutritional Practitioner by the Institute of Holistic Nutrition

CNS: Certified Nurse Specialist

CPC: Certified Professional Counselor

CPT: Certified Poetry Therapist

CR: Certified Rolfer by the Rolf Institute

CST: Certified Structural Therapist

CSW: Certified Social Worker

CTP: Certified Trager Practitioner

CTPM: Certified Trigger Point Myotherapist

CVA: Certified Veterinary Acupuncturist

DAc: May indicate advanced (Doctor) training in acupuncture (or DAC). Used in some states for licensed acupuncturist (LAc)

DACS: Diplomat of the ICA Council on Applied Chiropractic Sciences

DAMS: Doctor of Ayurvedic Medicine and Surgery

DC: Doctor of Chiropractic

DCH: Doctor of Clinical Hypnotherapy

DHANP: Diplomat of the Homeopathic Association of Naturopathic Physicians

DHMS: Diplomat of Homeopathic Medicine and Surgery

DHOM: Diplomat of Homeopathic Medicine

DHt: Diplomat in Homeotherapeutics by the American Board of Homeotherapeutics

Dip ABT: Diplomat in Asian Bodywork Therapy

Dip Ac: Diplomat in Acupuncture

Dip CH: Diplomat in Chinese Herbology

Dip OM: Diplomat in Oriental Medicine

Dipl ABT: Diplomat in Asian Bodywork Therapy by the National Certification Commission for Acupuncture and Oriental Medicine Certification

Dipl Ac: Diplomat in Acupuncture by the National Certification Commission for Acupuncture and Oriental Medicine Certification

Dipl CH: Diplomat in Chinese Herbology by the National Certification Commission for Acupuncture and Oriental Medicine (NCCAOM) Certification

Dipl OM: Diplomat in Oriental Medicine by the National Certification Commission for Acupuncture and Oriental Medicine (NCCAOM) Certification

DNBAO: Diplomat in National Board of Acupuncture Orthopedics (NBAO)

DO: Doctor of Osteopathy

DOM: Doctoral Degree in Oriental Medicine (Doctor of Oriental Medicine)

DSW: Doctor of Social Work

DTR: Dance Therapist Registered

GCFP: A guild-certified Feldenkrais practitioner by the Feldenkrais Guild

HHP: Holistic Health Practitioner by the California Bureau of Private Post-Secondary Vocational Education (BPPVE)

HMD: Homeopathic Medical Doctor

LAC: Licensed Acupuncturist

LCSW: Licensed Clinical Social Worker

LicAc: Licensed Acupuncturist (also LAc)

LICSW: Licensed Independent Clinical Social Worker

LMT: Licensed Massage Therapist

LN: Licensed Nutritionist

LNC: Licensed Nutritionist Counselor

MAc: Master of Acupuncture by the Accreditation Commission for Acupuncture and Oriental Medicine

MATI: Designates teaching members of Alexander Technique International

MD: Medical Doctor

MDH: Medical Doctor of Homeopathy

MFCC: Marriage Family and Child Counselor

MHC: Mental Health Counselor

MH: Master Herbalist by the American Herbalists Guild

MBW: Master Bodyworker by the California Bureau of Private Post-Secondary Vocational Education (BPPVE)

MOM: Master's Degree in Oriental medicine from the International Institute of Chinese Medicine by the Accreditation Commission for Acupuncture and Oriental Medicine

MS: Masters of Science degree (also Master's degree in Traditional Oriental Medicine)

MSN: Master of Science in Nursing

MSW: Master of Social Work

MSTCM: Master of Science in Traditional Chinese Medicine

MSTOM: Master of Science in Traditional Oriental Medicine

MT: Massage Therapist

MTOM: Master's Degree in Traditional Oriental Medicine

NASTAT: Member of the North American Society of Teachers of the Alexander Technique

NC: Diploma in Nutritional Consulting by the Alive Academy of Natural Health

NCAD: Nationally Certified Addiction Counselor

NCADC: Nationally Certified Alcohol and Drug Counselor

NCTMB: Nationally Certified Therapeutic Massage and Bodywork

ND: Naturopathic Doctor or Doctor of Naturopathy

NMD: Doctor of Naturopathic Medicine

NT: Nutritional Counselor

OBT: Oriental Bodywork Therapist

OMD: Oriental Medical Doctor or Doctor of Oriental Medicine

PhD: Doctor of Philosophy (Generic)

PP: Polarity Practitioner

PsyD: Doctor of Clinical Psychology

QME: Qualified Medical Evaluator

RAC: Registered Acupuncturist

RCT: Registered Craniosacral Therapist

RD: Registered Dietician

RDT: Registered Dance Therapist

RHN: Registered Holistic Nutritionist (not a state officiated registration) by the Edison Institute of Nutrition (EIN)

RHom: Registered with National Union of Professional and Trained Homeopaths RMT: Registered Massage Therapist

RN: Registered Nurse

RNC: Registered Nutritional Consultant

RNCP: Registered Nutritional Consultant Practitioner

RPP: Registered Polarity Practitioner by the American Polarity Therapy Association (APTA)

RPT: Registered Poetry Therapist

RSHom, NA: Registered Member of the North American Society of Homeopaths (NASH)

ST: Somatic Therapist

LICENSED PROFESSIONS

CHAPTER 1

CHIROPRACTIC MEDICINE (DC)

The founding principles of chiropractic medicine were established during the turn of the twentieth century by Daniel David Palmer, a man with broad understanding of anatomy, physiology, and osteopathy yet no official medical training. One underlying belief of his time was that a unifying "great secret" held the key to health and illness. Palmer believed he had discovered this panacea after two remarkable incidents using hands-on joint manipulation, which resulted in an apparent cure for one patient's deafness and another's heart trouble. Palmer concluded that the metaphysical "innate intelligence" of the body expressed itself through the nervous system and that health could be optimized by ensuring an unimpeded flow of life force. The key was to keep the vertebrae in proper alignment, which is why most Americans today associate chiropractors with spinal adjustments. While joint manipulation may date as far back as the ancient Egyptians, and at least to Hippocrates circa 400 B.C., chiropractic medicine differs from these earlier traditions due to its high degree of adjustment precision.

Palmer founded the first chiropractic college, Palmer School of Chiropractic, in 1897, and he soon found himself in a lifelong squabble with the prevailing allopathic medical establishments. After being prosecuted for practicing medicine without a license, Palmer sold his school to his son, B.J., and headed west to establish more chiropractic schools. Father and son argued for years about how the discipline should be taught, and there was no resolution when the elder Palmer died in 1913. Though the elder founded chiropractic medicine, his son B.J. Palmer is credited with developing chiropractic into a powerful political force as well as a respected medical modality. B.J. created the Universal Chiropractic Association in order to resist legal attacks from the American Medical Association (AMA), and successfully marketed it as a healing modality that integrates science, art, and philosophy.

Until the 1980s, the AMA considered it "unethical" for a medical doctor to collaborate with a doctor of chiropractic (DC). But a lengthy and well-publicized court battle in 1987 determined the AMA guilty

THERE ARE primarily two schools of thought in chiropractic philosophy. The original and traditional version believes that precise adjustments of spinal misalignments (or subluxations) can prevent and treat nearly all health ailments. The other philosophy is more modern and inclusive. It believes that there are other reasons for good or ill health beyond joint alignment and optimal life force.

of illegitimate conspiracy against the profession. The AMA now reports that chiropractic medicine "has a reasonably good degree of efficacy," and MDs and DCs collaborate with increasing frequency. Most insurance companies provide at least partial payments for chiropractic services, making it an attractive choice for those desiring greater acceptance within the medical mainstream. Chiropractics enjoy being primary healthcare providers and, by far, are the most recognized integrative health providers in the United States.

There are primarily two schools of thought in chiropractic philosophy. The original and traditional version believes that precise adjustments of spinal misalignments (or subluxations) can prevent and treat nearly all health ailments. Such adjustments of the vertebrae allow for optimal flow of an intelligent, spiritual life force throughout the nervous system of the person receiving the adjustment, just as Daniel Palmer intended. A chiropractor following this orthodox, vitalistic methodology is known as a "straight." The other philosophy is more modern and inclusive. It believes that there are other reasons for good or ill health beyond joint alignment and optimal life force. These more mainstream practitioners are known as "mixers," and they promote healing techniques in addition to joint manipulation, including advice on nutrition, herbal medicine, supplements, and psychology, among other holistic modalities. Mixers make up the majority of chiropractors in the United States, and its philosophy is widely adopted at chiropractic schools. A subtype of mixers called "reformers" practice joint manipulation—often along with allopathic modalities—solely for the treatment of joint pathologies.

It is scientifically understood that nerves from the spinal cord emerge from small holes in the protective spinal vertebrae. A spinal subluxation can therefore cause pain at various points throughout the body due to pinching of the spinal nerves. Realigning the vertebrae with a manual adjustment, or with any one of a variety of adjustment tools, can offer immediate or delayed relief from such pain. What is more controversial is the "straight" belief that the function of every organ, including the function of the brain and psyche, can be directly improved by joint adjustments. Even more controversial is the belief that these joint adjustments allow for a spiritual, intelligent life force to flow optimally throughout a patient's nervous system.

Preparation for joint adjustment is essential to treatment. A patient ideally receives a soft tissue massage around painful areas of the back and the rest of the body. This massage may be done by a practitioner's hands or with help from a heating pad (or a cold compress for acutely inflamed areas), electrical muscle stimulation, massage chair/bed, or traction roller pads. The intent is to loosen chronically contracted muscles so that an adjusted joint is not quickly re-misaligned by a spasming muscle. Following soft tissue preparation, diagnosis of spinal or other joint misalignment is performed. This diagnosis occurs while the patient's joints are stationary (static palpation) or moved by the chiropractor (motion palpation). Once the chiropractor understands which joints are misaligned and in which directions, he or she then treats the joints as levers and adjusts them into proper position.

The following general adjustment methods are commonly used, among many others, depending on the needs of the client and the training of the practitioner. No one method has proven to be best, and every chiropractor has his or her personal favorites.

- **Toggle Drop:** The chiropractor uses his or her hands to firmly press on an area of the spine. Then, with a quick, precise thrust, the spine is adjusted. This is done to increase vertebral mobility only where it is needed, leaving properly positioned joints stable and unmoved.

- **Lumbar Roll** (a.k.a. "Side Posture"): The chiropractor positions the patient on his or her back, then twists the patient's lower body to one side or the other. The practitioner then applies a quick and precise thrust to the lower vertebrae in order to help realign the entire spine. Usually two thrusts are given, one to each side of the patient's lumbar area.

- **Release Work**: The chiropractor applies gentle pressure using his or her fingertips to separate the vertebrae.

- **Table Adjustments**: The patient lies on a special table with sections that drop down several inches.

The chiropractor applies a quick spinal thrust at the same time the underlying section drops down. The dropping of the table allows for a less forceful adjustment without the potentially injurious twisting positions that can accompany other techniques.

- **Instrument Adjustment**: This is often the gentlest method of adjusting the spine. The patient lies on the table face down while the chiropractor uses a spring-loaded "activator" instrument to perform the spinal adjustments. The activator moves much more quickly than a hand and so less force is needed to provide a successful adjustment. This technique is often used to perform adjustments on animals, too.

Modern mixers also use a diverse group of medical modalities with which to diagnose or treat their patients, including:

Lifestyle Counseling: To encourage patients to live an all-around healthy lifestyle, many chiropractors engage in lifestyle counseling with their patients. Topics of conversation include optimal nutrition, exercise, and stress reduction; the importance of self-esteem and spirituality for psycho-physiological well-being; avoidance of toxins such as tobacco, alcohol, other recreational drugs, environmental chemicals, and excessive prescription drugs; education regarding daily stretching routines, correct posture, and proper lifting techniques; improving interpersonal relations; and cultivating a supportive and fulfilling community life.

Applied Kinesiology: This subjective method is used by approximately 40 percent of DCs for the purpose of diagnosing areas of physical, psychological, and chemical imbalance. To accomplish this, a chiropractor (or other health practitioner, as this modality isn't exclusive to chiropractic medicine) chooses one or more muscle groups to test on a patient. For example, a doctor asks a patient to hold up his arm and resist when the doctor attempts to pull it down. If the patient resists smoothly and strongly, the nervous system has indicated that it is strong within this muscle group, as well as within any organ system that is believed to be functionally connected to the muscle group being tested. If the patient resists the doctor's downward pull in a spasmodic or weakened manner, then that patient's nervous system has indicated dysfunction within the related muscles and organ systems. After an immediate attempt to treat this condition, the same muscle group is again tested. If the chiropractor feels that the muscle group is now strong, the treatment is considered a success.

Using the same technique, some practitioners also believe that the appropriateness of specific medications can be deduced for patients. One common method for discovering this information is to first determine a subjective baseline reading for a strong muscle group in a patient's body. For example, the chiropractor feels a smooth, strong response from a patient's muscles when he attempts to push down the patient's arm. Next, a small amount of the tested medication is placed under the patient's tongue (or sometimes is simply kept in its container and held in the patient's hand) and the same muscle group is tested.

A strong response is interpreted to mean that this medication is appropriate for the patient; a staccato or weakened response means that the medication is inappropriate. Similar tests can be performed by way of verbal questioning, with baseline muscle strength assessed before a "yes" or "no" question is asked of the patient. If the muscle remains strong, that is a "yes" answer in the language of the patient's nervous system. If the muscle weakens, it is a "no." This is one basic methodology, and many more complex versions are also used.

There is understandable criticism surrounding applied kinesiology by the scientific community because its results are subjectively determined by the doctor doing the testing. Proponents agree that, because the testing is subjective, a client must choose an applied kinesiologist with care. And since many CAM diagnostic techniques are subjective in nature (pulse and tongue diagnoses within ayurvedic and traditional Chinese medicine, for example), subjectivity alone is not evidence of fraud or practitioner ignorance.

Magnet Therapy: Magnetotherapy harkens back to the days of Paracelsus, the groundbreaking sixteenth-century Swiss physician. David Palmer, the founder of chiropractic medicine, was a practitioner of magnetic healing and spiritualism before he focused his attention on joint subluxations. So it is no surprise that modern chiropractors also employ magnet therapy in an attempt to treat musculoskeletal pain, as well as many other ailments. In using magnets for healing purposes, unipolar or multipolar magnetic devices are placed over body areas in need and are often taped into place so that patients are able to literally wear their therapeutic magnets after treatment.

It isn't scientifically understood why a magnetic field would assist in the healing process; however, it has been suggested that improved circulation, altered nerve function, and increased alkalinity of body fluids may play a role. Until 1997, it was easy to debunk magnet therapy because no supportive scientific research existed. But a double-blind study performed at Baylor University concluded that patients undergoing magnetic therapy experienced a decrease in pain compared with the placebo group, forcing skeptics to take a closer look at the healing potential of magnetic fields upon the human body.

X-rays: Many DCs prefer having objective, technological backup support beyond their usual manual diagnosis of joint subluxations. X-rays are an excellent medium for this service, as they give clear illustration of bone positioning, deterioration, abnormal growth, and other signs of bone health and pathology. Even within the field of chiropractic x-ray analysis, there is wide variation among DCs regarding the importance of x-rays versus manual palpation. Some chiropractors draw intricate, protracted lines along the vertebral angles of x-rays in order to chart short- and long-term treatment courses.

Others are only concerned with bone pathology, such as arthritis and cancer, in order to avoid potentially worsening such patient ailments with nearby joint adjustments. Nearly all doctors appreciate the clear snapshots of the internal human framework that have only been available to us since the discovery of x-rays in 1895 (coincidentally the same year that David Palmer introduced chiropractic to the medical world). Demonstrating to patients improved joint structure and validating the practitioner's manual diagnosis by way of x-ray photography is also a time-honored method of improving patients' confidence in their physicians, regardless of their specific academic degree.

Electromyography: Some chiropractors prefer to take objective measurements of patients' muscle tension. As such, electromyography's more of a ruler than a technique. Using a surface electromyograph to measure muscle tension before and after treatment gives both doctor and patient greater confidence in treatment direction. To measure relative muscle tension, electrodes are placed along either side of a joint, typically the vertebrae. Because electricity flows at different rates through a relaxed muscle versus a contracted one, levels of muscle tension can be measured during each treatment session as well as over the course of weeks or months. Chronically contracted muscles are often considered a general indication of both musculoskeletal and psychological well-being. By demonstrating improved muscle relaxation via an objective, machine-provided measurement, chiropractors can convince themselves and their patients that applied soft tissue and joint adjustments have been successful at promoting overall health.

CAREER AND TRAINING

All signs point toward chiropractic medicine remaining a lucrative and satisfying career choice for individuals desiring to work within the field of complementary medicine. Chiropractors typically earn a relatively low income as they build their medical practices but gradually reach an average income of greater than $100,000 per year, according to 2005 statistics. Of the more than 50,000 chiropractors in the United States, the vast majority are in private (solo or group) practices. The remaining DCs tend toward teaching, research, or patient care within hospitals.

Chiropractic emphasizes preventive care, healthful lifestyle changes, and a drug-free, noninvasive approach to healing. This is appealing to more and more individuals seeking an alternative to drug- and surgery-oriented allopathic medical treatment. Chiropractic adjustments are also increasingly respected as an effective way to prevent and treat back pain, as well as an assortment of other musculoskeletal maladies. Because these ailments tend to occur at a greater rate within the geriatric population, the elderly of

America will be seeking chiropractic care well into the future. Already back pain affects 60 to 80 percent of the U.S. population, with an estimated national expenditure of at least $20 billion due to healthcare costs and lost productivity. These numbers are only likely to increase, as are the existing majority of individuals who seek out chiropractic medicine instead of allopathic medicine when they are troubled with back pain.

Every state in the nation allows chiropractors to become primary care providers upon meeting local educational and examination requirements that vary state by state. Each state licensing board requires at least two years of undergraduate education (with some requiring a bachelor's degree), as well as the completion of at least ninety semester hours from a four-year program at an accredited chiropractic college. Once these requirements are completed, graduates may sit for the comprehensive test administered by the National Board of Chiropractic Examiners (NBCE). Individual states may also require graduates to pass their own board exams, though the testing material is similar to that of the national exams.

Once graduates pass these board exams, they are given the title of doctor of chiropractic (DC) by the licensing state. To retain their licenses, as with most every medical profession in every state, chiropractors must maintain some form of continuing education. It is also common for DCs to earn postgraduate degrees and certifications in subspecialties within chiropractic. This helps to differentiate a clinician's offering and can result in added prestige and success.

WHERE CHIROPRACTORS PRACTICE

A little over half of chiropractors work in private practice. Others may work in a holistic health clinic or in a progressive allopathic hospital environment. Most work independently, though some share their practice with other chiropractors who complement their specialty. Alternatively, chiropractors may share their practice with different integrative healers, such as massage and occupational therapists, orthopedic physicians, podiatrists, reflexologists, and osteopaths.

Chiropractors typically work in clean, comfortable offices averaging a forty-hour workweek. Sole practitioners are able to set their own hours but often must work evenings or weekends in order to accommodate their clients. Seldom will you find even a small town in America without at least one chiropractor.

DEGREES, LICENSURE, ACCREDITATION, AND CERTIFICATION

Because chiropractic medicine is well established, there are many different types of certification programs for licensed practitioners. All students of chiropractic receive their DC licensure after completing an Association of Chiropractic Colleges-accredited program and passing the NBCE examination. Further accolades, research projects, and/or certification programs are not necessary to hold legal practice, yet they often increase a practitioner's area of expertise as well as his or her reputation in the chiropractic community.

Index of Chiropractic Degrees

- **DC:** Doctor of Chiropractic
- **MS:** Master of Sciences
- **PhD:** Doctor of Philosophy

Diplomate Programs

Diplomate programs are usually offered by chiropractic schools or professional chiropractic organizations as postgraduate advanced programs of study These individual programs, with the acronyms spelled out below, may be thought of as private certification programs. They do not have a legal impact on a practitioner's profession, and they are only available to professionally licensed chiropractors. Often postgraduate training is followed by an intensive examination from a national board of senior specialists. The following are just a small sampling of advanced topics in chiropractic medicine which can be pursued at institutions and associations of higher learning and research:

- **DACS:** Diplomate of the ICA Council on Applied Chiropractic Sciences

- **DIBAK:** Diplomate of the International Board of Applied Kinesiology

- **DACBOH:** Diplomate of the American Chiropractic Board of Occupational Health

- **DACBR:** Diplomate of the American Chiropractic Board of Radiology

- **DABCI:** Diplomate of the American Chiropractic Board of Chiropractic Interests

- **DABCO:** Diplomate of the American Chiropractic Board of Chiropractic Orthopedists

- **DACNB:** Diplomate of the American Chiropractic Neurology Board

- **CCSP:** Certified Chiropractic Sports Physician

- **DACBN:** Diplomate of the American Clinical Board of Nutrition

- **DACS:** Diplomate of Applied Chiropractic Sciences

- **DICCP:** Diplomate of the ICA Council on Chiropractic Pediatrics

- **ACRB:** American Chiropractic Rehabilitation Board

- **DPhCS:** Diplomate of Philosophical Chiropractic Standards

- **AACA:** Diplomate of the American Academy of Chiropractic Acupuncture

EDUCATION REQUIREMENTS

To become a licensed chiropractor in the United States, you must complete a four-year graduate education program at an institution accredited by the Association of Chiropractic Colleges. Prospective students of chiropractic must meet minimal undergraduate requirements in order to gain admittance to a chiropractic college. In most cases, an undergraduate degree is strongly recommended—chiropractic programs require a minimum of ninety semester hours of college credits including courses in English, psychology, social science, biological science, chemistry, and physics. These standards are determined by the Council on Chiropractic Education. Some

programs allow students to fulfill requirements for a bachelor's degree by combining the basic science courses contained in the first two years of the chiropractic program in addition to prerequisite courses such as chemistry and biology. However, well over half of chiropractic students enter school with a bachelor's degree.

Upon admission, a student must complete 4,200 hours of classroom instruction. The first two years focus on the basic sciences (anatomy, advanced biology, and physiology) and core adjustment techniques. The third year focuses on clinical sciences, such as diagnostic radiology, physical diagnosis, and clinical neuromusculoskeletal diagnosis, while the fourth year primarily involves patient care experience through a clinical externship with classes on chiropractic theory and ethics. Upon successful completion of a chiropractic program, graduates sit for the National Board of Chiropractic Examiners (NBCE) Test, which leads to a DC degree.

National Board of Chiropractic Examiners

Upon completing all of these required programs, students are eligible to sit for a four-part comprehensive test administered by the National Board of Chiropractic Examiners. Some states supplement the national board test with their own version, yet the essential cores of these tests are ostensibly identical. The test, as well as the entire chiropractic program, is rigorous and academic—students must be well versed not only in chiropractic diagnosis but also in chemistry, biology, anatomy, minimal physics, and medical history.

State-based Variations

Every state in the U.S. recognizes chiropractic medicine as a legitimate field of medical care. As a result, all states require chiropractors to meet satisfactory educational and examination requirements before they can receive a state-specific license to practice. Chiropractors can only practice in states in which they are licensed; however, some states have agreements permitting licensed chiropractors to more easily obtain licensure in a different state without further examination, provided their educational, examination, and practice credentials meet state specifications.

Most state boards require two years of undergraduate education (although many states are moving toward a four-year bachelor's requirement) and the completion of a four-year program at an accredited chiropractic college with ninety semester credit hours.

After receiving a degree, the now qualified doctor of chiropractic must apply for state licensure to practice. Contact information for various state chiropractic associations is listed later in the chapter.

Continuing Education

Licensed DCs are required to participate in continuing education activities such as postgraduate studies, professional seminars, or publishing research. In general, DCs are required to have at least of seventeen hours of continuing education hours per year in order to qualify for state licensure renewal. Like any healthcare professional, chiropractors maintain the integrity of their field by requiring its practitioners to stay current in research, knowledge, and therapeutic technique. These postgraduate and continuing education programs are usually offered at chiropractic institutions. There is a multitude of acronyms that can be added to your name after completing these programs, as increasing your expertise benefits your status in the community as well as the success of your practice.

ORGANIZATIONS

American Chiropractic Association
www.amerChiro.org/index.cfm

The ACA is the largest lobbying, public relations, and professional chiropractic association worldwide. The ACA, boasting approximately 18,000 members, was responsible for spearheading reach-out programs to victims of Hurricanes Katrina and Rita.

International Chiropractic Association
www.chiropractic.org

The ICA, representing about 8,000 practitioners worldwide, was established in 1926 by Dr. B.J. Palmer and is the oldest and one of the largest international chiropractic associations. The ICA hosts several conventions every year.

The National Association for Chiropractic Medicine
www.chiromed.org

The NACM is a consumer advocacy association of chiro-

practors who seek to legitimize the utilization of professional manipulative procedures in mainstream medicine. Founded by chiropractors who were concerned about its scientific legitimacy, the NACM lobbies to limit the scope of chiropractic practice to dealing exclusively with irrefutable scientific facts.

Association of Chiropractic Colleges
www.chirocolleges.org

The ACC provides worldwide leadership in chiropractic education as the formal accrediting body of all chiropractic schools in the United States. Additionally, via the enhancement of scholarly activity, the ACC fosters financial, physical, and legislative efforts in chiropractic medicine.

National Board of Chiropractic Examiners
www.nbce.org/index.html

Established in 1963, the NBCE is the sole testing agency for the chiropractic profession. Further information about the NBCE test may be found above.

World Chiropractic Alliance
www.worldchiropracticalliance.org

Members of the WCA, which was founded in 1989 as a nonprofit organization, are self-announced professional "watchdogs" and advocates of the chiropractic profession. Today, the WCA is the only major chiropractic organization that passionately fights for the rights of subluxation-based doctors.

Foundation for Chiropractic Education and Research
www.fcer.org

Founded in 1944, the FCER is the oldest and most respected chiropractic research-funding institution in the world. The FCER is also responsible for several publications that highlight cutting-edge chiropractic research.

Council on Applied Chiropractic Sciences
www.chiropractic.org/councils/cacs/CACS.htm

The CACS is a networking association dedicated to the philosophy, science, and art of chiropractic medicine. Through a vast practitioner-based network, the council seeks to deepen the general public's understanding of chiropractic care and dispel popular myths about chiropractic medicine. It also offers several postgraduate programs (available only to members) in various specialties and sponsors an annual national conference.

Council on Chiropractic Education

www.cce-usa.org

The CCE, a subdivision of the ACC, consists of a board of expert practitioners who will determine the future course of chiropractic education in the United States. If a school is not accredited by the ACC (via the CCE), it is not a legally recognized college of chiropractic medicine (and therefore cannot professionally certify its students).

Council on Chiropractic Guidelines and Practice Parameters

www.ccgpp.org

The CCGPP, founded in 1995, takes care of examining all existing guidelines, parameters, protocols, and best practices in American chiropractic medicine, focusing on the interplay between patient care and professionalism. Essentially bringing the holistic philosopher, the skeptical scientist, and the pragmatic practitioner together, the CCGPP's main objective is to meet the needs of the patient.

Federation of Chiropractic Licensing Boards

www.fclb.org

Established in 1926, the FCLB is one of the oldest chiropractic organizations in the United States. This nonprofit corporation serves as a forum for the discussion of chiropractic issues, usually dealing with maintaining uniform standards across different types of chiropractic practice. The FCLB is also the largest contributor to the CIN-BAD (Chiropractic Information Network-Board Action Databank) system—a technological forum that offers member boards and subscribers access to a database of chiropractic regulatory boards.

Congress of Chiropractic State Associations

www.cocsa.org

The COCSA, which acts as a liaison between the various chiropractic state organizations (listed below) and individual practitioners, was formed in the late 1960s. It holds many state-wide conventions at various times during the year, including an annual convention with all state-based organizations.

PEER-REVIEWED PERIODICALS

Journal of Chiropractic Education

www.journalChiroed.com

The American Chiropractor Online

www.theamericanchiropractor.com

Chiropractic Economics

www.chiroeco.com

Chiropractic Research Journal

www.cinahl.com

Journal of Manipulative & Physiological Therapeutics

ww3.us.elsevierhealth.com/jmpt

Journal of the American Chiropractic Association

www.amerchiro.org/index.cfm

Journal of Chiropractic Humanities

www.journalchirohumanities.com

Includes editorials and provocative debates within the chiropractic profession.

Journal of Sports Chiropractic and Rehabilitation

www.acasc.org

Today's Chiropractic Lifestyle

www.todayschiropractic.com

Topics in Clinical Chiropractic

www.chiro-online.com/interadcom/topicsfr.html

ONLINE RESOURCES

Chiro Web

www.chiroweb.com

Chiro Access

www.chiroaccess.com

Johns Hopkins Intelihealth

www.intelihealth.com

A new program in conjunction with Harvard University that promotes communication within integrative medicine.

Mantis Database

www.healthindex.com

The largest source of osteopathic, chiropractic, and manual medical literature in the world.

Medscape

www.medscape.com/home

A comprehensive resource for studies in integrative medicine.

POSTGRADUATE PROGRAMS IN CHIROPRACTIC MEDICINE

In addition to the required continuing education hours that DCs must obtain yearly in order to renew their state licenses, DCs may obtain optional postgraduate education and training in a variety of specialty areas. These specialty programs are offered at accredited U.S. chiropractic colleges. Accredited U.S. chiropractic colleges offer two types of specialty programs: part-time postgraduate training and full-time residency training. The former, which is less time consuming, may be of-

fered as a night class, whereas the latter is a more intense, more demanding course of study.

Figure 1 illustrates a sampling of some common postgraduate programs from a variety of different institutions, as well as their requirements for diplomate status, which are largely determined by the institutions that offer training. After completing a particular postgraduate program, practitioners are able to extend their specialties to new horizons. To find a more comprehensive list of postgraduate opportunities in your area, contact the nearest accredited chiropractic college, or one of the various chiropractic research associations.

Figure 1

Area	Description of Program Requirements	Eligibility after Completion
Radiology	A three-year, full-time residency program. Residents must spend time in the radiology departments of cooperative teaching hospitals and imaging centers.	Eligible to sit for the exam by the American Chiropractic Board of Radiology to obtain diplomate status (DACBR)
Family Practice	A three-year, full-time residency program involving instruction in advanced diagnostic skills, nutritional therapy, intravenous therapy, injectable nutrients, preventive medicine techniques, lifestyle changes for health promotion, and treatment techniques.	Eligible to sit for exam to become a diplomate of the American Board of Chiropractic Internists (DABCI)
Orthopedics	A three-year, full-time program (nonresidency) that focuses on all conditions affecting the neuromusculoskeletal body systems. Emphasis is placed on the diagnosis and chiropractic management of orthopedic conditions, which is particularly relevant in chiropractic practice.	Eligible to sit for the exam for diplomate status with the American Board of Chiropractic Orthopedists (DABCO)
Clinical Sciences	A three-year, full-time program (nonresidency) where residents are involved in the areas of clinical practice, teaching, and research with opportunities for interdisciplinary studies in cooperative teaching hospitals and medical centers.	Eligible to sit for the American Board of Chiropractic Orthopedists (ABCO) and the College of Chiropractic Sciences (Canada) Fellowship (FCCS) examination
Family Practice	300-hour nonresidency program that focuses on patient assessment, identification of early signs of disease, prevention of disease, application of diagnostic modalities in the clinical setting, and use of appropriate lifestyle and nutritional therapies that will benefit the patient. Equivalent in education to the residency program but with less field experience.	Eligible to sit for exam to become a diplomate of the American Board of Chiropractic Internists (DABCI)

Area	Description of Program Requirements	Eligibility after Completion
Clinical Neurology	A 300-hour program that prepares chiropractors to serve the public and other healthcare providers as a neurological specialist or consultant who is trained to diagnose and attend disorders of the human nervous system without the use of drugs or surgery.	Eligible to sit for the Certification Examination in Neurology given by the American Chiropractic Neurology Board to obtain diplomate status (DACNB)
Sports Chiropractic	A 320-hour program that emphasizes the total care of the injured athlete. It encompasses industrial, community, intramural, and recreational athletes who participate in sports activities and are at risk of sustaining sports-related injuries.	Eligible to sit for the exam to become a Certified Chiropractic Sports Physician (CCSP)
Nutrition	A 300-hour program centered on development of advanced knowledge, skills, and abilities in the use of nutrition in the practice of chiropractic.	Eligible to sit for the exam to become a diplomate of the American Clinical Board of Nutrition (DACBN)
Chiropractic Occupational Health and Applied Ergonomics	A 300-hour program that provides doctors with the information and skills to be effective professional consultants to corporate clients within their communities. This is a particularly advanced academic chiropractic degree.	Eligible to sit for the exam to become a diplomate of the American Chiropractic Board of Occupational Health (DACBOH)
Applied Chiropractic Sciences	A 360-hour program designed to enhance and advance the expertise and application of both classic chiropractic care approaches and emerging technologies. It provides a comprehensive correlation of clinical protocols that are presented in the context of subluxation-based chiropractic models of care.	Eligible to sit for the exam to become a diplomate of Applied Chiropractic Sciences (DACS)
Orthopedics	A 384-hour program that extends the ability of a chiropractor to diagnose, treat, and manage conditions or disorders of the musculoskeletal system.	Eligible to sit for the exam given by the American Board of Chiropractic Orthopedists to obtain diplomate status (DABCO)
Pediatrics	A 360-hour program that is designed to offer the materials and tools to handle the issues, concerns, and practice protocols relevant in caring for children and pregnant women.	Eligible to sit for the exam to earn diplomate of the ICA Council on Chiropractic Pediatrics (DICCP) status
Rehabilitation	A 300-hour program that prepares doctors to become specialists who are not only experts in manipulation but know how to transition from passive to active care and how to evaluate the biobehavioral component of musculoskeletal illness.	Eligible for the exam given by the American Chiropractic Rehabilitation Board (ACRB)
Applied Kinesiology	Via the International College of applied Kinesiology (www.icak.com/)	Diplomat of the International Board of Applied Kinesiology

Area	Description of Program Requirements	Eligibility after Completion
Philosophical Chiropractic Standards	A 320-hour program that addresses the appeal for graduate-level training with the unique tenets of chiropractic philosophy. Courses are typically lecture intensive.	Eligible to sit for the exam given by the ICA Council on Chiropractic philosophy to obtain diplomate in Philosophical Chiropractic Standards (DPhCS) status

There are many other areas of postgraduate study in chiropractic medicine, including but not limited to: physiological therapeutics, occupational health and applied ergonomics, spinal manipulation under anesthesia, and applied kinesiology. General research is also a large part of the practice and may also be a valid form of continuing education. The International Chiropractic Association is perhaps the best resource for more information on postgraduate research. Teaching at a chiropractic college or giving a guest lecture at a colloquia are other ways that licensed chiropractors may satisfy their continuing education requirement.

EDUCATIONAL INSTITUTIONS

To become a professional chiropractor in any state, the law requires candidates to attend and graduate from an accredited institution. The Association of Chiropractic Colleges is responsible for accrediting and regulating chiropractic education in the United States. All the following chiropractic schools have been formally reviewed and endorsed by the ACC. If a school is not accredited by the ACC, it will not necessarily be able to professionally certify chiropractors in the United States.

Cleveland Chiropractic College: Kansas City
Kansas City, Missouri
www.clevelandchiropractic.edu

Cleveland Chiropractic College: Los Angeles
Los Angeles, California
www.clevelandchiropractic.edu

Life University College of Chiropractic
Marietta, Georgia
www.life.edu

Life Chiropractic College West
Hayward, California
www.lifewest.edu

Los Angeles College of Chiropractic of the Southern California University of Health Sciences
Whittier, California
www.scuhs.edu

Doctor of Chiropractic Degree Program in the College of Professional Studies of the National University of Health Sciences
Lombard, Illinois
www.nuhs.edu

New York Chiropractic College
Seneca Falls, New York
www.nycc.edu

Northwestern College of Chiropractic of the Northwestern Health Sciences University
Bloomington, Minnesota
www.nwhealth.edu

Palmer College of Chiropractic
Davenport, Iowa
www.palmer.edu

Palmer College of Chiropractic West
San Jose, California
www.palmer.edu

Parker College of Chiropractic
Dallas, Texas
www.parkercc.edu

Sherman College of Straight Chiropractic
Spartanburg, South Carolina
www.sherman.edu

Texas Chiropractic College
Pasadena, Texas
www.txchiro.edu

University of Bridgeport College of Chiropractic
Bridgeport, Connecticut
www.bridgeport.edu/chiro

Western States Chiropractic College
Portland, Oregon
www.wschiro.edu

EXAMPLES OF RESEARCH TOPICS IN CHIROPRACTIC MEDICINE

RAND. 1991. *The Appropriateness of Spinal Manipulation for Low Back Pain.*

Report to the Committees on Armed Services and Appropriations. December 1993. *CHAMPUS Chiropractic Demonstration*, prepared by the Office of the Assistant Secretary of Defense for Health Affairs.

U.S. Department of Health and Human Service Agency for Healthcare Policy and Research. December 1994.Clinical Guideline: No. 14: *Acute Low Back Problems in Adults: Assessment and Treatment.*

Monograph of the Quebec Task Force. April 1995. *Whiplash: Associated Disorders.*

Harvard Symposium on Alternative Medicine. April 1995. *What the Scientific Literature Tells Us About the Use of Spinal Manipulative Therapy for Back and Neck Pain.*

Hansen, John P. and Futch, Daniel B. March 1997. Chiropractic Services in a Staff Model HMO, Utilization and Satisfaction. *HMO Practice,* vol. 2, no. 1, pp. 39–42.

DuVall, Charles E., Jr. 1997. Wiley Expert Witness Update: *New Developments in Personal Injury Litigation*, Chapter 2, Chiropractic Medicine: Myth, Reality, and the Expert Witness. Wiley Law Publications, John Wiley & Sons, Inc.

OSTEOPATHIC MEDICINE (DO)

Osteopathic medicine was introduced to the world in 1874 by Andrew Taylor Still, MD, who had for more than ten years consolidated osteopathy's philosophies and techniques from more ancient bone adjusting medical modalities. He was dissatisfied with the allopathic medicine of his time, especially after serving in the Union Army of the American Civil War and seeing two of three soldiers die from infectious diseases such as measles, mumps, and whooping cough. He was also frustrated in trying to quell Native American epidemics upon his return home and helplessly watched his wife and six of his children die from a variety of infectious diseases.

Still devised a drugless, surgery-free system of medicine that was not meant to be an alternative to allopathy. Instead, he wanted to complement the use of "heroic" allopathy for acute trauma with a gentler, holistic method for diagnosis and treatment of almost all other ailments. Seeking a panacea was common for medical practitioners of the 1800s, and Still's panacea was the correction of patients' musculoskeletal deviations toward an anatomical ideal. He claimed that nearly all diseases could be cured by way of repositioning misaligned ribs, vertebrae, or any other joint in need of alignment. Still believed that, by performing accurate joint manipulations, any doctor could optimize the flow of spiritual "nerve force" throughout a patient's entire body. In Still's mind, and in the minds of all "vitalists" like him, this unimpeded flow of life force was the one essential for human health.

Still's intent was to improve upon allopathic medicine. Yet he was immediately labeled a charlatan by his MD peers and a channeler of the devil by church authorities. He became a traveling physician and experienced enough success that he was able to establish the first osteopathy school in the United States. The American School of Osteopathy (now the A.T. Still University, Kirksville College of Osteopathy) was founded in 1892 in Kirksville, Missouri. One year later, Daniel David Palmer visited Still for treatment. By 1895, Palmer announced that he was introducing to the world chiropractic medicine, a system of therapeutics

OTHER THAN additional training in musculoskeletal diagnosis and manipulation, present-day osteopaths and MDs study and practice much the same kind of medicine. This means that most osteopaths are no longer truly holistic doctors. Osteopathy is included in this volume because any DO has the option of practicing in a traditional, vitalistic manner that acknowledges the importance of healing body, mind, and spirit with equal emphasis.

very similar to osteopathy ("curing via the bones"). Still was proud of the differences in his school's curriculum versus those of most allopathic schools of his time. He refused the State of Missouri's offer to grant graduating students an MD degree instead of a DO. More than two decades then passed with doctors of osteopathy (DOs) remaining arch rivals of allopathic medical doctors (with MDs being called "regulars" at this point in time).

A major occurrence in U.S. medical history occurred in 1910 when the infamous Flexner Report was released, under the auspices of the American Medical Association (AMA) and the Carnegie Foundation. In 1908, the AMA had requested that the Carnegie Foundation publish a report on the status of medical education within the United States. Education expert and Johns Hopkins University graduate, Abraham Flexner, was hired for the job. He proceeded to visit the 155 U.S. medical schools then in existence. In his report, Flexner stated that the majority of medical schools in the U.S. offered education and hygiene standards far below those deemed professionally appropriate. Using Johns Hopkins Medical School as his model, Flexner outlined his allopathically biased guidelines to be applied to all U.S. medical schools. Most of these guidelines are still followed to this day. The Flexner Report was fully accepted by federal and state medical authorities. The result was that by 1935 only sixty-six U.S. medical schools remained, none of which were allowed to teach any classes on vitalism, herbalism, naturopathy, homeopathy, or any other alternative medical system or philosophy.

The field of osteopathic medicine was required to follow suit, and only those schools willing to change to a more allopathic curricula were allowed to survive. DOs and MDs continued their bitter disputes until the 1970s, even though their university training began to appear very similar. Vitalism was simply unacceptable to the materialistic AMA. After first being stripped of their degrees, California DOs were offered in 1962 MD degrees by the state for a nominal fee. Although osteopaths were allowed membership into the AMA starting in 1969, it wasn't until 1974 that California once again allowed osteopaths to practice as DOs rather than as MDs.

It is rare for a medical system to so radically alter its protocols and practices within such a short period of time. From 1874 until at least 1910, all osteopaths were practicing vitalists as described above. After 1910, osteopaths began to undergo training similar to regular MDs because of the Flexner Report. The result is that today there is often no difference in patient experience between visiting a DO and an MD, unless the DO in question has remained a traditional osteopath. The percentage of traditional versus "allopathic" osteopaths continues to decline, especially since traditional schools of osteopathy are few in number. Approximately 6 percent of osteopaths today use traditional techniques with a majority of their patients.

Other than additional training in musculoskeletal diagnosis and manipulation, present-day osteopaths and MDs study and practice much the same kind of medicine. This means that most osteopaths are no longer truly holistic doctors. Osteopathy is included in this volume because any DO has the option of practicing in a traditional, vitalistic manner that acknowledges the importance of healing body, mind, and spirit with equal emphasis. As a prospective student, if you wish to practice traditional osteopathy, be sure to attend a school that emphasizes a traditional osteopathic curriculum (as noted below). However remember that this is the exception rather than the norm.

Traditional osteopathy is a health care system that places the highest priority on a patient's musculoskeletal system, including the bones, muscles, joints, ligaments, and tendons. It believes that a properly aligned musculoskeletal structure leads to optimal functioning of the entire "body-mind." This occurs because proper structural alignment leads to optimal blood and lymph flow, as well as optimal nerve transmission. Proper functioning of the circulatory and nervous systems then allows for ideal flow of the non-physical healing power of nature. Belief in this spiritual healing power is termed "vitalism." The original version of osteopathy is one of the most influential western medical systems to base its philosophy on vitalism versus "materialism," the belief that physical forces are all that truly exist. In vitalistic systems such as osteopathy, it is the spiritual force that makes the human organism one that is always self-regulating and self-healing. Removing the barriers to this vital force are all that is required to ensure that healing occurs easily and automatically.

A doctor of osteopathy (DO) is trained to diagnose and treat all diseases via assessment and correction of musculoskeletal misalignments. Because of their expertise in anatomy, traditional DOs are able to detect even subtle deviations in a patient's physical structure. They then adjust these abnormalities by using a variety of more than one hundred different manual manipulation techniques, which are collectively called "osteopathic manual medicine." It is important to understand that an osteopath does not intend to merely improve the functioning of the bones and muscles. Instead, osteopaths seek to prevent and treat every type of illness, from heart disease to hemorrhoids, by way of focusing attention solely upon the musculoskeletal system. No matter whether you visit a traditional DO because you have a cold or a cancer, your diagnosis and treatment will be based on how well your musculoskeletal structure matches the ideal human anatomy.

It is well understood scientifically that impingement of a nerve or spasming of a muscle due to spine or rib misalignment may cause pain that can be quickly relieved by manually realigning the misplaced joint. However, Still and the traditional osteopaths noticed something altogether different. They determined that a pathology as distant as a lung infection could be quickly cured by adjusting a misaligned sacrum. Or a chronic digestive could be healed by adjusting a misplaced collarbone. This is confounding to present-day materialists, but vitalists believe that any obstacle to the flow of life force anywhere in the body can result in pathology within any sector of a patient's internal workings. There is no scientific research proof validating this traditional osteopathic belief. However, another vitalistic system, the acupuncture of traditional Chinese medicine (TCM), has recently been accepted by the AMA. MDs now take approved continuing education classes in medical acupuncture. Vitalistic systems of medicine should, therefore, not be written off simply because there is no research to support them. In the case of TCM, it has taken thousands of years to achieve some degree of scientific backing. Traditional osteopathy is only 200 years old and may yet be embraced by the scientific community. Few traditional osteopaths remain,

however, and there is little interest in the modern osteopathic community regarding research into vitalism or practice of joint manipulation as the sole form of medical treatment.

TECHNIQUES

There have been hundreds of osteopathic manual medicine techniques devised since Still's initial hands-on musculoskeletal manipulations. The following practices represent those used most frequently by modern osteopaths who still choose to perform traditional osteopathic adjustments:

Hands-on Contact: Not an actual technique, but an important philosophy to emphasize. Traditional osteopaths believe that patient healing begins once touch has been initiated. DOs may begin an exam by gently rapping on the soft tissue over the heart and lungs, for example. Regardless of what information is received by the doctor from this practice, if the DO's touch is perceived by the patient as skillful and soothing, then a potentially healing bond is already being formed between doctor and patient. From a DO's perspective, the more touch the better during every patient visit.

Soft-Tissue Technique: This method involves rhythmic stretching, deep manual pressure, and traction applied to the muscles and fascia surrounding any joint—but especially the vertebrae. Chronically tense musculature is relaxed, blood and lymph flow is stimulated and brought into balance, and patient anxiety is lessened.

Myofascial Release Treatment (MRT): Fascia is a weblike system of connective tissue that surrounds and fuses with all the muscles of the human body. If the fascia is misaligned, often the muscles and bones are misaligned as well. Since osteopaths believe that misaligned muscles and bones are a direct cause of almost all pathology, releasing tight fascia is an important part of preventing and treating illness. DOs either force the muscle and fascia (myofascia) into place with direct MRT or instead guide dysfunctional tissue along a path of least resistance until release occurs with indirect MRT.

Cranial Osteopathy: Just as fascia surrounds muscles, so does another form of connective tissue surround the brain and the rest of the central nervous system (CNS) from the skull to the sacrum. Within this connective tissue flows the cushioning cerebrospinal fluid (CSF). In the 1930s, William Sutherland, DO, invented the technique of cranial osteopathy. Using this technique, DOs gently hold a patient's head in order to sense the subtle, wavelike fluctuation of CSF around the spine and brain. They also try to detect the synchronized movements of the skull and the sacrum. This dual flow is termed the cranial rhythmic impulse (CRI). Balancing CRI is believed to improve the overall health of patients because the CNS controls the functioning of every organ, muscle, and nerve in the human body. The merits of cranial osteopathy are highly debated within the field of modern osteopathy due to its lack of supportive science. A more popularized version of cranial osteopathy is craniosacral therapy. This is basically cranial osteopathy for nonosteopaths and was named by John Upledger, DO, when he began teaching this technique to nonmedical students.

Lymphatic Techniques: A little known circulatory system parallels the bloodstream. This is the lymphatic system, and it circulates filtered blood through lymph nodes as a major part of our immune system. If patients have reduced lymph flow, they are more susceptible to infection. Unlike the bloodstream, lymphatic fluid requires regular physical activity and muscle contraction in order to flow properly. Since many patients are excessively sedentary, a practitioner can stimulate lymph flow by hands-on pressure application. Some lymphatic techniques use heavy manual pressure and some use light pressure. "Manual lymphatic drainage" is performed by gently stroking the skin with slow motions that attempt to match the equally slow pulsations of lymph flow. Strokes always move from the center of the body toward the periphery in order to drain central lymph nodes and encourage lymph flow from the periphery back to the center. Many health improvements beyond greater immunity are claimed for the proper use of lymphatic techniques, none of which have been scientifically proven.

Thrust Techniques: These techniques were originally introduced to Americans by Still and the traditional osteopaths, although most people connect these practices with the more popular offshoot of osteopathy: chiropractic medicine. Thrust techniques involve a practitioner applying a high velocity, low-pressure manual push upon a joint to restore appropriate joint position and mobility. Blood/lymph circulation and nerve transmission are believed to simultaneously improve, leading to greater overall body-mind health via optimal flow of life force. Musculoskeletal pain, range-of-motion restriction, and asymmetry are often quickly reduced or eliminated. Thrust techniques are the most scientifically proven of all traditional osteopathic modalities regarding pain relief and structural repositioning.

Muscle Energy Technique: Traditional osteopathy prides itself on being a holistic health care system that takes a complete body approach to all diagnosis and treatment. Before using muscle energy technique, the osteopath assesses joint mobility from head to toe and focuses treatment on the most movement-restricted segments. When a specific joint is to be treated, the DO directs the patient to isometrically contract a specific muscle connected to the joint being treated while the DO applies a precise counterforce. Muscle energy technique is believed to help mobilize restricted joints and relax chronically contracted musculature while normalizing nerve transmission.

Strain/Counterstrain: Discovered in 1955 by Lawrence Jones, DO, this technique first involves palpating for tender points and then placing the patient in the position that gives greatest relief from his or her overall physiological pain. The patient remains in this position for several minutes with help from the DO, relaxing or stretching chronically contracted musculature. Upon return to normal posture, patients often report a lessening of pain and an improvement in mobility. Strain/counterstrain is commonly used on patients too fragile, or in too much pain, for therapies such as thrust techniques. An updated version is termed positional release therapy.

Visceral Manipulation: A system of manual manipulation of the abdominal organs performed to loosen tightened organ ligaments. These ligaments may tighten after physical, chemical, thermal, or emotional trauma. Organ positioning and function may then be altered to such an extent that body-mind function as a whole is compromised. Gentle but deep massage of internal organs such as liver, kidney, and intestines helps the DO locate and correct altered ligaments. Improved digestion, joint mobility, and stress reduction are some of the claims made for successful visceral manipulation. Though practiced for several hundred years dating back to Tibetan folk healers and European "bonesetters," visceral manipulation was incorporated into osteopathy in 1971 due to the updating influence of Jean-Pierre Barral, DO. This technique departs from Still's initial focus on health improvement solely via the human musculoskeletal system. It is another example of how osteopathic medicine has changed since its inception in 1874.

CAREER AND TRAINING

By 2009, there will be twenty-nine osteopathic medical schools in the United States. They are all accredited by the American Osteopathic Association (AOA), which since 1897 has been the primary certifying body for American DOs. Accreditation from the AOA is officially recognized by the U.S. Department of Education. Applicants to osteopathic medical school are required to have earned a four-year undergraduate degree, including one year of coursework in English, general chemistry, organic chemistry, biology, and physics. Applicants must also receive above average scores on their MCAT (Medical College Admission Tests) exam. Similar to "regular" medical school, the first two years of the four-year osteopathic college training program are focused upon lecture coursework such as anatomy, physiology, and biochemistry. During the final two years the focus of coursework switches to clinical training, including pharmacology, patient case intake, and hands-on osteopathic manual medicine (OMM). Preventive medicine and a whole-body approach to patient wellness are taught in schools emphasizing traditional osteopathy.

After students have graduated from osteopathic medical school, they must complete a rotating twelve-month internship, which exposes them to the broadest possible array of clinical conditions such as emergency medicine, family medicine, and obstetrics. DOs then spend two to six more years in a residency program, focusing on specialties such as psychiatry, pediatrics, or sports medicine. Note the lack of traditional musculoskeletal focus within the abovementioned internships and residencies, as osteopathic manual medicine continues to fall out of favor within osteopathic training facilities.

Following the above-mentioned postgraduate studies, DOs must pass state medical board examinations to receive licenses from those states in which they are planning to practice. All fifty states offer DO licensure to qualified applicants. In order to retain their state medical license(s), DOs must complete 120 credit hours per year of continuing medical education. It is within the arena of postgraduate training that traditionally oriented practitioners typically receive advanced training in manual medicine techniques.

Family osteopaths earn a high salary, ranging from $75,000 to $150,000 per year. They make up 46 percent of DOs nationwide. Specialized osteopaths earn even more, with pediatrics and internal medicine being the two most popular specialties. Overall the median income for DOs is $160,000 per year, nearly identical to MDs. Only 1 percent of DOs currently claim traditional osteopathy, using osteopathic manual medicine (OMM), as their chosen area of specialization. So even though osteopaths originally treated all medical conditions using OMM techniques alone, now they treat all medical conditions, or their chosen specialties, using mostly allopathic techniques favored by MDs. The vast majority of DOs are in solo and group practice, although there is also the option of full- or part-time teaching and research.

The number of graduating osteopaths is growing quickly in the United States because so many student applicants are not being accepted into their preferred MD training programs. Between 1980 and 2005, there was a 250 percent increase, from around 1,000 per year to 2,800 per year. This number is predicted to reach 5,000 per year by 2015. The absolute number of U.S. osteopaths is projected to increase from the present number of around 60,000 to an all-time high of approximately 100,000 in 2020. This change should also result in an increase in the percentage of U.S. physicians who are osteopaths (currently at 6 percent). And in only six years, from 2002 to 2008, the number of osteopathic medical schools will have increased from nineteen to twenty-nine. Already one in five U.S. medical students is attending an osteopathic medical college.

The burgeoning growth of osteopathy is occurring in the midst of an American population that is greatly unaware of both the definition, and the scope of practice, of an osteopathic doctor. But this shouldn't be a major problem for the prospective student, since all fifty states license DOs and there is a projected shortage of primary care physicians into the foreseeable future. Osteopaths are now accepted as equally skilled medical practitioners at nearly all institutions that employ MDs, especially since the majority of DOs have abandoned the traditional techniques that differentiated them from "regulars."

A greater concern for the holistically inclined student is that the hands-on techniques so important to traditional osteopathy are widely criticized by members of the mainstream medical community. Frequent education of patients and medical peers regarding osteopathic principles will be required of traditional osteopaths during the course of their careers. As a prospective student, you must decide whether the high status and income likely to result from a DO degree is worth the osteopathic training that has been diluted from a holistic, preventive, hands-on approach toward one that is often indistinguishable from an MD's materialistic allopathic training.

Relevant Degrees

- **AAMA:** Member of the American Academy of Medical Acupuncturists. Open only to medical doctors (MD) and doctors of osteopathy (DO)

- **DHt:** Diplomate in Homeotherapeutics (also DHT). By the American Board of Homeotherapeutics. Available only to MDs (medical doctors) and DOs (doctors of osteopathy)

- **DO:** Doctor of Osteopathy

WHERE PRACTICED

The career opportunities for an osteopathic physician are as varied as they are for an allopathic doctor. Because osteopaths are legally approved to prescribe pharmaceutical drugs, they can be found in all areas of modern medicine—from pediatrics to neurosurgery. In keeping with its holistic roots, however, most DOs choose to practice within primary care, which includes family practice, gynecology, obstetrics, and internal medicine. Additionally, osteopaths tend to have an area of expertise—whether it be surgical, manipulative, nutritional, or medicinal—which they pursue in their postgraduate studies through certification and diplomate programs.

As DOs are trained extensively in human anatomy, particularly in the musculoskeletal system, it is not uncommon to find osteopaths practicing in sports medicine, where they oversee entire sports teams and have physical therapists and massage therapists on their staffs. Osteopaths may also start their own private practice or work in conjunction with holistic and allopathic doctors. Because their training is comprehensive and their knowledge vast, a career as an osteopath tends to be flexible and is a central addition to a comprehensive wellness center.

DEGREES, LICENSURE, ACCREDITATION, AND CERTIFICATION

A doctor of osteopathy is educated in the United States as a fully licensed physician or surgeon, practicing a combined scope of modern and traditional medicine. The curriculum for osteopaths is rigorous. As with many other health professions, the basic DO degree is required to gain state licensure. Additionally, there are various types of postdegree certifications and specialties including: RCT (registered craniosacral therapist), AAMA (member of the American Academy of Medical Acupuncturists), and DHT (diplomate in homeotherapeutics certified by the American Board of Homeotherapeutics). The American Association for Colleges of Osteopathic Medicine, the accrediting body for osteopathic schools, endorses twenty-five osteopathic schools in the United States.

EDUCATION REQUIREMENTS

To become a DO in the United States, you must graduate from a school of osteopathic medicine. Osteopathic schools are similar to medical school. They are four- to five-year programs: the first two years focus on foundation coursework, while the third and fourth years focus on hands-on clinical training and diagnosis. You can expect osteopathic medical school to be just as demanding as allopathic medical school. Due to the program's academic rigor, a high GPA and MCAT (Medical College Admission Test) score are required. Three to four years of undergraduate training with a background in science is the minimum requirement, and a collegiate degree in the hard sciences (biology, chemistry, anatomy) is recommended. As a result, most students of osteopathic medicine earn some kind of undergraduate, master's, or doctorate degree before applying to medical school.

To become a licensed osteopath and to be granted legal permission to practice in a particular state, the applicant must pass state medical board examinations. These are the same tests that allopathic doctors undergo. While each state has its own experiential prerequisites before starting a practice, typically four years of training plus three to eight years of residency clinical work are required.

Allopathic vs. Osteopathic

There are significantly more MDs practicing medicine than DOs in the United States. The Bureau of Labor statistics calculated that, as of 2006, there were more than 633,000 practicing MDs compared to only 59,000 osteopaths. Because a DO degree is medically comparable to a MD degree, the two are often equated. While it is true that osteopathic physicians can prescribe all forms of medication, conduct surgery if trained, and pursue all medical specialties that MDs can, there are characteristic differences between the two professions. Osteopathic education includes several units on the musculoskeletal system that is not found in allopathic curricula. Additionally, osteopaths often seek postgraduate training in any number of complementary and alternative techniques such as medical acupuncture, craniosacral therapy, and ortho-bionomy. Therefore, osteopaths can be a fine example for the aspiring integrative practitioner.

Figure 2 illustrates differences in education, licensing, and career trajectories between DOs and MDs. While the particular tracks are remarkably similar, DOs have more internship opportunities, a greater choice of residency programs, and a more extensive medical school curriculum.

Figure 2

	Allopathic Medicine (MD)	Osteopathic Medicine (DO)
Pre-Medical Requirements	• Biology (8 semester credit hours) • Physics (8 semester credit hours) • Inorganic Chemistry (8 semester credit hours) • Organic Chemistry (8 semester credit hours) • MCAT examination • Bachelor's degree strongly recommended	Same
Medical School	Four-year program	Four-year program (plus additional training in musculoskeletal system and manipulative medicine)
Internship(s)	Three available tracks: • *Medicine* • *Surgery* • *Transitional Year*	The AOA suggests a rotating year, which includes many different specialties at an AOA-approved site.
Residency Programs	Specialty Dependent—three (family practice) to seven years (neurosurgery) *Examples:* pediatrics, internal medicine, surgery, psychiatry, obstetrics, geriatrics, cardiology, and ophthalmology	Same

	Allopathic Medicine (MD)	Osteopathic Medicine (DO)
Licensing	Requirements vary by state. Regulated by American Medical Association.	Requirements vary by state. Contact the American Osteopathic Association for more information.
Postgraduate Certification	Usually sub-specialties (e.g., prenatal surgery) or complements to specialties.	Examples include: • Craniosacral Therapy • Medical Acupuncture • Ortho-Bionomy • Homeotherapeutics • Manual Lymphatic Drainage • Naprapathy • Various other diplomate programs • Also includes all programs open to MDs

Financial Information

Family osteopaths earn from $75,000 to $150,000 per year. Specialized osteopaths can earn more, depending on their field of expertise and the institution in which they practice.

Internships and Residency Programs

After graduating, DOs are required to serve a one-year internship to enhance clinical skills in various disciplines. Described as a rotating year, internships shift the aspiring osteopath around, exposing the doctor to many different types of medicine. More extensive information on these internships, which must be approved by the AOA, may be found on the association's Web site: www.osteopathic.org. The goal of these programs is to ensure that osteopaths are prepared to enter the field of medicine in both a holistic and allopathic way. After the internship, DOs fulfill a residency program (varying from two to eight years) in a specific area of medicine.

Postgraduate Studies and Continuing Education

As with other medical professions, osteopaths are required to take continuing education to maintain licensure. These requirements are usually regulated by the state osteopathic institutions listed below. As a point of reference, osteopaths must take up to forty-five hours of continuing education a year, or 125 hours during a three-year period.

Continuing education courses are offered by accredited osteopathic schools and include topics such as acupuncture, anesthesiology, cardiology, dermatology, obstetrics/gynecology, internal medicine, infectious diseases, nutrition, and pediatrics.

ORGANIZATIONS

American Osteopathic Association
www.osteopathic.org

Founded in 1897, the AOA is a member association that represents more than 61,000 osteopathic physicians. It serves as the primary licensing body for DOs and is also responsible for running the American Association of Colleges of Osteopathic Medicine (AACOM)—the main accrediting organization of osteopathic schools. It conducts research on the osteopathic profession and is responsible for defending osteopathic ethics and policies.

American Academy of Osteopathy
www.academyofosteopathy.org

The AAO is a medical membership society focused on educational integrity in osteopathic medicine. The mission of the AAO is to teach, advocate, and research the art and philosophy of osteopathic medicine. Most academy members specialize in osteopathic manipulative medicine.

American Association of Colleges of Osteopathic Medicine
www.aacom.org

Founded in 1898, the AACOM is the sole accrediting body for osteopathic colleges in the United States. Today, the organization represents the students, faculty, and administration at all accredited osteopathic medical programs. The AACOM, in conjunction with the AOA, is also responsible for cooperating with osteopathic state departments to maintain continuity in credentialing, continuing education requirements, and integrity in the field.

American College of Osteopathic Family Physicians

www.acofp.org

The ACOFP seeks to promote excellence and leadership in osteopathic family medicine through equality education and responsible advocacy. Its goals are to increase the number of students selecting AOA-approved family practice residency programs, to increase the size of ACOFP membership, and to increase the interaction between the ACOFP and osteopathic colleges.

American College of Osteopathic Internists

www.acoi.org

The mission of the ACOI is to advance the practice of osteopathic internal medicine. Through excellence in education, advocacy, research, and the opportunity for service, the ACOI strives to enhance the professional and personal development of the family of osteopathic internists.

American College of Osteopathic Surgeons

www.facos.org

The ACOS is committed to assuring excellence in osteopathic surgical care. Like many others of its kind, it is an advocacy, networking, and educational organization dedicated to improving the osteopathic profession. The ACOS also is an excellent resource for graduate education programs in surgical medicine.

American Osteopathic College of Dermatology

www.aocd.org

The purpose of the ACOD is to improve the standards in the practice of osteopathic dermatology and to promote a general understanding of the nature and scope of services rendered to hospitals, clinics, and the public by osteopathic dermatologists. The ACOD has served as a mediator between public health clinics and practitioners since 1957. To date, approximately 282 physicians have been certified by the ACOD. Members include full-time physicians, aspiring dermatologists in residency programs, and student members.

National Board of Osteopathic Medical Examiners

www.nbome.org

The NBOME assesses the competency of health care disciplines relevant to osteopathic medicine. It serves the state licensing agencies via administering examinations that test potential osteopaths' medical knowledge. It also issues the COMLEX examination, which is currently the national standard test for the osteopathic profession. Students of osteopathic medicine must pass this exam before they can become a full-fledged practitioner.

American Osteopathic Academy of Sports Medicine

www.aoasm.org

The **AOASM** is the oldest primary care-based sports medicine specialty. It was formed in 1984 to fulfill the mission of a branch of the healing arts profession that utilizes a holistic, comprehensive approach to the prevention, diagnosis, and management of sport- and exercise-related injuries, disorders, dysfunctions, and disease processes.

American Osteopathic Foundation

www.aof-foundation.org

The AOF supports initiatives that enhance the osteopathic profession, including programs that advance the quality of public heath and recognize excellence in the area of osteopathic research. The AOF is a nonprofit organization, guided by a practitioner board of directors that offers scholarships, research grants, and networking opportunities for osteopathic students and practitioners. Its most recent project is the creation of the Osteopathic Research Center located at the University of North Texas Health Science Center.

PEER-REVIEWED PERIODICALS

Journal of the American Osteopathic Association

www.jaoa.org

International Journal of Osteopathic Medicine

www.intl.elsevierhealth.com/journals/ijos

Osteopathic Medicine and Primary Care

www.om-pc.com

An online scientific journal published by BioMed Central.

The Cranial Letter

www.cranialacademy.com/mbrben

A journal dedicated exclusively to osteopathy in the cranial field.

Inter Linea: The Journal of Osteopathic Philosophy

www.interlinea.org

The International Journal of Osteopathic Medicine

www.sciencedirect.com/science/journal/17460689

The Journal of Osteopathic Medicine
www.sciencedirect.com/science/journal/14438461

Osteopathic Family Physician News
www.acofp.org/membership/ofpn/current

Osteopathic Hospital Leadership

The Popular Osteopath
The oldest osteopathic journal.

ONLINE RESOURCES

Mantis Database
www.healthindex.com
The largest source of osteopathic, chiropractic, and manual medical literature.

The Osteopathic Home Page
www.osteohome.com
General consumer information about osteopathic medicine.

Osteopathic Literature Database
www.ostmed-dr.com
A digital repository for articles about osteopathic medicine.

The Student Doctor Network: Osteopathy
www.osteopathic.com
A good general resource for many forms of medicine, especially osteopathy.

Family Health Radio Series
www.fhradio.org
Started by the Ohio University College of Osteopathic Medicine, it offers a daily series of short minute radio programs on everyday health issues.

EDUCATIONAL INSTITUTIONS

Osteopathic schools are frequently part of larger academic institutions. The following directory begins with the larger institution and then lists its corresponding osteopathic college.

A.T. Still University
Kirksville College of Osteopathic Medicine
Kirksville, Missouri
www.atsu.edu/kcom

A.T. Still University
School of Osteopathic Medicine in Arizona
Mesa, Arizona
www.atsu.edu/soma

Midwestern University
Arizona College of Osteopathic Medicine
Glendale, Arizona
www.midwestern.edu/azcom

Midwestern University
Chicago College of Osteopathic Medicine University
Downers Grove, Illinois
www.midwestern.edu/ccom

Des Moines University
College of Osteopathic Medicine
Des Moines, Iowa
www.dmu.edu/com

Philadelphia College of Osteopathic Medicine
Philadelphia, Pennsylvania
www.pcom.edu

Kansas City University of Medicine and Biosciences
College of Osteopathic Medicine
Kansas City, Missouri
www.kcumb.edu/kcolleges/com/com

Lake Erie College of Osteopathic Medicine
Erie, Pennsylvania
www.lecom.edu

Lake Erie College of Osteopathic Medicine (Bradenton Campus)
Bradenton, Florida
www.my.lecom.edu/bradenton

Lincoln Memorial University
DeBusk College of Osteopathic Medicine
Harrogate, Tennessee
www.lmunet.edu/dcom

Michigan State University
College of Osteopathic Medicine
East Lansing, Michigan
www.com.msu.edu

Nova Southeastern University
College of Osteopathic Medicine
Fort Lauderdale, Florida
www.medicine.nova.edu

The New York Institute of Technology
New York College of Osteopathic Medicine
New York, New York
www.iris.nyit.edu/nycom

Oklahoma State University Center for Health
Sciences
College of Osteopathic Medicine
Tulsa, Oklahoma
www.healthsciences.okstate.edu

Ohio University
College of Osteopathic Medicine
Athens, Ohio
www.oucom.ohiou.edu

Pikeville College School of Osteopathic Medicine
Pikeville, Kentucky
www.pcsom.pc.edu

Pacific Northwest University of Health Sciences
College of Osteopathic Medicine
Yakima, Washington
www.pnwu.org/s_services

Rocky Vista University
College of Osteopathic Medicine
Parker, Colorado
www.rockyvistauniversity.org

Touro College of Osteopathic Medicine
New York, New York
www.touro.edu/med
(Additional campuses in California and Nevada)

University of Medicine and Dentistry of New Jersey
School of Osteopathic Medicine
Stratford, New Jersey
http://som.umdnj.edu

University of New England
College of Osteopathic Medicine
Biddeford, Maine and Portland, Maine
www.une.edu/com

University of North Texas Health Science Center at
Fort Worth
Texas College of Osteopathic Medicine
Fort Worth, Texas
www.hsc.unt.edu/education/tcom

Edward Via Virginia College of Osteopathic
Medicine
Blacksburg, Virginia
www.vcom.vt.edu

Western University of Health Sciences
College of Osteopathic Medicine of the Pacific
Pomona, California
www.westernu.edu/xp/edu/home

West Virginia School of Osteopathic Medicine
Lewisburg, West Virginia
www.wvsom.edu/gate.cfm

CHAPTER 3

ACUPUNCTURE AND TRADITIONAL CHINESE MEDICINE (LAC)

HISTORY

Chinese medicine is one of the oldest continuously used medical systems in the world. It is probably second only to East Indian ayurvedic medicine in this regard. Just as the native martial arts and spiritual philosophies of India spread north to China by way of mutual trade and exploration around 600 B.C., so did ayurvedic principles and practices likely have great influence upon the formulation of Chinese medicine. There are now sizeable differences between the martial arts and spiritual beliefs of China and India, and also between their medical systems. This is because their medical systems are based upon local religious ideologies that support the respective medical philosophies.

As Shamanism is based upon the religion of Animism, and as ayurvedic medicine is based upon the Indian religions of Yoga and Hinduism, so is Chinese medicine based upon Taoism and Buddhism (itself originally an atheistic offshoot of Indian Yoga as a spiritual protest against the superficialities of Hinduism). It is wise for the prospective student of natural medicine to keep in mind that there are few clear dividing lines between most ancient belief systems, especially medicine. Instead, proponents of one medical system borrowed from, and contributed to, the future philosophies and protocols of neighboring medical systems.

The two most important foundations for Chinese medicine are Yin/Yang and Wu Xing, also known as the Five Elements. Both of these concepts are attempts to describe the inherent flow of vital force that animates the natural world, from which humans are believed to be inseparable. Both Yin/Yang and Five Element theory were conceived of thousands of years ago by the Chinese, though the even older Rig Veda scripture of India speaks of the original earth, water, and fire elements of both ayurvedic and Chinese medicine. It is believed by some that

THE TWO most important foundations for Chinese medicine are Yin/Yang and Wu Xing, also known as the Five Elements. Both of these concepts are attempts to describe the inherent flow of vital force that animates the natural world, from which humans are believed to be inseparable.

the first Chinese medicine text, *Basic Questions of Internal Medicine*, was written by the legendary Yellow Emperor around 3000 B.C. It is also believed that the foundation behind the Taoist-based *Book of Changes*, or *I Ching*, were invented by the legendary Fu Xi around the same time. But the exact dates of inventions within Asian medical systems are not really known.

Since it isn't vital for the prospective student to know in which exact centuries these ancient practices were first conceived, let's fast forward from 3000 B.C. to 300 B.C., when both Yin/Yang and Five Element philosophy were firmly in place within Chinese medicine. Taoism and Confucianism were flourishing throughout China, with religion, philosophy, and medicine fully fused. Learning to remain even minded amidst the inherent changes of dualistic nature (Yin/Yang) is seen as desirable and healthful. Behaving honorably, for the good of one's family and society, is insisted upon. Keeping the body whole, including abstinence from surgery, is believed to offer a person the best chance at reaching the ancestral heavens. The basics of how to maintain health, via balancing the Five Elements that manifest as the human body-mind and the rest of the universe, is taught from childhood onwards in homes and schools.

Yin and Yang are the two opposing and complementary forces inherent in nature, as conceived by the ancient Taoists. Yin is the shadowy, cool, passive, feminine, consuming night, and includes that half of the universe that most closely correlates to these qualities. Yang is the light, warm, active, masculine, productive daytime, which represents the other half of the universe. But Yin and Yang are not mutually exclusive. As seen in the popular circular Yin/Yang symbol, the "taichitu," Yin always contains a dot-like seed of Yang and Yang always contains the seed of Yin. Yin and Yang are also relative, since one object may seem Yin-like in comparison to a second object, but Yang-like in comparison to a third object. Throughout the universe, and in all its seeming individual parts, there is a constant flow of life energy ("chi" or "qi") that appears as relatively Yin or Yang to a human observer. And neither Yin nor Yang can exist without the other.

A human being is viewed as a microcosmic equivalent of the macrocosmic universe. The same forces of Yin/Yang (and the Five Elements) are fully at play in both the individual and the cosmos. In order to manifest health, the individual must instinctively or intuitively cooperate with nature and not attempt to impose upon it ignorant willfulness and selfish desires. Ideally, individuals must feel themselves as an extension of nature and not as separate entities. Compassion, moderation, humility, noninvasiveness, spontaneity, kindness, and emptiness are some of the qualities most respected within this paradigm. Successful balance with the Tao, or the way of nature, results in gradual, effortless enlightenment. Simultaneously, it also results in effortless well-being, as it assists the life force to flow in a harmonious manner throughout the invisible meridian channels that flow through the human body from head to fingers and toes.

A sage or doctor can diagnose an individual's relative attunement with the Tao by observing external appearance, quality of movement, vocal timber, body aroma, etc. Most importantly, they can assess health by observing their patients' tongues and by feeling for the shallow and deep pulses at their patients' wrists. Tongue and pulse qualities reveal the relative flow of Yin and Yang throughout the human organ systems, themselves classified as either relatively Yin or Yang. Pressure, heat, or puncturing upon skin points along the meridian channels alters the flow of life force and rebalances Yin and Yang toward their proper amounts and locations. Herbs, foods, meditations, massages, physical exercises, and proper placement of objects within the patient's external environments contribute to the same. The goal is to re-establish the harmonious dynamic equilibrium of energy flow between patient and universe—viewed as one inseparable, omnipresent Tao.

The Elements constitute one of the earliest descriptions of the human organism. It originated with the ayurvedic texts of India that promoted the concept of life being a mixture of earth, water, and fire. By the time of Aristotle circa 400 B.C., ayurveda had added two more elements originating out of fire: air and ether. The Greeks agreed with these additions, although the earlier Hippocratic medical system left ether out of the mix. Buddha in 500 B.C. also ignored the concept of an ether element within his four element system, and when his teachings entered

China, they encountered Taoist thought. The Taoists apparently already had in place their own system of the elements, and like ayurveda, they decided upon five elements: earth, water, fire, and two new ones—wood and metal. In the Taoist system, air was considered an equivalent to the life force, comparable to ayurveda's prana. But the Taoists determined that it wasn't truly an element. Instead it became chi, the vital force that animates the other elements and can be accurately assessed as it flows through the human meridian channels.

Just as every part of the macro- and microcosmic universe can be categorized as relatively Yin or Yang, the same can be said for every part of the universe being classified as being most like one or more of the Five Elements. Also, the same diagnostic methods of patient observation, including tongue and pulse diagnosis, reveal a similar relative balance of the Five Elements within each person. Because Taoism views nature as a constant flow of energy, the Five Elements are also called the Five Movements or the Five Phases. In China, practices as diverse as warfare, astrology, music, and, of course, medicine have all relied heavily for inspiration upon the flowing five element system from at least 300 B.C. until the more materialistic twentieth century.

From the time that the first known silk scrolls illustrating meridian channels were written around 300 B.C., throughout numerous dynasties and global upheavals, Chinese medicine was improved upon, systematized, and specialized, until every known human medical condition had guidelines for treatment. It became a mature medical system with a foundation as solid and complete as the world religions that supported it. When Buddhism was overlaid upon Taoism and Confucianism in the first century, it brought ayurveda-like protocols from India and meshed them with existing Chinese traditions. Modern day Tibetan Buddhist medicine currently illustrates the full effect of this Yogic ayurveda upon Taoist Chinese medicine, as it made its way north into China.

Despite periods of stagnation and withholding of potentially helpful medical information by teachers promoting competing schools of thought, Chinese medicine guided the health and well-being of China until 1911. At this time a variety of cultural forces resulted in the final Chinese monarchy being overthrown by revolutionaries intent upon forging a democratic republic. Since Chinese medicine was associated with the social system being overthrown, it was officially condemned for being naïve and unscientific despite millennia of constant use within China. Chinese medicine was quickly replaced in urban areas by allopathic medicine, which revolutionary leader chiang Kai-Shek believed would impress the western governments whose help he needed.

The unofficial ban on Chinese medicine continued past the communist revolution of 1949, led by Mao Zedong. In the mid-1950s, Mao began to encourage the return of Chinese medicine, in the form of an integrative medicine in conjunction with allopathy, as there were simply too few allopaths to treat 400 million Chinese citizens. Mao officially encouraged Chinese medicine practitioners to participate as "barefoot doctors" treating the vast rural population. At the same time, allopaths would also be trained in Chinese medicine.

Because there were so many contradictory texts and procedures, a consolidated system, based partially on new scientific research, was put in place and given the new name, *traditional Chinese medicine* (TCM). Many Chinese medicine doctors complain to this day that the finest medical knowledge within Chinese medicine was thrown away due to this attempt at integrative modernization. Since the 1950s there have been ups and downs for TCM practitioners in China. Sometimes they have been lauded as maintainers of a noble tradition. At other times, they have been persecuted as traitors to the new People's Republic of China.

TODAY'S CHINESE MEDICINE

Currently there are approximately a third of a million TCM practitioners in China, approximately the same number as in 1952. Despite this apparent growth stagnation, there has been significant change regarding acceptance for TCM practitioners. Since the early 1950s, the number of TCM facilities has grown—there are now more than 2,500 TCM hospitals instead of just 20; 250,000 TCM hospital beds instead of 225; and 70 TCM research institutions versus zero. Clearly TCM has reached critical mass in modern, capitalistic China. Comparable perhaps to modern naturopaths in the United States who have fused traditional naturopathy with allopathic diagnostic skills, TCM practitioners in China combine Chinese medicine with modern allopathy. In the U.S., however, Chinese medicine has a different history with different results.

Americans had little awareness of nonallopathic medical systems until the counterculture revolutions of the late 1960s. This is despite the fact that many foreign immigrants had for centuries practiced the medical systems of their home countries in cities across America. Even before Asian immigration, French physicians had imported some acupuncture techniques into the American colonies from French Asian colonies in the 1700s. And the 1901 version of *Gray's Anatomy* listed acupuncture as a worthy treatment for sciatic nerve pain. In the late 1960s, many progressive Americans began to idealize foreign belief systems, especially if the foreign vitalistic philosophies (such as Taoism) more closely aligned with their own.

In 1971, a *New York Times* reporter traveling with the Nixon administration suffered an attack of appendicitis in Peking. Impressed by the integrative TCM treatment that he and his fellow patients received while hospitalized, the reporter wrote of his experience for millions of American readers. At a press conference soon afterwards, Secretary of State Henry Kissinger mentioned that he and President Nixon were interested in the healing potential of acupuncture. Nearly overnight, Americans became interested in the medicine (and martial arts) from the Chinese culture. Licensed MDs in America had always been allowed to perform acupuncture with no training. In 1973, Nevada became the first state to license nonphysician acupuncturists. The number of states with similar licensure has now grown to more than forty. There are currently only ten states in the United States that do not regulate the profession. Acupuncturists from the followings states are therefore *not* eligible to sit for the National Certification Commission for Acupuncture and Oriental Medicine's Acupuncture Modules Exam: Alabama, California, Delaware, Kansas, Louisiana, Mississippi, North Dakota, Oklahoma, South Dakota, and Wyoming. California provides its own exam, considered at least as challenging as the exam offered by the NCCAOM.

The main difference between TCM in the U.S. and TCM in China is that American practitioners tend to avoid the use of allopathic methods whereas TCM practitioners in China are often simultaneously trained in allopathy and continue to offer fully integrated services throughout their careers. "Integrated allopathic traditional Chinese medicine" is common in Chinese hospitals and clinics. In the U.S., most TCM practitioners have solo practices instead. There has also been an increase in the number of American MDs who learn acupuncture, usually via the more materialistic training involved in the certification for medical acupuncture. Chinese medicine has finally found mainstream acceptance in both the East and West, despite reservations regarding the religious beliefs that form its foundation. Although Chinese medicine has been diluted to such an extent that it is sometimes invisible during an appointment with a modern TCM practitioner, the continued presence of any version of Chinese medicine is a testament to the elegance and efficiency of its ancient techniques.

TREATMENT

Traditional Chinese medicine practitioners identify excesses or deficiencies of Yin, Yang, chi, and the Five Elements that comprise the whole of a patient. They also identify external pathogens that differ greatly from those described in the West. Diagnosis occurs by way of sensing every aspect of a patient's body-mind: looking, listening, smelling, tasting, touching, and especially analyzing the patient's tongue and radial pulses. Though style and technique will vary from practitioner to practitioner, doctors will usually examine the skin, complexion, bony structure, smells, sounds, mental state, superficial preferences (colors, foods, season), emotional traits, tongue, pulses, demeanor, and body build of a patient.

It is not uncommon for doctors to conduct a full in-depth health history. Conversely, it is not uncommon for practitioners to give rapid assessments or conduct a diagnostic analysis with little or no communication with their patients (sometimes due to a language barrier). Some practitioners use written questionnaires in their diagnostic work, while others use extensive oral interviews. One example of a TCM diagnosis might be: "cold damp *bi* syndrome affecting the hand tai yang and yang ming channels with underlying liver and kidney emptiness." An allopathic medical student needs to learn a new set of words, affectionately termed, "medical-ese." TCM students must not only learn new words, including rudimentary Mandarin; they must also learn an entirely new medical paradigm.

Few patients exhibit perfect balance, so a TCM practitioner can almost always find reasons for treating even persons who feel well. Once the patient's energetic imbalances are determined, the doctor applies in-office acupuncture, acupressure, or moxibustion to specific points on the skin that correspond to the most important junctions of chi along the body's meridian channels. The doctor then rechecks the patient's pulses to determine whether the treatment has begun to work. The pulses reflect the relative balance of energy flow in the meridians, with each meridian approximating the function of its similarly named organ system. Often a patient is sent home with an herbal formula (tea, powder, pellet, etc.) that will continue the energy balancing work begun in the doctor's office.

Dietary recommendations might also be made, since each food is relatively Yin or Yang and is also composed of unique Five Element constitutions. The patient might receive massage specific to his or her needs or be sent energy from the hands of a doctor practicing chi Gung. External pathogens are acknowledged within TCM, although they are usually classified by words and concepts such as "cold," "wind," and "damp heat." If healing is successful within the realm of Chinese medicine, the patient will experience relief from his or her presenting ailment, and the doctor will declare that the patient has approached more harmonious energetic balance with his or her internal and external environments.

CHINESE MEDICINE CONCEPTS

Three Jiaos or Three Burners. This is an organ system not recognized by Western physiology. It is mostly energetic, with no corresponding physical organ. It perhaps most closely correlates with the lymphatic system and the metabolism and elimination of food and air. The location of the top burner is from chest to diaphragm, the middle burner is from diaphragm to navel, and the lower burner is from navel to pubic bone. The relative health of this organ system is detected especially via pulse diagnosis. This system is mentioned to illustrate that to learn TCM is to learn a foreign language of life processes that can be confounding to the Westerner. It will also help to understand the details of "Zang-fu" below.

Zang-fu is the Chinese name for Yin/Yang philosophy applied to the interconnected functions of the major "organ systems" in the human body. There are six Yin organ systems (heart, liver, spleen, lung, kidney, pericardium) collectively termed "zang," and six Yang organ systems (small intestine, large intestine, gallbladder, urinary bladder, stomach, and the Three Jiaos) collectively termed "fu." Since Chinese medicine originated at a time long before exact organ function was understood, these classifications do not correlate with the current Western understanding of organ function. For example, the Chinese "Lung" not only is responsible for dispersing chi to the rest of the body from inhaled air, but it also governs the skin and hair. The Chinese "Liver" adds governing sinews and tendons to its digestive and detoxifying functions. That is why the Chinese capitalize the Zang-fu organ systems in order to illustrate their difference from the modern understanding of the organs themselves. Each Yin or Yang Zang-fu organ is also classified as either earth, water, fire, wood, or metal.

This is where duality and the Elements meet within Chinese medical philosophy. Each organ has another corresponding organ, one that is the opposite Yin/Yang polarity but of the same Element. Each Elemental organ pairing then has another pairing that healthfully inhibits it and one more that healthfully stimulates it. TCM doctors use this system of thought in conjunction with their hands-on diagnosis and the patient's complaints to create an individualized treatment plan. All organ systems have corresponding meridians that are accessible via acupuncture. They are also influenced by herbal medicine, diet, and every other treatment modality.

Elegant treatment. Within Chinese medicine, the alleged goal is always "elegant" treatment, which is the least amount of force for the greatest therapeutic benefit.

Meridians are channels for the vital force called "chi." They flow along the surface of the body, and twelve of them correspond to each of the Zang-fu organ systems. These channels are interconnected, one fusing into the next. They do so in a manner that correlates with the way in which each of the Five Elements influences the others within the Zang-fu hypothesis. In general, they flow from the tips of the fingers up the arms to the head and torso, alongside the knees and nose, and down to the tips of the toes. There are approximately twenty meridians and from four hundred to two thousand major and minor acupuncture points that lie along the interconnected meridian trail. No body of scientific research has validated the existence of chi meridians.

Occasionally researchers from the East or West will claim that they have discovered meridian-like channels flowing through a specific body area, such as the connective tissue that surrounds all muscles in the body. No supportive studies confirm these findings. This lack of physical scientific proof for meridians shouldn't necessarily convince a skeptic that all of TCM is based on false premises. Cultures as far apart as India and the Mayan/Incan empires had their own medical systems touting accessible meridians and chi points.

EFFECTIVENESS

Traditional Chinese medicine practitioners believe that every ailment can be successfully treated with acupuncture. Western scientists have so far acknowledged that acupuncture can assist with treating only a fraction of known human ailments. There is grudging acceptance of TCM and acupuncture within allopathic medicine, necessitated by scientific validation of acupuncture's effectiveness. Along with this acceptance usually comes the refutation of TCM philosophy since it runs counter to the Western understanding of anatomy, physiology, and cosmology.

A consensus panel convened by the National Institutes of Health in 1997 concluded that there is evidence for acupuncture treatment being effective for postoperative and chemotherapy nausea and vomiting, nausea of pregnancy, and postoperative dental pain. The twelve-member panel also concluded in their statement that there are a number of other pain-related conditions for which acupuncture may be effective as an adjunct therapy or as an acceptable alternative. It was judged that there is less scientific validation for treating the following ailments: addiction, stroke rehabilitation, headache, menstrual cramps, tennis elbow, fibromyalgia (general muscle pain), low back pain, carpal tunnel syndrome, and asthma. However, such treatments are still scientifically significant, with patient relief occurring at rates higher than random placebo insertion of acupuncture needles.

The World Health Organization meanwhile recognizes acupuncture and Chinese medicine's ability to treat some forty common disorders including:

- Gastrointestinal disorders, such as food allergies, peptic ulcer, chronic diarrhea, constipation, indigestion, gastrointestinal weakness, anorexia, and gastritis.

- Urogenital disorders, including stress incontinence, urinary tract infections, and sexual dysfunction.

- Gynecological disorders, such as irregular, heavy, or painful menstruation; infertility in women and men; and premenstrual syndrome.

- Respiratory disorders, such as emphysema, sinusitis, asthma, allergies, and bronchitis.

- Disorders of the bones, muscles, joints, and nervous system, such as arthritis, migraine headaches, neuralgia, insomnia, dizziness, and low back, neck, and shoulder pain.

- Circulatory disorders, such as hypertension, angina pectoris, arteriosclerosis, and anemia.

- Emotional and psychological disorders, including depression and anxiety.

- Addictions, such as alcohol, nicotine, and drugs.

- Eye, ear, nose, and throat disorders.

- Supportive therapy for other chronic and painful debilitating disorders.

TECHNIQUES

Modern acupuncturists may discount all of the above philosophy and technique and simply needle pre-specified meridian points that have been determined to reduce the symptoms presented by patients. This is the case with medical acupuncturists. Modern Chinese "patent" medicines may also be prescribed in a similar manner to allopathic medications, by matching a Western disease label with a premixed herbal formula. This is a distortion of TCM philosophy and practice, however. At its core, TCM is a system primarily dedicated to balancing energy flow and only secondarily to symptom alleviation.

Current acupuncture techniques include those developed in Korea, Japan, Tibet, Vietnam, and other countries influenced by TCM.

General acupuncture is the puncturing of the skin at specific chi points believed to help regulate the flow of vital force and bring into relative balance the Yin/Yang and Five Element forces that determine health and well-being. Sharp stones, bones, bamboo, and metal have all been used as needles in the past. Currently, hair-thin metal needles are in vogue since they cause the least amount of pain to the patient. Once a doctor has determined which chi points must be stimulated, needles are inserted with a quick thrust and given a gentle twist. The patient, and especially the practitioner, can usually feel if a needle has been inserted correctly and the chi activated. Patients often feel this activation as a slightly annoying mild energy jolt. Doctors feel the needle "tugged" into the patient by the activated chi. Needles are left in place for several minutes to a half hour, and some doctors give inserted needles several more gentle, stimulating twists during the full treatment session.

Auricular acupuncture is a specialized needling therapy that focuses solely on acupuncture points upon the outer ears. It was practiced in previous centuries by both the Chinese and the Plains Indians of North America (who apparently used porcupine quills). There are approximately 120 acupuncture points on each ear, and proponents believe that all energetic imbalances can be treated via the ears alone. This is because every major meridian is believed to

cross the ear on one side or the other. Others say that an inverted diagram of a human fetus placed over the ear allows needling to influence corresponding areas of the human body represented by the fetus mapping. This is reminiscent of the "holographic" beliefs behind reflexology and iridology. Research has been mixed regarding claims made for diagnosis solely via ears, hands, feet, or eyes. The modern doctor of auriculotherapy uses either tiny metal needles or electric/laser stimulation. Medical acupuncturists favor this therapy for treating all forms of drug dependence, including nicotine, alcohol, opiates, and cocaine.

Medical acupuncture is defined by the American Board of Medical Acupuncture as "the medical discipline having a central core of knowledge embracing the integration of acupuncture from various traditions into contemporary biomedical practice." In practice, this means that the practitioner ignores most of the Taoist cosmology and medical hypotheses behind TCM and instead memorizes specific needling protocols for specific diseases or symptoms. Over the last two decades, this technique was created for MDs, DCs, and DOs who want to use acupuncture because of its proven effectiveness much the same way physical Hatha Yoga is practiced separate from its original spiritual philosophy. Needling points may be based on traditional point location, or simply upon what segment or area of the body is experiencing symptoms. Chinese medicine and TCM doctors both criticize medical acupuncturists for heavily diluting Chinese medical theory and practice.

Korean hand acupuncture is a misnomer, since most of the time treatments are done via hand massage upon the hands' meridian chi points. A doctor may also use tape-on acupressure pellets, heat stimulation, or sometimes tiny metal needles. Developed by Dr. Tae Woo Yoo in 1971, it is one of many offshoots from standard TCM-based acupuncture. Hand acupuncture is similar to acupressure and could be considered the Korean version of hand reflexology. Similar to auriculotherapy, it is believed that the entire TCM acupuncture meridian trail is represented on the hands alone. It is especially convenient for use with children and others who fear needles.

Acupoint therapy is a Swedish extension of akupunkt massage, a type of bodywork that is loosely based on TCM. Founded by Willy Penzel, a German MD during World War II, akupunkt massage uses a metal pen instead of acupuncture needles. At the core of akupunkt massage is pen pressure along the Yin and Yang aspects of the meridians and their associated chi points. This system illustrates how divergent from TCM some acupuncture systems have become.

Sonopuncture (a.k.a. acutonics or phonophorese) is a modern blend of New Age belief and TCM techniques. Using the traditional meridian model for the human body, sonopuncturists use sound rather than pressure or needles upon acupuncture points in order to stimulate chi and subsequent healing. The primary tool in a sonopuncturist's practice is a specialized tuning fork said to be tuned according to the physics and harmonics of the solar system. It is one of the most distant derivations of TCM, although Chinese medicine did include music therapy as one method of treatment.

Chinese herbs. The use of herbs for medical purposes probably outdates acupuncture in classical Chinese medicine. Each item of the universe has been classified by the Chinese as being relative Yin or Yang, and as being composed of varying amounts of the Five Elements. This is especially convenient when applied to herbs, since they can be ingested, smeared, inhaled, insufflated (snorted), and generally made to effectively impact the entire human organism. A TCM doctor uses single herbs, standard herbal combinations, or newly devised formulas to influence chi and blood flow and to alter Yin, Yang, and Five Element ratios within the Zang-fu organ systems.

These herbs often come in the form of teas that must be cooked for an hour or more per day. This is annoying to many Americans with little spare time, and the teas are frequently unpleasant in taste. For these reasons, herbal tablets are more and more commonly used. Since herbs are taken several times a day, they are usually the primary medicine for those patients whose doctors make use of herbal medicine. Acupuncture then becomes a secondary medication because patients rarely choose to go to a doctor's office for treatment more than a few times per week. Doctors may choose to apply tape-on metal balls to acupuncture points to continue treatment between office visits. But tape-on point treatment isn't considered very potent compared with concentrated herbal teas and pellets.

Chi kung (a.k.a. qi gong) is the cultivation and use of the vital life force. It is a direct analogue to the breath-oriented meditations of the Indian Yoga religions, as well as to the Hatha Yoga movements practiced by Yogis for balanced energy flow, flexibility, psychosomatic health, and ease of remaining in meditation posture. Buddhists carried their Yoga-based protocols into China during the first century. There they intermixed with Taoist systems of breathwork and movement. Both religions believe that control of the vital force via breathwork and movement is nearly essential in order for individual enlightenment to occur.

Chi kung usually combines deep diaphragmatic breathing with energy flow visualization for the purpose of improving the practitioner's spiritual health, body-mind well-being, and martial arts skills. It is also used clinically for the purpose of sending healing energy directly into a medical patient. Within TCM, a doctor can train patients to self-heal via their own chi kung practice. They may also offer patients more potent chi kung treatments derived from the doctor's more skilled practice. Chi kung practitioners send healing chi into a patient via visualization, placement of hands upon the patient's body, or directing of energy into the patient from hands located just above the patient's body.

Until recent times, all Asian systems of spirituality, medicine, and martial arts were closely guarded secrets that remained within strict student-teacher lineages. Currently, chi kung lessons are easily found, even at your local YMCA. Tai chi chuan martial arts classes are founded in chi kung practice, although students may never be told they are doing anything other than a relaxing Chinese dance. Medical chi kung treatment has been officially recognized as a standard medical technique in Chinese hospitals since 1989. It is sometimes included in the curriculum of major universities in China.

After years of debate, the Chinese government

decided to officially manage chi kung through government regulation in 1996 and has also listed this medical modality as part of its National Health Plan. A vast amount of scientific research has been done in China over the last fifty years. The results suggest that chi kung is nearly a panacea. Whether this is due to the stress reduction effects of breathwork and meditation, or due to specific control of a vitalistic force, is a difficult medical question to answer.

Fire cupping. Various folk medicines have incorporated this technique, including those from Persia, Mexico, Russia, Vietnam, and Greece. There is no conclusive proof regarding where this technique was invented, but the earliest mention seems to be from Plato circa 360 B.C. Fire cupping involves using a flame to create vacuums inside small glass cups and then placing the cups directly on a patient's body. The vacuum causes the skin to be pulled toward the cup, and the patient simultaneously feels the warmth from the extinguished, vacuum-creating fire.

World cultures have used this technique for the relief of musculoskeletal pain and for treatment of respiratory illnesses such as bronchitis and the common cold. TCM adds to this treatment list by claiming that cupping reduces chi stagnation or sluggishness in the flow of chi. To rebalance chi flow, cups are placed over chi-stagnated meridian points or over regions experiencing a lack of vital force. Cups are commonly placed along the meridians of the back, as the skin is less sensitive here and there are many accessible chi points. Medicated oils are sometimes placed at the cupping sites to augment healing and create a better vacuum seal. Vivid maroon welts remain for around a day following treatment. There has been little scientific research testing this memorable form of acupressure.

Chinese medical massage is considered to be one of humankind's oldest healing arts. Every culture has evolved systems of therapeutic bodywork that reflect their unique belief systems regarding cosmology, medicine, and physical intimacy. The Chinese inevitably united their massage practices with the philosophical foundations of Chinese medicine as a whole. Massage may occur at specific chi points in order to affect the Five Element organ systems at their respective meridians. Massage may also be applied in a specific Yin or Yang manner to impact the body-mind in a more general way. Still another approach is to apply hands-on chi kung treatment directly through a patient's skin. The five primary massage types within traditional Chinese medicine include the following:

- **Amno, press and rub,** is used for rejuvenation and health maintenance. Commonly performed as self-help home care, in martial arts and general sports therapy, and as an adjunct to chi kung.

- **Tuina, push and grasp,** is a sophisticated medical massage used to treat injuries, joint and muscle problems, and internal disorders as classified by TCM.

- **Infant tuina** is one of the primary ways in which the Chinese treat babies and young children. The points and channels used can be quite different to the standard ones used within TCM, reflecting the evolution and alteration of chi flow within a growing organism.

- **Dian Xue, point press,** is familiar to Americans as acupressure. The technique uses simple, held pressure techniques, especially upon meridian chi points. It is both a home remedy and a replacement for acupuncture.

- **Wai Qi Liao Fa, curing with external chi,** is healing by direct transmission from chi kung practitioners, presumably after years of training and discipline.

Moxibustion is a specialized herbal treatment involving chi point stimulation. "Moxa" refers to the mugwort (*Artemesia vulgaris*) herb. "Bustion" is the act of burning, as in combustion. Burning aged and fluffed mugwort upon or above chi points is believed to predate acupuncture by many centuries. This process may also be used to warm and stimulate chi and blood flow within general body regions versus within specific chi points and their corresponding meridians and organ systems.

Acupuncture is believed to have superseded moxibustion around 200 B.C. But moxa is still commonly used today. Modern forms include processing the moxa into a solid stick form for ease of usage. The more ancient fluffed version can also be burned on top of an inserted acupuncture needle in order to create an intensified healing effect. To prevent scarring, sometimes moxa is burned on top of a slice of ginger placed upon the skin. Moxibustion is considered preferable to acupuncture for chronic illness, for physically or energetically weak individuals, and for the elderly.

CAREER AND TRAINING

During the last thirty-five years, traditional Chinese medicine has remained the most popular "foreign" medicine in the United States.

Americans now react nonchalantly to the concept of having tiny needles stuck into their bodies to stimulate an invisible force that is reputed to help relieve many symptoms. Insurance companies are increasingly willing to cover routine series of acupuncture treatments for a variety of disorders but it depends on the company and policy. Most Americans don't understand the subtle Taoist spiritual science behind their treatment before receiving acupuncture. And many Western acupuncturists are of the medical variety who don't believe in the existence of chi. Still, in a diluted form, TCM has come a long way toward mainstream acceptance in the U.S.

In 2002, the National Institutes of Health released a survey that found that some 8.2 million American adults had tried acupuncture at some point in the lives, and that 2.1 million of them had used it in the previous year. A Food and Drug Administration study found that Americans made 12 million visits to acupuncture practitioners.

WHERE PRACTICED

Most acupuncturists have a private practice. Others work in a hospital, clinic, or increasingly within a holistic spa setting.

DEGREES, LICENSURE, ACCREDITATION, AND CERTIFICATION

In 1973, Nevada became the first state to license nonphysician acupuncturists. Previously, only licensed doctors—regardless of their training in oriental medicine—could legally practice acupuncture. It was not uncommon for doctors with no formal training in acupuncture to start a practice with little knowledge of its methods or philosophy. Before the existence of advocacy groups such as the National Certification Commission for Acupuncture and Oriental Medicine, acupuncture was an unlicensed and unrestricted profession. Although even today licensure for acupuncture and Chinese medicine is not currently available in every state, forty states regulate the profession with a nationally administered exam given only after candidates have completed an accredited graduate program.

Currently, most states regulate and license acupuncturists. The National Certification Commission for Acupuncture and Oriental Medicine (NCCAOM) is responsible for standardizing professional requirements among the various states—through both accrediting training programs and administering tests—but some states issue their own certification exam and may have different licensure requirements. To best understand the laws in your state, consult the Web site of your state board, which can be found in the lists below.

EDUCATION REQUIREMENTS

To gain certification in acupuncture, according to the NCCAOM, currently the largest national accrediting body for acupuncture, oriental medicine, Asian bodywork, and Chinese herbology, students must meet all the requirements under any one of three formal training venues: 1) formal education at an accredited program (typically three years); 2) apprenticeship, which is defined as training completed under a preceptor who assumes responsibility for the theoretical and practical education of the apprentice (ranging from three to six years); or 3) a combination of apprenticeship and formal education. Most practitioners recommend the third realm of education because it fuses both academic and empirical knowledge of the profession. Once one of the three avenues has been satisfied, applicants are allowed to sit for an examination which, if passed, will grant them national certification as a licensed acupuncturist. Certification in oriental medicine, Asian bodywork, and Chinese Herbology operate in a similar fashion but with slightly different requirements. For more specific educational requirements in any of the Asian therapies, consult the NCCAOM's Web site: www.nccaom.org

Financial Information

An acupuncturist's gross annual income in 2006 ranged from $30,500 to more than $105,000 per year, depending on the practice. This is clearly a huge range from which to gauge your future income. Practitioners who worked in hospitals usually earned $65,000 per year, while practitioners who worked for nonprofit organizations tended to make under $35,000. Some students may choose to follow their hearts alone and attend a program that they know will probably not reap a solid return on investment. As a student of TCM, your head can rest assured (more than with many CAM therapies) that you will be employable and accepted by the allopathic community.

Postgraduate Studies and Continuing Education

There is a plethora of continuing education and postgraduate studies for practitioners of traditional Chinese medicine and acupuncture. Through research programs, seminars, educator programs, and membership organizations, practitioners can expand their practice. Some states require a form of continuing education after practitioners finish school, which may take the form of teaching, taking classes, attending conferences, or doing research. Below are just a few continuing education programs in acupuncture; there are many others, which may be found by contacting your state's licensed board or any of the Accreditation Commission for Acupuncture and Oriental Medicine's accredited acupuncture programs. For more information regarding the specific continuing education requirements in your state, contact your local state board. Contact information is listed at the end of this chapter.

CONTINUING EDUCATION ONLINE COURSES

https://healthcmi.com

This Web site offers online continuing education programs for acupuncture practitioners.

Acupuncture Foundation of Canada Institute
Toronto, Canada
www.afcinstitute.com

The Art and Science of Acupuncture
Miami, Florida
www.cam.med.miami.edu

Acupuncture Training Program
Valhalla, New York
www.nymc.edu/cpm

Chinese Acupuncture for Physicians: Scientific Basis and Practice
Los Angeles, California
www.chineseacupunctureforphysicians.com

McMaster University School of Medicine
Hamilton, Canada
www.acupuncturecourses.com

Medical Acupuncture for Physicians
Berkeley, California
www.HMIeducation.com
Organizations

National Certification Commission for Acupuncture and Oriental Medicine
www.nccaom.org

Established in 1982, the NCCAOM is a nonprofit organization with a mission to establish, assess, and promote recognized standards of competence and safety in acupuncture and oriental medicine for the protection and benefit of the public. It is responsible for administering several different examinations and works with state boards to standardize licensure requirements

The Accreditation Commission for Acupuncture and Oriental Medicine
www.acaom.org

The ACAOM is the national accrediting agency, recognized by the United States' Department of Education, which accredits master's-level programs in both acupuncture and oriental medicine. Currently, it accredits fifty schools and colleges in the United States.

The American Association of Acupuncture and Oriental Medicine
www.aaaomonline.org

The AAA's goal is "to promote excellence and integrity in the professional practice of acupuncture and oriental medicine, in order to enhance public health and well-being." It is responsible for educating legislators, regulators, and public health care providers regarding the benefits of acupuncture and oriental medicine.

The American Organization for Bodywork Therapies of Asia
www.aobta.org

The AOBTA is a nonprofit, professional membership organization representing instructors, practitioners, schools, programs, and students of Asian bodywork therapy.

The Council of Colleges of Acupuncture and Oriental Medicine
www.ccaom.org

The mission of the CCAOM is to advance acupuncture and oriental medicine by promoting educational excellence within the field. The philosophy of the council is based on respect for the broad range of traditions of acupuncture and oriental medicine and a commitment to academic freedom. It offers a membership network, newsletters, job announcements, and other resources for practitioners.

The Federation of Acupuncture and Oriental Medicine Regulatory Agencies
www.faomra.com

Created after two years of conversations with acupuncturists around the United Sates, the federation provides an organization through which membership agencies and practitioners can network. The goal of the federation is ultimately to protect the public through concise communication about licensure, practice, regulatory activity, and professional disciplinary action relevant to both acupuncture and oriental medicine.

Council of Acupuncture and Oriental Medical Associations
www.acucouncil.org

Founded in the late 1970s, the CAOMA is an umbrella organization of oriental medicine professional membership organizations advocating for excellence in the education and practice of oriental medicine as a primary health care profession.

National Acupuncture Detoxification Association
www.acudetox.com

The NADA is a nonprofit association that conducts training and provides public education about the use of acupuncture as an adjunctive treatment for addictions and mental disorders.

The American Academy of Medical Acupuncture
www.medicalacupuncture.org

The purpose of the American Academy of Medical Acupuncture is to promote the integration of concepts from traditional and modern forms of acupuncture with Western medical training and thereby synthesize a more comprehensive approach to health care. The academy has a separate board certifying body for MDs, a membership organization, and a list of approved training programs for medical acupuncture.

The Society for Acupuncture Research
www.acupunctureresearch.org

The SAR is a research group that promotes scientific inquiry into oriental medicine systems (including acupuncture, herbal therapy, and body-oriented modalities). It emphasizes clinical efficacy and theoretical foundations in a combined effort to help nationally legitimize the practice of oriental medicine.

PERIODICALS

Acupuncture & Electro-Therapeutic Research
www.cognizantcommunication.com/filecabinet/

An international journal from Cognizant Communications Corporation.

Acupuncture in Medicine
www.medical-acupuncture.co.uk/aimintro.htm

Published twice a year and is included in many medical databases, including Medline.

Acupuncture Today
www.acupuncturetoday.com

A monthly industry newspaper that provides timely information on the latest news, research, and other issues affecting the acupuncture and oriental medicine profession.

American Journal of Acupuncture
acupuncturejournal.com

Blue Poppy Press On-line Chinese Medical Journal
www.bluepoppy.com

A free online journal dedicated to clinical audits and research reports in Chinese medicine.

Chinese Journal of Information on TCM
www.cintcm.ac.cn/journal-e.html

Sponsored by the (People's Republic of China) State Administration of TCM. Published by the National TCM Information and Library Coordination Committee, in conjunction with the Institute of Information on TCM of the China Academy of TCM. Web site features subscription information only.

Chinese Journal of Integrated Traditional and Western Medicine
www.relaxingnaturalhealth.com/journal.html

Published by the Chinese Association of the Integration of Traditional and Western Medicine and the China Academy of Traditional Chinese Medicine.

Clinical Acupuncture & Oriental Medicine
www.harcourt-international.com/journals/caom

An International peer-reviewed acupuncture journal that provides an authoritative and international source of clinical and professional information for the global community. This journal focuses on the clinical issues in acupuncture and oriental medicine.

Medical Acupuncture
www.medicalacupuncture.org/aama_marf/journal/

A journal for and by physicians. Published by the American Academy of Medical Acupuncture.

Tho Journal of Chinese Medicine
www.jcm.co.uk

Features in-depth articles on the treatment of diseases by acupuncture and Chinese herbal medicine, articles on different aspects of Chinese medicine theory and practice, and abstracts of clinical articles taken from The Journal of TCM.

The Medicine Buddha
www.themedicinebuddha.com

An e-zine on acupuncture, Chinese herbal medicine, and Eastern healing techniques. Targeted mostly toward consumers.

The Pulse
www.pulsemed.org/pulse-of-oriental-medicine.htm

Hundreds of articles about acupuncture, Chinese herbs, diseases, and conditions. Includes explanation of Chinese concepts and medical research.

World Journal of Acupuncture-Moxibustion
tcm.medboo.com/wjam/index.htm

The official publication of World Federation of Acupuncture-Moxibustion Societies (WFAS). Co-sponsored by WFAS and Institute of Acupuncture & Moxibustion, China Academy of Traditional Chinese Medicine.

ONLINE RESOURCES

Acupuncturists Career Center
www.acupuncture-schools.us/index.cfm

Great information on picking the right acupuncture program for you.

Acupuncturists Without Borders
www.acuwithoutborders.org

Acupuncturists Without Borders was formed in September 2005 in the immediate aftermath of Hurricanes Rita and Katrina. Now AWB has volunteer projects for professional acupuncturists all over the world. It recently began a project to help veterans returning from Iraq and Afghanistan cope with conditions incurred at war.

Natural Healers.com
www.naturalhealers.com/qa/acupuncture.html

A career guide to general statistics and nuances of professional acupuncture practice. This resource also includes useful information about the various state-based requirements for licensure in detail.

EDUCATIONAL INSTITUTIONS

There are approximately 150 schools (with more than forty accredited) for acupuncture and oriental medicine in the United States. The following programs are only those accredited by ACAOM:

Acupuncture Master's Programs

Academy for Five Element Acupuncture
Gainesville, Florida
acupuncturist.edu

Academy of Chinese Culture and Health Sciences
Oakland, California
www.acchs.edu

Academy of Oriental Medicine at Austin
Austin, Texas
www.aoma.edu

Acupuncture and Integrative Medicine College, Berkeley
Berkeley, California
www.aimc.edu

Acupuncture and Massage College
Miami, Florida
www.amcollege.edu

American Academy of Acupuncture and Oriental Medicine
Roseville, Minnesota
www.aaaom.edu

American Institute of Alternative Medicine
Columbus, Ohio
www.aiam.edu

American College of Acupuncture and Oriental Medicine
Houston, Texas
www.acaom.edu

American College of Traditional Chinese Medicine
San Francisco, California
www.actcm.org

Arizona School of Acupuncture and Oriental Medicine
Tucson, Arizona
www.asaom.edu

Asian Institute of Medical Studies
Tucson, Arizona
www.asianinstitute.edu

Atlantic Institute of Oriental Medicine
Fort Lauderdale, Florida
www.atom.edu

Bastyr University
Seattle, Washington
www.bastyr.edu

Colorado School of Traditional Chinese Medicine
Denver, Colorado
www.cstcm.edu

Dongguk Royal University
Los Angeles, California
www.dru.edu

Dragon Rises College of Oriental Medicine
Gainesville, Florida
www.dragonrises.edu

East West College of Natural Medicine
Sarasota, Florida
www.ewcollege.org

Eastern School of Acupuncture and Traditional Medicine
Montclair, New Jersey
www.easternschool.com

Emperor's College of Traditional Oriental Medicine
Santa Monica, California
www.emperors.edu

Five Branches University: College of Traditional Chinese Medicine
Santa Cruz, California
www.fivebranches.edu

Florida College of Integrative Medicine
Orlando, Florida
www.fcim.edu

Institute of Clinical Acupuncture and Oriental Medicine
Honolulu, Hawaii
www.orientalmedicine.edu

Jung Tao School of Classical Chinese Medicine
Sugar Grove, North Carolina
www.jungtao.com

Mercy College: Program in Acupuncture and Oriental Medicine
New York, New York
www.mercy.edu

Midwest College of Oriental Medicine
Campuses in Chicago, Illinois, and Racine, Wisconsin
www.acupuncture.edu/midwest/

Minnesota College of Acupuncture and Oriental Medicine
Bloomington, Minnesota
www.nwhealth.edu/edprogr/mcaom.html

National College of Natural Medicine
Portland, Oregon
www.ncnm.edu

New England School of Acupuncture
Campuses in Newton, Massachusetts, and Watertown, Massachusetts
www.nesa.edu

New York College of Health Professions
Syosset, New York
www.nycollege.edu

New York College of Traditional Chinese Medicine
Mineola, New York
www.nyctcm.edu

Oregon College of Oriental Medicine
Portland, Oregon
www.ocom.edu

Pacific College of Oriental Medicine
Campuses in San Diego, California; New York, New York; and Chicago, Illinois
www.pacificcollege.edu

Phoenix Institute of Herbal Medicine and Acupuncture
Phoenix, Arizona
pihma.edu/

Samra University of Oriental Medicine
Los Angeles, California
www.samra.edu

Santa Barbara College of Oriental Medicine
Santa Barbara, California
www.sbcom.edu
www.acupuncturetoday.com/schools/santabarbara.php

Seattle Institute of Oriental Medicine
Seattle, Washington
www.siom.edu

South Baylo University
Anaheim, California
www.southbaylo.edu

Southern California University of Health Sciences
Los Angeles, California
www.scuhs.edu

Southwest Acupuncture College
Campuses in Albuquerque and Santa Fe, New Mexico, and Boulder, Colorado
www.acupuncturecollege.edu

Swedish Institute School of Acupuncture and Oriental Studies
New York, New York
www.swedishinstitute.org

Tai Sophia Institute
Laurel, Maryland
www.tai.edu

Texas College of Traditional Chinese Medicine
Austin, Texas
www.texastcm.edu

Touro College: Graduate Program in Oriental Medicine
New York, New York
www.touro.edu

Traditional Chinese Medical College of Hawaii
Kamuela, Hawaii
www.tcmch.edu

Tri-State College of Acupuncture
New York, New York
www.tsca.edu

University of Bridgeport
Bridgeport, Connecticut
www.bridgeport.edu

University of East West Medicine
Sunnyvale, California
www.uewm.edu

World Medicine Institute
Honolulu, Hawaii
www.acupuncture-hi.com

Yo San University of Traditional Chinese Medicine
Los Angeles, California
www.yosan.edu

Oriental Medicine Master's Programs

The Doctor of Acupuncture and Oriental Medicine (DAOM) degree is the highest formal educational credentialing available in the field of acupuncture and Oriental medicine in the United Stated. Recognized and accredited by the Accreditation Commission for Acupuncture and Oriental Medicine, a doctoral degree can open several doors for a licensed acupuncture, including increased stature, hospital credentialing, research opportunities and increased income. A doctoral degree in acupuncture and Oriental medicine, through the following programs, is equivalent to a PhD-type degree. The DAOM degree is not equivalent to an allopathic doctoral degree. DAOM practitioners are legally allowed to practice acupuncture but their medicinal responsibilities have a much more limited scope.

Bastyr University
Seattle, Washington
www.bastyr.edu

Oregon College of Oriental Medicine
Portland, Oregon
www.ocom.edu

The cost of education is generally $6,000 to $12,000/year for tuition and supplies. Schools accredited by the Accreditation Commission for Acupuncture and Oriental Medicine are able to offer federal student loans.

State Acupuncture Institutions

Alabama Association of Oriental Medicine
www.acuphysician.com

The Acupuncture and Oriental Medicine Association of Alaska
www.acupuncturealaska.com

Arizona Society of Oriental Medicine and Acupuncture
www.azsoma.org

California State Oriental Medical Association
www.csomaonline.org

United California Practitioners of Chinese Medicine
www.ucpcm.org

Acupuncture Association of Colorado
www.acucol.com

Connecticut Society of Acupuncture and Oriental Medicine
www.csaom.org

Florida State Oriental Medicine Association
www.fsoma.com

Chinese Medical Association of Georgia
www.cmaga.com

Hawaii Acupuncture Association
www.hawaiiacupuncture.org

Idaho Acupuncture Association
www.idahoacupuncture.org

Illinois Association of Acupuncture and Oriental Medicine
www.ilaaom.org

Indiana Association of Acupuncture and Oriental Medicine
www.iaaom.org

Maine Association of Acupuncture and Oriental Medicine
www.maaom.org

Maryland Acupuncture Society
www.maryland-acupuncture.org

Acupuncture and Oriental Medicine Society of Massachusetts
www.aomsm.org

Michigan Association of Acupuncture and Oriental Medicine
www.michiganacupuncture.org

Acupuncture and Oriental Medicine Association of Minnesota
www.aomam.org

Mississippi Oriental Medical Association
www.missippiacupuncture.org

Acupuncture Association of Missouri
www.missouriacupuncture.org

Nebraska Oriental Medicine Association
www.omahahealingarts.com

New Hampshire Association for Acupuncture and Oriental Medicine
www.nhaaom.org

New Jersey Association of Acupuncture and Oriental Medicine
www.njaaom.net

Acupuncture Society of New York
www.asny.org

North Carolina Association for Acupuncture and Oriental Medicine
www.ncaaom.org

Ohio Association of Acupuncture and Oriental Medicine
www.oaaom.org

Oklahoma Acupuncture Association
www.okacupunctureassociation.org

Oregon Acupuncture Association
www.oregonacupuncture.org

Association for Professional Acupuncture In Pennsylvania
www.acupuncturepa.org

Rhode Island Society of Acupuncture and Oriental Medicine
www.risaom.org

Tennessee Acupuncture Council
www.tenneseeacupuncturecouncil.com

Texas Association for Acupuncture and Oriental Medicine
www.taaom.org

Texas Association of Acupuncturists
www.taoa.org

Vermont Association of Acupuncture and Oriental Medicine
www.vaaom.org

Acupuncture Society of Virginia
www.acusova.com

Washington Acupuncture and Oriental Medicine Association
www.waoma.org

Wisconsin Society of Certified Acupuncturists
www.acupuncturewisconsin.org

CHAPTER 4

ALLOPATHIC MEDICINE (MD)

Medicine known as "allopathic" has been with us for only two centuries, despite its much longer tradition. During the 1790s, Samuel Hahnemann, MD, was developing the radical principles of vitalistic homeopathic medicine in his German motherland. He quickly roused the ire of fellow MDs, who were called "regulars" at the time. Facing heavy criticism from his peers, Hahnemann coined the derogatory phrase "allopathy" as an approximate opposite to "homeopathy."

Allopathy is Greek for "different cures like," which probably doesn't seem too insulting to the average reader. Homeopathy, on the other hand, means "like cures like," because Hahnemann believed he had discovered this fantastic principle: a miniscule amount of a substance which when taken orally in a large dose would cause overt symptoms in a healthy person but when taken as a micro-dose would paradoxically relieve these same symptoms in a suffering patient. Since allopaths practiced the opposite philosophy—using fever-lowering substances to decrease a patient's dangerously high body temperature, for example—Hahnemann felt that his fellow MDs were misguided, even delusional.

He was adamant that his new medical system was the one to use, despite thousands of years of human healing at the hands of doctors who were not homeopaths. He also was convinced that MDs were *creating* disease via their suppression of patients' symptoms, because these symptoms, he reckoned, were the body's way of ridding itself of disease. He felt these suppressed symptoms would later return to patients in much more severe variations as their diseases worsened energetically—even if they appeared to improve observationally. Hahnemann was further troubled by the wretched side effects of some of the staple medical modalities used by allopaths of the day—including bloodletting; bowel purging via irritant laxatives; and the mixture of opium, myrrh, viper's flesh, and sixty-two other ingredients in a panacea-like preventive medicine called "theriac." Needless to say, this is not the allopathic medicine we recognize today.

Meanwhile, seminal practitioner Andrew Taylor Still, MD (founder

A NEW era of medicine has arrived. You now have more than thirty American medical schools to choose from that will allow you to combine allopathic and holistic training. As a student choosing a career in medicine, consider becoming a pioneer in the field of integrative medicine to bring humankind one scientific step closer to the ever-elusive ultimate medical truths.

of osteopathic medicine, 1874); Daniel David Palmer (founder of chiropractic medicine, 1895); and Benedict Lust, ND (founder of naturopathic medicine, 1902) were also rebelling so strongly against the "regulars" that they proselytized for their own competing medical systems. These proposed alternative systems were always in some way a return to the perennial vitalistic philosophy that has been the cornerstone of all healing modalities from all cultures—except that of allopathic medicine.

Allopathy is just a name. This same system of medicine evolved into recognizable form hundreds of years earlier, when the guidelines for modern, materialistic, scientific, "evidence-based" research methodology were first being understood around the time of the European Renaissance around the sixteenth century. The four steps of the scientific method were simple enough: observe, hypothesize, predict, and test. If your belief could not be tested, then it was simply an opinion, no better than any other—invisible vitalistic forces included. Only things that could be detected, weighed, and measured could be tested, and this meant that materialism would become nearly a religion in its own right to these new scientists (even as many scientists continued to practice their favorite, immeasurable religious dogmas within their private lives).

This gets to the philosophical heart of empiricism, its incredible usefulness, and its limitations. Ultimate descriptions of truth are impossible because new hypotheses and measuring technologies will almost surely continue to be developed by scientists over the next thousands of years. Even invisible forces such as radio waves and x-rays were originally impossible to measure and, thus, to believe in. So from any present vantage point, scientists of earlier times show their occasional arrogant tendency to "throw the baby out with the bathwater" due to the inherent limitations of their measuring devices. At their best, scientific beliefs are simply more accurate explanations for observable phenomena. But they are not ultimate truths.

The Western cultures of Europe were first confronted with the exhilarating and frightful news that the earth was no longer the center of an infinite universe. Invisible atoms, and not the five elements of nature (earth, air, water, fire, ether), were the basic building blocks of creation. Blood circulated in a loop throughout the body, rather than in two, disconnected, one-way compartments as was thought at the time. Times were changing; everything seemed up in the air.

The cutting-edge minds who were inspired by this myth-dispensing knowledge derived from science wanted it applied to almost every human craft. Medicine was one of the first crafts to test out the modern scientific methodology, since medical knowledge meant power over illness, life, and death. Immediately, some of the god-like cultural idols of Europe, such as Aristotle and Galen, were found to have major inaccuracies in their understanding of the human body. These intellectual pillars had been held up as the truth for millennia. But these new scientists embraced rigorous logic and new technologies instead of superstition and dogma.

Although ancestral geniuses were frequently correct, enough mistakes were unearthed by newer scientific protocols that now every previously held system of entrenched belief was open to question. Within the medical world, this meant that the dogma of illness being caused by spirit possession, evil spells, and energetic imbalances of invisible substances floating in and around the human body-mind had to be questioned, too. Treating illness via exorcisms, Shamanic soul retrievals, or the manipulation of patients' purported elemental imbalances with grandmothers' herbs began to seem like absurd hypotheses to those scientific medical practitioners who needed to be able to observe and measure something in order to believe in it. Even the traditional concept of humanity as a melding of body, mind, and spirit was derided since only the body was tangible and measurable. Scientific allopaths desired the simplest physical solution to a problem, rather than the holistic, multidimensional diagnoses and treatments preferred by the vitalists.

As the centuries progressed, the materialistic, scientific allopathic mind-set began to win over larger and larger segments of the Western world. Ironically, the treatments used by science-oriented allopaths were often more debilitating than the diseases they were supposed to treat. Allopaths embraced the very measurable effects of their bloodletting, purgative laxatives, oral mercury, and theriac, while shunning gentler, often less aggressive forms of traditional folk medicine.

There was plenty of contradiction to go around. The new allopaths believed in balancing Hippocrates' elemental humours up until the eighteenth century. During American colonial times, they believed that illness was caused by an imbalance of acid and alkaline, or tension and relaxation, and that miasmas of putrefied airs were the main culprit for disease. Even when diseases were understood to be somehow contagious, the same debilitating treatments were used for almost every ailment. It wasn't until the mid-nineteenth century that specific treatments for specific illnesses became commonplace. So, despite their lip service to science, the very unscientific day-to-day practices of the allopaths left open the door for competing "alternative" medical practitioners wanting the public's favorable attention.

Ironically, the medical modalities shunned by previous allopaths are now having some of their ideas scientifically verified, while the allopathic methods believed (by allopaths) to be more scientifically sound in earlier centuries are now viewed as having been tragically and morbidly unsound. George Washington was one of the many victims of bloodletting, however well intentioned, following a simple respiratory illness.

Then again, no one said the scientific method is perfect. It's only a more accurate route toward knowledge than shared cultural beliefs and religious guesswork. In the seventeenth century, an advanced microscope was used to discover microorganisms, and some of these infinitesimally tiny life forms were shown to produce predictable symptoms in susceptible hosts. Although vitalists insisted that patients' resistance to disease was more important than the presence of microorganisms, immunity could not yet be scientifically measured, and Louis Pasteur's germ theory of disease had won over the majority of Western medical minds by the 1870s. By then Samuel Hahnemann had coined his pejorative "allopathy" to describe the philosophy of the "regular" MDs, and the allopaths, homeopaths, osteopaths, chiropractors, and naturopaths all proceeded to battle for medical supremacy within Europe and the United States for several decades hence.

With the establishment in 1904 of the Council on Medical Education by the well-funded and politically connected American Medical Association, the end of the battle (though not the war) for medical bragging rights was near. The AMA joined forces with the even wealthier Carnegie Association and arranged an official review of all the medical schools in the United States. Called the Flexner Report, it provided negative opinions on almost all schools not allopathic in orientation, as well as some of the more lackluster allopathic programs. Soon the U.S. Government agreed that approximately ninety out of the 155 U.S. medical schools in existence should be shut down. Not coincidentally, almost all of the remaining schools were scientific, evidence-based, materialistic, allopathic medical schools. The dominance by allopathic medicine in the twentieth century was made nearly inevitable by the pre-World War I discovery and distribution of mass-produced antibiotics and the continuing inventions of modern lifesaving emergency medical techniques, potent synthetic drugs, and intricate scientific explanations for a large number of human pathologies.

The spectacular successes of modern allopathy brought to humanity greater control over many of the oldest scourges of humanity, such as smallpox, polio, cataracts, bubonic plague, and venomous snakebite, to name but a few. But the scientific method insists that hypotheses and testing must continue so that failures in understanding can be openly challenged and changed without regard to history and tradition. Allopathic failures were inevitable given the ever-present limitations of technology, and these began to be widely advertised again during the heavily vitalistic, Western counterculture movements of the 1960s.

The same materialistic forces that were producing such inspiring medical treatments also seemed to be creating equally pathological conditions in their wake. The chronic, degenerative lifestyle diseases so familiar today, such as diabetes, cancer, and Alzheimer's disease, were shown to be quite resistant to allopathic treatment. And the ongoing science-based attempts to dominate nature and appreciate only the material and the measurable seemed to have also helped to create a Western culture more connected to corporations, chemicals, and commercials than to spirit and nature-based themes. The latter had been a major inspiration for all of the slower-paced cultures that preceded our mercurial culture, one based on speed, superficial faith, and general imbalance.

Perhaps science-obsessed allopaths took their own scientific dogma too unscientifically, since increasing criticism from the somewhat monolithic intolerance of the American Medical Association toward alternative medical philosophies did not inspire allopathic researchers to spend equal time and funding on nonallopathic answers to unsolved medical questions. One could blame human greed and power, or the seemingly ingrained human tendency to defend long-held beliefs (when shown a more accurate truth) rather than admitting (as would a hypothetical ideal scientist) lifelong error.

Whatever the reasons, allopathic acceptance has been exceedingly slow regarding even the possibility that certain aspects of vitalistic medical traditions may reflect truth in a greater way than does allopathy. Only in the last twenty years have we seen a large shift in the way the public views medical traditions from other cultures and traditions. In the United States, European-style naturopathy was resuscitated, chiropractic medicine became respectable, Chinese medicine began its ascent, transpersonal (spirituality-based) psychology arrived in Westernized form, and holistic mind-body-spirit medicine made its generic, though incredibly varied, return during the turbulent 1960s and 1970s. Ayurvedic medicine arrived in the 1980s, along with the mainstreaming of what came to be known as complementary and alternative medicine (CAM). A high percentage of Americans, never as scientifically minded as Europeans in general, began to use unproven CAM services yet not tell their allopathic physicians. Perhaps most MDs had become so rigidly intolerant toward any nonresearched or vitalistic medical approaches that level-headed conversations between CAM-using patients and allopathic physicians become nearly impossible.

Rebels exist within every group and rogue, open-minded, scientific MDs and medical research PhDs have existed in every decade. Starting in the late 1960s, MDs such as Andrew Weil, Elson Haas, Deepak Chopra, and many others began writing bestsellers and giving talks that challenged the knee-jerk criticism of CAM by their allopathic peers. In 1978, the American Holistic Medical Association was formed for holistically inclined MDs and DOs (osteopathic doctors) who desired greater contact with renegade kindred spirits. That same year, Bastyr University opened its doors to train naturopathic medical students who desired more science-based, sometimes allopathic, coursework to augment their instruction in vitalistic therapies. European medical researchers began churning out scientific data supporting the traditional use of many herbal medicines, as evidenced by the allopathic German "E" Commission report of 1993, which supported hundreds of herbal treatments for an even higher number of indications; and even the decades-long use of homeopathy by the English royal family was revealed.

Younger generations, exposed to multicultural beliefs from an early age, and older generations, wanting all available treatment options, began purchasing more and more CAM products and services and turned the natural products industry into a multibillion-dollar juggernaut. Then in 1998 the *Journal of the American Medical Association* (JAMA) reported that between 1990 and 1997 Americans' use of at least one CAM service per year had increased from 34 percent of the population to 42 percent. Even though many of these CAM users had merely taken multivitamins or received massages, hardly leaping from materialism to vitalism in the process, the allopathic world received this news article as a bombshell. Also in 1998, JAMA reported that prescription drugs, taken as directed, killed approximately 106,000 Americans each year, making them the third leading cause of death after cardiovascular disease and cancer. Compounding these revelations is the well-documented health profiteering of current corporate health maintenance organizations (HMOs), pharmaceutical corporations, and insurance companies that process the vast majority of doctor-patient visits in the United States.

Never before has there been so much overall dislike of the U.S. medical system by both practitioners and patients alike. Fairly or not, it is the inhumane heartlessness of scientific extremists who get blamed for the formation of the three-headed monster of HMO-Big Pharma-insurance, which tends to prioritize quarterly profits over compassionate patient care. Allopathic medicine never had all the best medical solutions all of the time, nor should it have been scientifically expected to.

The stage is now set for Western medicine to give

serious scientific attention to contrasting medical beliefs and to begin scientifically fusing allopathic and CAM modalities into some type of evidence-based integrative medicine by putting an equal amount of research time and dollars into CAM treatment modalities. For now, we can appreciate smaller steps toward this goal. In 1994, hippie-in-hiding Andrew Weil, MD, helped to found the first of its kind: the Program in Integrative Medicine (PIM) at the University Medical Center at the University of Arizona in Tucson. It offers residential and research fellowship programs and operates an outpatient clinic. Its forward-thinking principles include: emphasizing health prevention over disease treatment; focusing on nutrition and botanical medicines for both preventive and disease treatments; and including mind-body interventions to complement conventional synthetic drug and surgery protocols. PIM also operates an annual nutrition and health conference and a botanical medicine conference. As of 2005, more than 250 MDs, DOs, physician assistants, and nurse practitioners had completed the program.

Since the founding of PIM, academic instruction in integrative medicine has grown rapidly. There are now thirty-one academic medical centers that offer integrative medicine programs, including the Mayo Clinic, Harvard Medical School, and Georgetown, Duke, and Columbia universities. A truce seems to be coming between the competing medical modalities that vied for supremacy at the beginning of the twentieth century.

In the year 2000, Harvard Medical School established the Division for Research and Education in Complementary and Integrative Medical Therapies. Its main priorities are to "1) structure scientific research involving complementary and integrative medicine therapies according to traditional investigative and evaluative techniques, including controlled clinical trials; 2) share evidence-based resources across Harvard Medical School and its teaching affiliates; 3) coordinate educational programs and policy development in such areas as credentialing, referrals, and co-management of patient care; and 4) develop criteria in order to responsibly recommend the use or avoidance of herb/supplements and other complementary therapies."

These and similar trends demonstrate a serious commitment to unearthing the wealth from non-allopathic sources, even if it is being applied to the materialistic analysis of largely vitalistic therapies. At least allopaths are now willing to accept almost any treatment as their own, as long as it can pass the test of science, as evidenced in this quote by Daniel Federman, MD, from the Program in Integrative Medicine: "When research using standard methods of assessment has demonstrated effectiveness, there should be no need for the term complementary; and when it does not, support for such claims should be withdrawn."

A new era of medicine has arrived, as allopathic medical science looks in two directions for the first time. One direction is toward honing technologies such as those providing insight into manipulating the human genome for the prevention and treatment of many diseases. The other direction is toward the ancient folk wisdom of the collective human psyche, as represented by all of the nonscientific, anecdotally based medical systems that predated allopathy. Although the effects may seem subtle in your life at the present time, as a prospective student of integrative medicine, you now have more than forty American medical schools to choose from that will allow you to combine allopathic and holistic training. While China began in the 1950s to integrate its allopathic and traditional Chinese medicine treatments within its medical schools, the current integration of U.S. medicine is a watershed moment for medicine across the globe due to the much greater influence of American culture worldwide. As a student choosing a career in medicine, consider becoming a pioneer in the field of integrative medicine to bring humankind one scientific step closer to the ever-elusive ultimate medical truths.

WHAT EXACTLY IS ALLOPATHIC MEDICINE?

Allopathic medicine is simply the use of medical agents in opposition to a patient's disease symptoms employed to treat these same symptoms. Using anti-inflammatory drugs to reduce inflammation is allopathy by definition. But most medicines throughout time have been allopathic under this definition. Shaman opposed their patients' disease-causing demons by fighting them in the netherworlds; traditional osteopaths and chiropractors push misaligned bones in the opposite, not the same, direction as their misalignment; and ancient Indian and Chinese practitioners opposed imbalance of a patient's internal Elements by prescribing herbs that pushed the disease process in the balancing, opposite direction. Ancient anti-inflammatories such as the herb turmeric are found to be just as allopathic as is aspirin when tested with scientific methodology. So allopathy is neither inherently modern nor materialistic. There have always been plenty of vitalistic allopaths practicing medicine on planet Earth.

The only true nonallopaths are the homeopaths who coined and embraced the term and who believe in the veracity of "like cures like," where a large dose of a substance that causes a symptom in a healthy person is used in an infinitesimally tiny dose as a treatment for that same symptom. This is such a radical belief that no other system of medicine has ever made it the cornerstone of their philosophy. Homeopaths may appreciate gentler medical systems such as ayurveda more than they do modern Western medicine, but ayurveda still follows the allopathic model (use a "watery" herb to quench a "fiery" disease) more closely than the homeopathic one. So the most helpful question is not "what is the definition of allopathic medicine?" because that becomes an umbrella term covering a huge array of medical traditions. A better question might be: how does integrative medicine compare to the ideal model of a scientific, evidence-based, nonbiased allopathic model?

The principles of integrative medicine (once called "holistic") began to be seriously considered in the 1970s with the founding of the American Holistic Medical Association, a membership organization for MDs and DOs "seeking to practice a broader form of medicine than what was (and is) currently taught in allopathic medical schools."

Holistic medicine is defined as *the art and science of healing that addresses the whole person—body, mind, and spirit. The practice of holistic medicine integrates conventional and alternative therapies to promote optimal health and to prevent and treat disease.* Holistic medicine has attempted to integrate the best of modern-day technologies with the wisdom of the practice of medicine from the past. It represents the next stage in the evolution of health care, a true synthesis of ancient and modern. Like all evolutionary movements in history, it has been met with strong skepticism and sometimes downright hostility from those entrenched in conventional medicine.

THE PRINCIPALS OF HOLISTIC MEDICINE

The following twelve principles of holistic medical practice were established by the American Holistic Medical Association:

1. Optimal health. This is the primary goal of holistic medical practice. It is the conscious pursuit of the highest level of functioning and balance of the physical, environmental, mental, emotional, social, and spiritual aspects of human experience, resulting in a dynamic state of being fully alive. This creates a condition of well-being regardless of the presence or absence of disease.

2. The healing power of love. Holistic health care practitioners strive to meet the patient with grace, kindness, acceptance, and spirit without condition, as love is life's most powerful healer.

3. Whole person. Holistic health care practitioners view people as the unity of body, mind, spirit, and the systems in which they live.

4. Prevention and treatment. Holistic health care practitioners promote health, prevent illness, and help raise awareness of dis-ease in our lives rather than merely managing symptoms. A holistic approach relieves symptoms, modifies contributing factors, and enhances the patient's life system to optimize future well-being.

5. Innate healing power. All people have innate powers of healing in their bodies, minds, and spirits. Holistic health care practitioners evoke and help patients utilize these powers to affect the healing process.

6. Integration of healing systems. Holistic health care practitioners embrace a lifetime of learning about all safe and effective options in diagnosis and treatment. These options come from

a variety of traditions and are selected in order to best meet the unique needs of the patient. The realm of choices may include lifestyle modification and complementary approaches as well as conventional drugs and surgery.

7. Relationship-centered care. The ideal practitioner-patient relationship is a partnership that encourages patient autonomy and values the needs and insights of both parties. The quality of this relationship is an essential contributor to the healing process.

8. Individuality. Holistic health care practitioners focus patient care on the unique needs and nature of the person who has an illness rather than the illness that has the person.

9. Teaching by example. Holistic health care practitioners continually work toward the personal incorporation of the principles of holistic health, which then profoundly influence the quality of the healing relationship.

10. Learning opportunities. All life experiences including birth, joy, suffering, and the dying process are profound learning opportunities for both patients and health care practitioners.

If you compare this list of principles with the seven principles of naturopathic medicine you will see a significant degree of overlap. In fact, only two of the seven naturopathic principles are not overtly represented here: "Do no harm" and "Treat the cause (versus merely the symptom)." Yet someone practicing the style of medicine as mentioned in holistic medicine principle, "the healing power of love," would inherently bring minimal harm to a patient. And though naturopaths tend to disagree with them here, MDs usually feel that they, too, often try to treat the deepest cause of a patient's illness. They cut out malignant tumors and kill bacteria-causing infections with antibiotics.

They also, among many examples, often suppress skin rashes with topical steroids rather than encourage patients to detect potential rash-causing allergens in their daily diet. Regardless, the American Holistic Medical Association saw no reason to list the obvious benefit of treating the cause of illness within its holistic principles because it believed that this was already the unspoken norm. Physicians can make the accurate claim that most patients are satisfied with quick symptom relief versus lifestyle changes that might heal them at a deeper level but that require willpower to enact. In other words, they simply give their customers what they want.

So we seem to have come to a point in time at which there is no apparent difference between the principles of naturopathic or holistic allopathic medicine. Neither expresses concern that patient treatments be scientifically proven. Naturopathic medicine turned toward evidence-based medicine in 1978, with Bastyr University's founding. The more than forty integrative medical school programs around the United States should have little argument with naturopathic/holistic medicine principles and protocols—especially if they have stood the test of scientific research. Hence, the desire for an integrative model.

So what is the difference between becoming a licensed naturopath versus an integrative practitioner. In a phrase: schooling camaraderie, income potential, and societal clout. If you are an undergraduate student who fully believes in naturopathic-holistic principles and are following a lifestyle patterned after them, you will find a much more nurturing experience attending a school still considered alternative and complementary. Most programs listed in this book fit this definition.

Most "mainstream" schools, such as those for MDs, DOs, RNs, NPs, and PAs, simply do not. At these schools, you will more frequently be viewed as an aberration, because integrative medicine is at a fledgling stage and the vast majority of instructors in the allopathic health fields are still more attracted to nonholistic, heavily technology-based, Western solutions. If you are either a brave soul willing to be conspicuously holistic, or a cowardly one willing to hide your true beliefs during your schooling process, attending a more materialistic, mainstream medical school may be for you.

This is because the income potential and societal influence for allopathic health practitioners, simply due to their degree power alone, are much greater than for their peers practicing the naturopathic, ayurvedic, Chinese, and other forms of overtly counterculture, nonallopathic medicine. If securing high status and income is important to you as a practitioner—and there is nothing inherently wrong with this—consider playing the percentages and becoming an integrative practitioner via mainstream routes.

However, if your heart calling to practice holistic medicine is more important than your pocketbook or your clout, consider schooling at institutions that are holistic from the ground up—rather than those that have just recently showed a tolerance toward holistic medicine such as the still very conservative Harvard Medical School. Whichever route you take, as an engaged practitioner, you will be part of a small minority of healers prioritizing integrative medical principles and continuing to assist in the never-ending evolutionary process of global medicine. Thank you for your participation and picking up this book.

TECHNIQUES

There are no techniques that belong to holistic integrative medicine per se. This is because, by definition, integrative medicine is a meshing of previous or current medical protocols that have shown themselves to be a preferred treatment choice. These preferences occur via the combination of scientific proof and strong empirical evidence (if scientific research has either not been performed or has been inconclusive).

It should be noted that approximately 50 percent of all medications used by allopathic physicians (MDs and DOs) do not have conclusive science supporting their use. They do have, however, clever marketing and insurance backing, which do not necessarily produce effective treatments at rates greater than "old wives" tales that CAM practitioners are criticized for accepting as the authority behind their medicaments.

Both allopathic and CAM medical systems allow their own versions of biased lobbyists to distract them from separating harmful and helpful treatment modalities. The samplings of categorical techniques that follow are thus derived from the overlapping subsets that make up the previously separate realms of scientific allopathy and empirical CAM. The great potential of integrative medicine can be sensed when looking at the broad comprehensive treatment modalities offered herein. What we need in order to manifest this potential are medical scientists devoted

to sharing their truth rather than defending their turf. Science and intuition must trump the very human instincts of territorialism and bias. While overcoming ingrained human nature, may we continue to stumble in the right direction.

Preventive medicine: When it comes to focusing on prevention, allopathic medicine has historically lagged behind CAM medicine. Usually following the lead of allopathy-based public health dictums, the area of preventive medicine in the allopathic world has often been limited to such generalities as: don't smoke tobacco, exercise regularly, wear your seatbelt at all times, follow the nutrition pyramid of the U.S. Department of Agriculture, cover your nose and mouth when you cough or sneeze, wash your hands frequently, drink eight glasses of water per day, sleep eight hours per night, get a yearly overall physical exam, etc. While there is certainly nothing wrong with such helpful guidance, it pales in comparison with the intricate and individualized daily preventive medicine applications that have been part of CAM for millennia.

Once a patient determines his or her energetic constitution at birth in the ayurvedic and Chinese medical systems, for example, from this day forward every meal can be used as preventive medicine specific to each person. Individual meals can be specifically prepared so that, on an energetic level, health is promoted and disease more easily avoided. Group meals can be made in a "tri-doshic," balanced elemental fashion so that they keep stable the energetics of each person eating the meal. At least a portion of these meals is often left uncooked, so that the vitalistic life force of living plant material can be directly absorbed by the meal taker. Meats are often diminished in importance to avoid unnecessary involvement in killing. Organic foods are encouraged so that the global community is less burdened by chemical toxins. When combined with the guidelines of scientific Western nutrition—with its understanding of macronutrients (proteins, carbohydrates, fats), micronutrients (vitamins, minerals, co-enzymes), fibers, food allergies and sensitivities (detecting and avoiding foods that stimulate symptom-causing immune responses)—and the ethos of organic, smaller balanced meals taken more frequently, a powerful integrative health synergy of nutrition results. Greater health promotion and disease prevention is the likely outcome.

Similar integrations are occurring in the realms of exercise, interpersonal relations, sleep, sex, career, within every category of life. Whereas allopathic prevention focuses on the general ("everyone should exercise regularly"), CAM specializes in the individualistic ("Mary should be swimming; John should be running; Hussein should be dancing"). Integrating allopathy and CAM allows the best of both worlds to combine and, practitioners hope, keeps the worst of both at bay.

Soon allopathic medicine will bring to us the new world of genetic medicine, which may someday help to prevent and treat nearly all human diseases. In the future, allopathy may become very individualized in its preventive medicine focus via testing an individual's genome and then making specific alterations to any parts of an individual's genome that are likely harbingers for future disease. CAM, for its part, has already developed some universals of preventive medicine to balance out its focus on the individual over the group. For example, in ayurvedic medicine, seasoning food with the combination of fennel, coriander, and cumin is considered to be health promoting for all diners regardless of their individual constitutions. Combine the best of preventive medicines from around the globe, and we are well on our way to a more healthful world.

Birth: Holistic allopaths are in the process of making their shift from un-nurturing, uniformly white hospital rooms; drug- and technology-obsessed practitioners; expectant mothers trapped in the supine position; and excessive caesarean sections mostly used to help keep doctors on their birthing schedules. Coming into vogue are soothing, multicolored, cushioned birthing environments that allow women and their guests to move about as needed; drugs and machines taking a second place to human nurturing; and an openness to birth positions (such as gravity-assisted squatting) other than the supine Western norm. Given that naturopathic midwives have used the latter techniques for decades, it can be rhetorically asked: how is integrative medicine any different than modern naturopathic medicine, which has

already integrated allopathy and CAM to those levels at which they are legally allowed?

Pediatrics: The worlds of allopathy and CAM have yet to come to agreement regarding the use of vaccinations for disease prevention in the young. Allopaths usually insist that vaccinations are helping to prevent many epidemic scourges, such as diphtheria and pertussis. CAM practitioners often believe that vaccines cause more harm than good, from mild allergies to seizures and autism. These latter practitioners feel that the decline in diseases worldwide is not from vaccinations but from improved hygiene, education, and other factors. Integrative medicine practitioners must thus keep an open mind regarding the truths behind vaccinations, and other controversial medical topics, while not demonizing those who believe differently from themselves.

Similar discrepancies exist in basic pediatric care. Allopaths usually choose to treat ear infections, for example, with prescription antibiotics, especially since many parents demand a quick fix. CAM practitioners prefer to detect and eliminate children's individual food sensitivities (especially to cow's milk, gluten, et al), and use milder herbal antibiotics that don't tend to destroy as many friendly bacteria in children's intestinal tracts. In this example, integrative medicine could be represented by the use of prescription antibiotics as a later resort.

First, the noninvasive treatment of eliminating likely food allergens from the child's diet could be performed. Gentler local herbal antibiotics could be used directly in the child's ears. Basic stress reduction techniques could be taught to parents and child alike in order that everyone's immunity is kept optimal. Acupuncture and an ayurvedic diet protocol could be recommended. If necessary, high-powered antibiotics could be used to stop the current infection, to be followed by holistic preventive care in the future. This pattern of using milder CAM techniques first, followed by more intense and invasive allopathic techniques later on (if needed) can be seen as a general template to be followed in most cases regarding human health.

Emergency medicine: The major area in which allopathic techniques should precede CAM techniques within integrative medicine seems to be emergency medicine. Allopathy specializes in the use of "heroic," lifesaving, cutting-edge technology especially appreciated by patients suffering from accidents, heart attacks, and other events that bring patients to the edge of life and death. In these situations, CAM techniques play a supporting role. The emergency room environment can be made more conducive to healing, using a variety of colors, sounds, and aromas that differ from the stark white and sterile versions common today. Herbal remedies can be used, externally and internally, at every stage of the healing process once life has been stabilized. Healing counselors can make their way from gurney to gurney, offering calming therapies to every patient. Each exiting patient can have a preventive health interview, to at least educate patients on how to avoid similar health emergencies in the future.

Acute illness: This covers the beginnings of any illness up to the point at which it becomes chronic approximately two weeks from its inception. Emergency medicine was discussed above, so here we discuss nonlife-threatening illness up to two weeks in duration. Here the "CAM first, allopathy second, if needed" template begins to show its benefits.

Take muscular pain of the back as an example. Allopaths typically prescribe drugs such as ibuprofen for back pain without attempting to determine whether or not the pain is due to vertebral misalignment. A CAM practitioner, such as a chiropractor (DC), traditional DO, or naturopathic doctor (ND), would instead perform a vertebral exam and realign any bones as necessary. This would treat the cause, as opposed to merely offering the temporary symptom relief for which allopaths are so criticized. This example can be extrapolated to many—though definitely not all—instances of acute illness. A general rule of thumb is to treat acute illness with at least equal amounts of CAM and allopathic therapies, if you do not choose to treat solely with CAM therapies at first before moving on to the addition of allopathy if needed.

Chronic illness: This category accounts for the vast majority of illness in the world, being made up of illness longer than approximately two weeks in dura-

tion. Think heart disease, diabetes, and cancer. These ailments normally have a large percentage of their causes based on day-to-day activities such as diet, exercise, and stress reduction. The U.S. Centers for Disease Control and Prevention (CDC) has reported that the key factors influencing an individual's chronic state of health have not changed significantly over the past twenty years. *Quality of medical care makes up only about 10 percent of this influence. Heredity accounts for 18 percent, and a patient's environment makes up 19 percent. Everyday lifestyle choices are 53 percent.* The decisions people make about their lives and their resulting habits are, therefore, by a great degree the largest factor in determining their state of wellness.

Which side of the medical spectrum specializes in lifestyle habits and wellness? CAM, of course. Allopathy specializes in lifesaving medicine, but comes in a distant second regarding wellness habits when compared with the variety of CAM systems covered in this book. Thus integrative medicine treatment for chronic illness quickly begins to look like CAM, with just a dash of allopathy on the side in the case of stubborn illnesses. Taking heart disease as our example, teaching patients proper approaches to diet, exercise, stress reduction, and meditation are all longstanding CAM techniques publicized by the integrative MD Dean Ornish. These lifestyle changing techniques are far more effective at controlling future heart attacks than are the prescription drugs and surgeries that still are the allopathic norm. A general approach to chronic illness is thus: rely heavily on CAM techniques for treatment of disease and promotion of health at all of life's levels—body, mind, spirit, interpersonal, community, and more. Allow allopathic treatments into play only if patients refuse to alter their lifestyles or if no progress is seen using CAM therapies after several months time.

Geriatric medicine: The average person in the U.S. is taking approximately fifteen prescription medications on an ongoing basis by the time they are sixty-five years old. *This has led to a situation in which even correctly used prescription drugs are the third leading cause of death in the U.S., behind cardiovascular disease and cancer.* While not all of these deaths occur among the geriatric set, the sheer number of medicines taken by the elderly combines with their greater susceptibility to drug reactivity to result in the highest level of prescription drug deaths happening within the geriatric age group. Yet this need not be the case, because most of the illness within the geriatric population is chronic illness.

We have already established that chronic illness is best treated with the milder CAM therapies that focus on lifestyle change as well as acupuncture, massage, herbal medicines, joint adjustments, etc. These therapies kill very few, yet it is the more convenient prescription drugs that are used first in almost all cases. This pattern is encouraged by HMOs and pharmaceutical and insurance companies that want quick results to reap quick profits. For integrative medicine providers, the task is thus to treat their geriatric population with as many CAM treatments as necessary, knowing that rarely are there lethal side effects from their various combinations. Use allopathic medicine for emergencies or for resistant individuals and diseases. By no means should another prescription drug be recommended unless the recommender has specifically determined that no harmful drug reactions will result between those that have been prescribed.

Psychiatry and psychology: It took allopaths until recently to acknowledge that patients' psychological status has any impact on their immune systems. When they finally "discovered" this fact in the 1970s, they even gave it a new name: psychoneuroimmunology. CAM practitioners no doubt looked at each other with a shrug and wondered both what took so long and what all the fuss was about. In general, allopathic medicine has also lagged far behind CAM systems regarding the importance of psychology in treating every patient complaint, not just those related to immunity. The dictum, "mind over body, soul over mind," is a CAM statement reflecting the relative importance of these three seemingly separate components. In fact, allopaths often choose to treat the psyche as if it is simply part of the body, suggesting prescription anti-depressants to millions but too rarely suggesting that they undertake rigorous psychotherapy to help reach the deeper roots of their illness (which can be time consuming, tiresome, and expensive). Healing the psyche is an area of difficult debate among the allopathic and CAM communities,

since patients' impatience with their own psychological demons easily combines with the impatience of HMOs and insurance companies to produce the ineffective world of the superficial quick fix.

Integrative providers must make sure that their patients are aware of the importance of healing their psyches from the seemingly unavoidable traumas of birth and childhood, as well as strengthening their adult psyches to manifest emotional maturity in their interpersonal relations. Any untreated neurosis, personality disorder, or psychosis in a patient makes it that much more likely that the physical form will break down as well, with the most extreme example being a psychotic individual not being able to maintain basic hygiene. Proper dietary choices, exercise, and stress reduction must wait until their psyche has been stabilized.

There are many approaches to healing the psyche, with talk therapy being one of the most used and perhaps one of the least effective. Instead, the integrative practitioner can recommend practices that don't allow patients to talk their way around their issues. Toward this end, "body-centered" psychotherapies—such as bio-energetics, hakomi, core energetics, and orgonomy—offer therapies at least designed for quicker and deeper psychological healing by releasing and retraining patients' physical responses to intense emotions.

Another approach is to encourage patients to learn and practice "mindfulness." Although this term is borrowed from Buddhism, it simply means to become consistently aware of one's own thoughts, emotions, breath, muscle relaxation, and activities in general. Remember that Buddhism underlies traditional Chinese medicine and that Buddhism is an offshoot of the Yoga religion that underlies ayurveda. These are the two great spiritual ancestors of CAM, and mindfulness plus meditation are the two basic practices suggested by them for deepest healing of the mind and spirit. If these two practices are ignored, physical well-being is difficult to maintain because the mind and the spirit are both untrained and unfulfilled. Integrative doctors can keep this in mind and recommend specific psychotherapies, mindfulness exercises, and meditations for those suffering patients.

Spiritual crises: Most allopaths do not acknowledge spiritual disease and, thus, are not much help if it arises. This is as opposed to CAM therapies, such as ayurveda, Chinese medicine, and naturopathy, which acknowledge spiritual health as being essential to psychological and physical health. One allopath who differs greatly from the norm is Stanislav Grof, MD. A psychiatrist from Czechoslovakia, Grof has dedicated his career to helping patients heal their minds and spirits. He became one of the preeminent psychedelic researchers of his day, using prescription LSD with hundreds of patients when that was still a legal approach to proactive and curative psychological treatment.

Grof switched to the use of deep breathing for helping patients access deep altered states of consciousness once LSD was made illegal in the mid 1960s. Finding that many patients reexperienced their birth trauma when performing this "holotropic breathwork," Grof hypothesized that many psychopathologies had their origin in the womb. Unpleasantries experienced during childhood and adolescence merely compounded the issues. He also determined that many psychopathologies, especially psychoses, were patients' unconscious attempts to manifest positive spiritual breakthroughs due to their deep-seated needs for spiritual awareness.

He developed procedures for helping patients through these "spiritual emergence" states without sedating them with prescription drugs or otherwise turning their spiritual drives into perceived pathologies. This is one example of how integrative medicine can be practiced when dealing with the spiritual realms. What is important is that the spiritual aspect of patients be acknowledged, so that patients do not feel embarrassed or inappropriate when discussing this part of themselves. Much lip service is given to the spiritual within integrative medicine, yet integrative practitioners usually spend the least amount of time learning about their own spiritual yearnings via spiritual practice compared with studying their own bodies and minds. Integrative practitioners can serve their patients best by becoming comfortable with all aspects of life equally, including body, mind, soul, sex, career, finances, family of choice, family of origin, community, and globe. Of these, CAM systems have been based upon one primary thing: the vitalistic "life force" that most represents the spiritual side of humankind. As an integrative medical provider, if you remember one thing, remember the spiritual health of your patients.

Community medicine: Human beings are gregarious by nature. Their relations with others, to a great extent, help determine the health and relative happiness of groups and individuals alike. Integrative practitioners make use of this knowledge by asking patients about the health of their relations with others. We do this as a way to determine future preventive or treatment measures that would otherwise be unavailable to us if we assume that patients live as isolated individuals.

This just-mentioned ignorant assumption is most often manifested by doctors who forget to inquire into patient relations as part of their medical diagnosis and treatment. Allopaths usually consider community in terms of "herd immunity"—how best to keep our overall population safe from diseases brought to it by the individual. Vaccinate; cover your mouth when you cough; wear condoms—all excellent fragments of advice. The adept integrative practitioner, however, adds the important elements of what the community brings to the individual, not merely how unhealthy individuals affect our community. A person's community begins with his or her housemates, related or not. It extends through neighbors, coworkers, and those individuals and groups that a person interacts with on a regular, or even one time, basis. *Patients manifesting rich fulfillment within their community of social support are the most likely to report overall happiness in life.*

Psychoneuroimmunology, positive psychology and the much older CAM traditions tell us that psychological happiness leads to both greater productivity and greater body-mind health, both at the individual and community level. Integrative practitioners inquire into the well-being of a patient's community life. They realize that their own relations with patients make up a not insignificant part of the equation around the sum total of a patient's well-being.

Environmental medicine: Remember from the CDC study that an astonishingly 53 percent of an average person's health is determined by lifestyle choices.

Broken down further, 19 percent of health is determined by one's environment; 18 percent by heredity; and 10 percent by quality of medical care.

Environment is thus the second most important factor regarding the health of the human race. Yet most practitioners, allopathic or CAM, rarely inquire into the nature of their patients' environments. Skilled integrative practitioners correct this oversight by ensuring that they understand especially their patients' home and work environments—the two places in which patients spend the vast majority of their time. Encouragement can be given to patients to keep their homes nontoxic and workplaces safe. Patients can be queried as to whether they enjoy or despise their usual environments. Anything can be done other than to ignore this crucial aspect of patients' lives.

In conjunction with a patient's usual environments is the patient's felt connection with his or her local natural surroundings and with the planet on which we live. Just a few hundred years ago, almost all of humanity lived in close proximity to nature, for better and worse. We have lessened the worst of that lethal proximity by overcoming natural forces such as smallpox and grizzly bears. However, we have not made up for what we've lost: those health-giving properties derived from frequent exposure to sunshine, fresh air, and pure water; and that combination of relaxation and awe that occurs when we turn off our technologies and immerse ourselves into a forest under the Milky Way. The integrative practitioner investigates a patient's connection with nature and his or her feelings of connectivity with the entire planet, not in order to moralize or criticize, but to encourage patients to connect with their natural planetary source for their greater well-being. We may pretend to be okay living 90 percent of our time indoors interacting with our inanimate inventions, but the speed of evolution begs to differ. We are part and parcel of nature, and the more time we spend within those parts *least* influenced by the good intentions of humankind, the more we will experience the health-benefiting properties that nature bestows.

In summary, integrative practitioners do not use any unique techniques of their own. They simply choose from the range of what is available by allopaths (primarily prescription drugs, surgery, and the gamut of laboratory and physical exams so familiar to readers exposed to conventional Western medicine) and CAM providers (all of the other techniques listed in this book, from massage to acupuncture to joint adjustments to homeopathic remedies and beyond).

This is not a denigration of integrative medicine but a celebration. Never before has a system of medicine been so open-minded toward using the best, most scientifically proven, most holistic of all modalities, regardless of source. As long as there is some evidence, and ideally the firmest scientific evidence, backing the use of a given medical modality, it will be considered as a possible medical modality by the integrative provider regardless of whether or not the modality in question is vitalistic or materialistic in nature. Medical utopia is far from here, but the inroads made by integrative medical providers over the last decade and a half give us a glimpse of the vast improvements to come.

CAREER AND TRENDS

The future looks extremely promising for students looking to combine an allopathic medical degree with CAM training in order to offer patients a specialization in integrative medicine. You will be graduating with one of the most respected degrees in the world (MD) and tempering the perceived shadow side of that degree with the very skills that tend to shine light just where it is needed.

Most people are aware that, although respected, MDs are also often considered to be arrogant, narrow-minded, abrasive, condescending, and curt. If allopathic medical students are not tending toward this stereotype before their U.S. medical training begins, the rigorous hierarchical regimen impressed upon them by well-meaning instructors does seem to produce an unusually high percentage of doctors who believe that evidence-based allopathic American medicine is the only medicine worth considering. Often all other systems of medicine are viewed with overt disdain, and even allopathic medicine practiced by other countries (from England to Mexico to Thailand) is perceived as inferior to our own. Even when presented with evidence that the U.S. medical system ranks quite low in effectiveness compared with most European countries, or that allopathic medicine in general is not as effective as another system regarding treatment for a similar ailment (versus chiropractic medicine for chronic back pain, for example), the allopathic American prejudice remains.

CAM systems are rightly criticized for their own flaws, notably excessive wishful thinking regarding techniques that flout the basic sciences. But narrow-minded condescension does not tend to be one of the typical flaws of the average CAM provider, if only because they are used to being called quacks and charlatans by the prevailing allopathic medical establishment. And while CAM students and practitioners often have prejudices against allopathic extremes, the open-mindedness that CAM students are encouraged to show toward other CAM modalities simply doesn't produce the unique insistence of superiority so commonly seen in allopathic practitioners.

By blending allopathic and CAM training, the open-mindedness so needed by allopaths is combined with the scientific rigor so needed by CAM practitioners. With proper training along with individual effort, you can manifest the traits of an ideal modern physician: intellectual astuteness, emotionally availability, spiritual depth, and the ability to offer effective medical treatments from across the spectrum of choices conjured up by insightful practitioners from time immemorial.

Students of integrative medicine may also choose to enter the burgeoning world of CAM research that is more often than not spearheaded by holistically inclined MDs. In 1991, the U.S. Congress legislated that the National Institutes of Health establish the Office of Alternative Medicine (OAM) in order to coordinate research on nonallopathic medical practices and to establish a CAM information clearinghouse for the general public. In 1998, Congress formed the National Center for Complementary and Alternative Medicine (NCCAM) to supercede the OAM, and the annual budget increased from $2 million per year to $68 million per year overnight. The NCCAM supports basic and applied CAM research and provides information to both health providers and the public. The first strategic plan of the NCCAM (2001–05) stressed investment in basic and clinical research, training, dissemination of findings, and integration of safe and effective practices. A second strategic plan (2005–09) is currently underway.

In its first five years, the center funded more than 780 projects at 123 institutions, resulting in over 700 scientific publications; enrolled nearly 40,000 participants in clinical protocols; and developed a database known as "CAM on PubMED" that lists nearly 400,000 articles on CAM-related subjects published in 45 languages from 70 countries.

By 1997, visits to CAM providers had increased 47 percent, to 625 million. Today, half of all adults use CAM treatments, creating a $30 billion growth industry. Health insurers, HMOs, and Fortune 500 companies are now endorsing many alternative treatments as part of their health benefits. The research budget of NCCAM has increased fifty-fold from its inception, to $100 million per year. Furthermore, with 70 percent of their generation routinely using CAM therapies, today's medical students increasingly demand education in this area despite continued resistance by medical school administrations.

Similar to the ever-increasing acceptance of interracial marriage, nonheterosexuality, religions other than Christianity within U.S. borders, and the realities of global warming, the arrival of integrative medicine has seemed to be inevitable to many, mostly CAM practitioners for several decades now. Yet progressive thinkers usually have to bide their time and perhaps suffer a few slings and arrows before the wheels of time lurch forward and the powerbrokers of the day affirm what the public and Mother Nature nearly always affirm before them. Diversity rules.

Whether the subject is art, politics, religions, or the culinary arts, if any group insists that only their way is the right way then everyone suffers from unnecessary mediocrity and blandness. Visionaries who state the seemingly obvious and request that all opinions be considered equally are often slandered and imprisoned because they dare attempt to wrest power and prestige from those in the ruling majority (or minority). Nowhere has this scenario played out as dramatically as in the field of medicine, perennially an arena of money and status for those who have been able to convince others that their healing ways are the only true healing ways. But time and technology tend to be great equalizers, and the allopathic victors of the medical wars that peaked in the early twentieth century are surveying a different terrain in this new millennia.

The next era of medicine will usher in a reconsideration of all past medical modalities and, of course, introduce brilliant new modalities into our longer, more healthful lives. As a student of integrative medicine, you will be one of the most potent of the current medical pioneers. Your MD status will give you near immediate worldwide acceptance. Your starting salary as a general practitioner will hover around $170,000; as a specialist, $300,000 is the norm. As an integrative doctor, your salary will likely be somewhere in between, so you will be okay financially despite a student loan burden of over $100,000.

Remember that even though more and more medical schools, instructors, and students are open to the concepts of integrative medicine, you as an incoming first year medical student will likely be viewed as somewhat askew by the majority of your peers and teachers if you openly espouse CAM therapies. Your instruction will be almost 100 percent allopathic, with only a few electives available in CAM philosophy and therapeutics. Actual integrative medicine studies will occur after your first four years of medical school, and probably after your internships and residencies as well. By this time, you will have been fully washed with the allopathic mind-set and may have to struggle to maintain determination and continue schooling in order to receive postgraduate training in integrative medicine.

Whereas naturopathic doctors must spend four years to practice their version of integrative medicine, as an allopath, you will have to attend almost ten years of training. But the vast difference in wealth and status that you will experience should lighten the psychological load for you along the way. In the future, the roads to an integrative medical degree, as well as the roads afterward, will be easier for every practitioner. In the meantime, choose your path wisely. Your sanity and pocketbook are both at stake.

WHERE PRACTICED

Holistic medical doctors are not limited to any particular type of practice. As fully licensed primary care physicians, they may open private practices in addition to holding full-time positions at hospitals or clinics. While some holistic allopaths may practice medicine in traditional Western locations, the United States is seeing a significant upwards trend in integrative health centers. These programs will often partner licensed and nonlicensed holistic practitioners with holistically oriented allopaths resulting in a fully inclusive health clinic. As of 2008, private practice is the most common professional methodology for self-identified holistic doctors.

EDUCATION STANDARDS AND THE LICENSING PROCESS

Note: The licensing and academic procedure for MDs in the United States is a long and complicated process. This short section will give you a good general idea as to the expectations and length of the process, but it is not a comprehensive account of all the requirements that it takes to become a doctor in the United States. The American Medical Association (www.ama-assn.org) is a good resource to supplement information provided in this section.

Undergraduate Requirements

Holistic doctors must undergo the same rigorous certification and licensure requirements that any conventional allopathic MD. The degree is no different between the two professions; while there are particular residency programs that are geared more toward holistic sciences, the academic standards, licensing examination, and relative training requirements are identical. To be eligible for medical school, a necessary requirement for all practicing physicians of any kind, students must earn an undergraduate BA or BS degree at an accredited college or university. Most medical programs recommend a strong emphasis or major program in the hard sciences, such as biology or chemistry, yet some students may enter medical school with other academic interests. The application process to medical school is fairly simple, much like undergraduate programs, but much more competitive. Most programs require students' college transcripts and/or the results of candidates' scores on the MCAT (Medical College Admissions Test), which is taken between undergraduate and graduate school. Consult later sections in this chapter to find a list of accredited medical schools.

Graduate Education Requirements

Upon completing a four- to six-year program at a medical school accredited by the LCME (Liaison Committee on Medical Education), students officially earn their doctor of medicine degree (MD), although they must complete additional training before practicing on their own as a physician. Newly licensed MDs *must* participate in a medical residency program accredited by the NRMP (National Resident Match Program). Residency programs typically last three to seven years, educating students under the supervision of senior physicians. The length of the program is usually determined by the depth of the specialty. Surgery, for example, is a longer program than family medicine. For a comprehensive list of available residency specialties, consult the AMA's Web site: www.ama-assn.org/ama/pub/category/2375.html.

Doctors who wish to become specialized in a particular field, such as gastroenterology (which is a subspecialty of internal medicine), must have training in a one- to three-year fellowship in which they work in close proximity to senior physicians. Fellowships are optional and not necessary to attain a state-regulated license to practice medicine, yet they are highly recommended for pursuing high standards in a particular field of medicine. For a listing of fellowship programs and specialty resources, consult the AMA's Web site at www.ama-assn.org/ama/pub/category/2997.html.

After students have completed graduate medical education, a full residency program, and any relevant fellowship/internship programs, they still must obtain a license to practice medicine from a state or jurisdiction of the United States in which they are planning to practice. To be eligible, MDs must apply to their respective state licensing boards and also register for a comprehensive exam that reviews their training.

A License to Practice Medicine

Pending the approval of their application, students are eligible to sit for the state-based examination that is commissioned by the USMLE (United States Medical Licensing Examination). Some states may have slightly different tests, but the USMLE's standard form is a three-step process, in which each successive section measures increasingly complex theories of medical knowledge. Upon passing the USMLE and all relevant state-based examinations, and approval of the state's medical board, candidates become fully fledged doctors and are granted a legal license to practice medicine, in a particular field of expertise (e.g., geriatrics, surgery, general practitioner). Additionally, the vast majority of physicians choose to become board certified, an optional voluntary process which ensures that a doctor has been tested to assess his or her skills in an area of practice. There are two levels of certification, which are available through twenty-four specialty medical boards. There are thirty-six medical specialties, including eighty-eight additional subspecialty fields. For more information about board certification, consult the American Board of Medical Specialties at www.abms.org.

Continuing Education

Like most regulated professions, medical physicians must continue their education in conjunction with practice in order to maintain their medical license. Many states require a certain number of CME (continuing medical education) credits per year to ensure that physicians' skills and knowledge fit within the current medical paradigm. There may also be additional CME requirements for doctors working within professional organizations and hospitals. For more information on your state's continuing education requirements for medical doctors, consult your local state board's Web site. For a sampling of continuing education seminars and classes, consult the AMA's Web site for CME at www.ama-assn.org/ama/pub/category/2797.html.

GENERAL MEDICAL ORGANIZATIONS

The American Medical Association
www.ama-assn.org

The AMA is the largest medical organization in the United States that is dedicated to promoting the art and science of medicine for the betterment of public health. The AMA, with its membership community, influence, and industry standards, is an essential part of the professional life of every physician. The AMA helps doctors help patients through a network of united physicians working toward the same goal of public health.

The National Resident Match Program

www.nrmp.org

The NRMP is a private, not-for-profit corporation established in 1952 to provide a uniform date of appointment to positions in graduate medical education. Its Web site contains many of the available fellowships and residency programs for graduate medical students who wish to gain a license to practice medicine.

The Liaison Committee on Medical Education

www.lcme.org

The LCME is the nationally recognized accrediting authority for medical education programs leading to the MD degree in U.S. and Canadian medical schools. The LCME is sponsored by the Association of American Medical Colleges and the American Medical Association.

The Association of American Medical Colleges

www.aamc.org

Representing 129 accredited medical schools in the United States, this nonprofit organization is an advocate for academic medicine, medical education, research, and general health care. The AAMC oftentimes acts as an intermediary between individual medical schools and larger accrediting/standardizing organizations.

The American Board of Medical Specialties

www.abms.org

The ABMS is a nonprofit organization that was established in 1933 to promote excellence and academic notoriety in medical science. Currently compromised of twenty-four medical specialty member boards, it is the preeminent entity overseeing the certification of specialist physicians in the United States. Member physicians can boast that they are "board-certified" in a particular area of medicine.

The United States Medical Licensing Examination

www.usmle.org

The USMLE provides states with a common evaluation system for applicants for initial medical licensure. It is sponsored by the Federation of State Medical Boards of the United States and the National Board of Medical Examiners. It is responsible for commissioning the standard test that medical students must pass in order to gain their licensure.

The American Medical Association's Links to other National Organizations

www.ama-assn.org/ama/pub/category/2642.html

Because there are many national boards and associations dedicated to the promotion of allopathic medicine that are not listed here, this meta link is a great resource for finding other not-for-profit research groups dedicated to excellence in allopathic medicine.

HOLISTIC MEDICAL ORGANIZATIONS

The American Holistic Health Association

http://ahha.org

Founded in 1989, the AHHA is the combined result of two national holistic medical associations. The AHHA encourages health care physicians and practitioners to incorporate holistic principles into their practice through educating both the patient and the doctor as to the positive results of a holistic approach. It publishes a newsletter, facilitates membership networks, and supports medical research in holistic therapies.

The American Holistic Medical Association

www.holisticmedicine.org

The AHMA supports holistic practitioners and holistic doctors nationwide. Founded in 1978, it brings physicians interested in holistic, integrated health care together so they can advocate effectively for the transformation of the health care system, encourage research, and network.

American College for Advancement in Medicine

www.acamnet.org

The ACAMA is a not-for-profit association dedicated to educating physicians and other health care professionals on the latest findings and emerging procedures in complementary, alternative and integrative medicine.

The American Board of Holistic Medicine

www.holisticboard.org

Founded in 1996, the mission of the ABHM is to establish and maintain the highest standards of medical care while assisting holistic physicians in their training. It provides intensive review courses for holistic physicians and evaluates the candidacy of applicants desiring certification as specialists in holistic medicine. This is the holistic version of the American Medical Association's Board on policy changes and legislation.

American Academy of Hospice and Palliative Medicine

www.aahpm.org

The Academy is the professional organization for physicians specializing in hospice and palliative medicine. Membership is also open to nurses and other healthcare providers who are committed to improving the quality of life of patients and families facing life-threatening or serious conditions.

American Academy of Medical Acupuncture

http://medicalacupuncture.org

The AAMA promotes the integration of concept from tradition and modern forms of acupuncture with Western medical training, effectively synthesizing a more comprehensive, integrative approach to health care.

Consortium for Integrative-Alternative Medical Arts

http://aihcp-norfolkva.org

This large nonprofit organization spearheads three smaller, more focused research initiatives and membership groups including: The American Integrative Medical Association, the Association for Integrative Health Care Practitioners, and the University of Integrative Health Sciences. Consult the above link for information on any of these groups.

The American Association of Integrative Medicine

www.aaimedicine.com

The AAIM was formed to establish a network of related integrative health care providers and raise awareness about the efficacy of and increasing trends toward integrative medicine. It has continuing education programs, information on conferences/seminars, diplomat programs, membership networks, and practitioner databases. It also is a useful resource to other holistic MD Web sites.

The Society for Integrative Oncology

www.integrativeonc.org

The SIO is a nonprofit, multidisciplinary organization founded in 2003 for health professionals committed to the study and application of complementary therapies and botanicals for cancer patients. By researching holistic approaches to current health problems, the SIO and other similar organizations are an important part of the holistic community.

The Institute for the Study of Health and Illness

www.commonweal.org/ishi/

The ISHI is an education and training center for holistically minded physicians who wish to renew their commitment to natural medicine. Since 1991, ISHI has offered a series of post-graduate Category 1 CME retreat workshops that enable physicians to find deeper satisfaction and meaning in the day-to-day practice of medicine.

HOLISTIC PEER-REVIEWED JOURNALS

Integrative Medicine: A Clinician's Journal
www.imjournal.com/im

Alternative Therapies in Health and Medicine
www.alternative-therapies.com/at

Advances in Mind-Body Medicine
www.advancesjournal.com/adv

NONPEER-REVIEWED PERIODICALS

Natural Solutions Magazine
www.naturalsolutionsmag.com

Alternative Health News Online
www.altmedicine.com

ONLINE RESOURCES

Holistic MD.com
www.holisticmd.org

This is the personal Web site of Dr. Michael I. Gurevich, a holistic psychiatrist who integrates contemporary treatment methods with traditional healing approaches developed long ago.

The Conscious Choice
www.consciouschoice.com/archive/holisticmd.html

This site is an article archive of Dr. Ronald Hoffman's work. Hoffman is the medical director at the Hoffman Center in New York Center and is a contemporary authority on holistic doctors and their methods of practice.

The Holistic Internet Community
www.holistic.com

David Lazaroff's personal Web site offers some interesting articles on holistic medicine; in particular, he addresses the future of the allopathic and holistic community. It also includes a store, archive, and practitioner directory.

BOOKS FOR DOCTORS OF HOLISTIC MEDICINE

The American Holistic Medical Association Guide to Holistic Health: Healing Therapies for Optimal Wellness by Larry Trivieri Jr.

Integrative Holistic Health, Healing, and Transformation: A Guide for Practitioners, Consultants, and Administrators by Penny Lewis

Integrative Health Care: Complementary and Alternative Therapies for the Whole Person by Victor S. Sierpina MD

Health and Healing: The Philosophy of Integrative Medicine and Optimum Health by Andrew T. Weil

Molecules of Emotion: The science Behind Mind-Body Medicine by Candace B. Pert

EDUCATIONAL INSTITUTIONS

Accredited Medical Schools with Integral Interests

The Liaison Committee on Medical Education (www.lcme.org) is the federally recognized accreditation commission for medical schools in the United States. If you find a program that is not accredited by the LCME, it is not officially recognized as a medical program in the United States. There are currently 129 accredited medical programs in the United States. The growing list below includes schools that have programs, classes, and research involving integrative medicine.

Boston University School of Medicine
Boston, Massachusetts
www.bumc.bu.edu

Case Western Reserve University School of Medicine
Cleveland, Ohio
http://casemed.case.edu

City University of New York Medical School
New York City, New York
http://med.cuny.edu

Columbia University College of Physicians and Surgeons
New York City, New York
www.cumc.columbia.edu/dept/ps

Emory University School of Medicine
Atlanta, Georgia
www.med.emory.edu

George Washington University School of Medicine
Washington, DC
www.gwumc.edu

Georgetown University School of Medicine
Washington, DC.
http://som.georgetown.edu

Harvard Medical School
Boston, Massachusetts
http://hms.harvard.edu/hms/home.asp

Indiana University School of Medicine
Indianapolis, Indiana
http://medicine.iu.edu

Johns Hopkins School of Medicine
Baltimore, Maryland
www.hopkinsmedicine.org

Medical College of Pennsylvania
MedicalCollegeofPennsylvania/tabid/1086/Default.aspx
Philadelphia, Pennsylvania
www.drexelmed.edu/Alumni/Colleges/

Michigan State University Kalamazoo Center for Medical Studies
Kalamazoo, Michigan
www.kcms.msu.edu

Mount Sinai School of Medicine
New York, New York
www.mssm.edu

Pennsylvania State University College of Medicine
Hershey, Pennsylvania
www.hmc.psu.edu/college

Rush Medical College
Chicago, Illinois
www.rushu.rush.edu/medcol

Southern Illinois University School of Medicine
Springfield, Illinois
www.siumed.edu

Stanford University School of Medicine
Palo Alto, California
http://med.stanford.edu

Temple University School of Medicine
Philadelphia, Pennsylvania
www.temple.edu/medicine

Tufts University School of Medicine
Boston, Massachusetts
www.tufts.edu/med/index_flash.html

Uniformed Services University of the Health Sciences
Bethesda, Maryland
www.usuhs.mil

University of Arizona School of Medicine
Tucson, Arizona
www.medicine.arizona.edu

University of California, Los Angeles School of Medicine
Los Angeles, California
http://dgsom.healthsciences.ucla.edu

University of California, San Francisco School of Medicine
San Francisco, California
http://medschool.ucsf.edu

University of Cincinnati School of Medicine
Cincinnati, Ohio
www.med.uc.edu

University of Louisville School of Medicine
Louisville, Kentucky
http://louisville.edu/medschool

University of Maryland School of Medicine
Baltimore, Maryland
http://medschool.umaryland.edu

University of Miami School of Medicine
Miami, Florida
www.med.miami.edu

University of Minnesota School of Medicine
Minneapolis, Minnesota
www.med.umn.edu

University of Rochester School of Medicine
Rochester, New York
www.urmc.rochester.edu/smd

University of Virginia School of Medicine
Charlottesville, Virginia
www.healthsystem.virginia.edu/internet/som

Wayne State School of Medicine
Detroit, Michigan
www.med.wayne.edu

Yale School of Medicine
New Haven, Connecticut
www.med.yale.edu/ysm

New Jersey Medical School
Newark, New Jersey
http://njms.umdnj.edu

CHAPTER 5

MENTAL HEALTH (MFT) (PHD) (PSYD)

"If we are ever to have anything resembling a comprehensive, inclusive, integral view of psychology and consciousness, there is one and only one thing that we know for sure: it will include all . . . schools [of thought]. Hundreds of thousands of decent men and women around the world are *already* practicing neuroscience, or psychiatric pharmacology, or meditation, or subtle energy research, or transpersonal psychology, or contemplation, or chaos and complexity theories. What's left of the four forces [in psychology] (behavioristic, psychoanalytic, humanistic, transpersonal) will survive . . . only by being taken up into a fully integral approach."

—CONTEMPORARY EAST-WEST PHILOSOPHER KEN WILBER

THE WESTERN and modern psychologist and psychiatrist may be the closest thing to the ancient Shamanic healers of our ancestral cultures from over 10,000 years ago.

The Western and modern psychologist and psychiatrist may be the closest thing to the ancient Shamanic healers of our ancestral cultures from over 10,000 years ago. The Shaman ("they who know") began their intense apprenticeships with Shamanic elders, who were usually themselves insightful, compassionate, spiritual, eccentric outsiders who had risked their sanity, and sometimes their lives, to heal themselves and to pass on their healing skills to others. Those destined to become a Shaman within a tribe were often misfits or black sheep, seeming to carry greater physical, psychological, and spiritual burdens of sensitivity and awareness compared with their peers.

Before beginning their hands-on training, apprentices might at first be initiated via a serious (often psychological) illness; by being struck by lightning and dreaming of thunder; by a near-death experience; by a "vision quest"; or by simply following an inner calling to become a Shaman. Shamanic "initiatory illnesses" are usually involuntary psychospiritual crises, or rites of passage, experienced by those to become Shaman. These episodes often mark the beginning of a time-limited episode of confusion or disturbing behavior during which the initiate might sing or dance in an unconventional fashion or have the experience of being "disturbed by spirits."

These symptoms are usually not considered to be signs of mental illness by interpreters within the Shamanic culture; rather, they are believed to be introductory signposts for the individual who is meant to take on the office of Shaman. Once drawn to study under their "in-tune" respected Shamanic elder, apprentices discover that every aspect of their lives becomes open for introspection, exploration, and transformation under the strict guidance of their older and wiser guide. An entire spectrum of learning is placed in front of the awe-struck student, as mere understanding of the physical world of nature—including hunting cycles, fertility enhancement, extensive herbal medicine, storytelling and historical poem recitation, weather prediction, and crop assistance—is found to be not nearly enough to fulfill the job description.

The Shaman is a healer who is expected to fully comprehend—and travel effortlessly throughout—not one, but three, separate but overlapping realms: the underworld, our middle world, and the upper world. Access to these worlds is available to the Shaman via many tools but only one main gateway—the axis mundi or "cosmic axis"—which is the backbone or ladder that links the three worlds. This gateway can only be accessed via voluntary or involuntary altered states of consciousness. Symbols of the Shaman axis mundi are prolific—from the upright human spine to church steeples and temple stupas, sacred mountains (Olympus and Zion), trees (Bodhi and Christmas), columns of smoke (incense and candles), medicine (the caduceus symbol for MDs and the serpent/kundalini symbol for ayurvedists), and fairy tales (Jack's beanstalk and Rapunzel's hair).

Although Shamanism itself is global, it is not a truly united belief system. There are simply a great many similarities between differing Shamanic cultures despite their differing philosophies. These philosophies can be seen reflected in the diverse tools used both alone and together in order to reach the desired Shamanic altered state(s) and help lay the foundation of the role played by modern counselors, psychologists, and psychiatrists.

In general, the Shaman traverses the axis mundi and enters the spirit world by effecting a transition of consciousness and entering into an ecstatic trance, either auto-hypnotically or (less commonly) through the use of potent psychotropic plant medicines. Some methods for experiencing trances include:

- **Tobacco:** used for spirit offering, improved concentration, and nourishing the Mariri spirit (below) that supposedly lives in a Shaman's phlegm

- **Drumming:** the fast-paced six to eight beat is associated with trance states in music

- **Dancing**

- **Singing**

- **Listening to or making music**

- **Icaros/Shamanic medicine songs**

- **Vigils:** sleep deprivation combined with prayer and ritual

- **Fasting:** drinking only water, or restricting certain food intake

- **Sweat lodges:** very hot group sauna with song and prayer

- **Vision quests:** solo wilderness trips without much food, water, or sleep

- **Mariri:** eating or smoking the spiritualized phlegm of a Shaman

- **Swordfighting/bladesmithing:** think samurai/jedi arts

- **"Power" or "master" plants:** used as incense or consumed for the purpose of healing oneself or others via attaining nonordinary or "altered" states of consciousness. Some include:

  » **Psychedelic mushrooms:** called "holy children" by Mazotec Shaman such as María Sabina; contains psilocin and psilocybin

  » **Cannabis (marijuana):** contains THC

  » **San Pedro cactus:** named after St. Peter (holding the keys to the gates of the Christian heaven) by the Andean people

  » **Peyote:** similar to San Pedro, also contains mescaline

» **Ayahuasca:** Quechua for "Vine of the Dead"; contains orally active DMT

» **Cedar:** especially as a "smudge" incense

» **Datura:** contains scopolamine and atropine

» **Deadly nightshade (also known as belladonna):** contains atropine

» **Fly agaric:** contains muscarine

» **Iboga:** contains ibogaine; used by central African Shaman

» **Morning glory seeds:** contains LSD amide

» **Sweetgrass:** especially as a "smudge" incense

» **Sage:** especially as a "smudge" incense

» **Salvia divinorum:** "Diviners' sage"; contains salvinorum

Once in the upper world, images such as climbing a mountain, tree, cliff, rainbow, or ladder; ascending into the sky on smoke; flying on an animal, carpet, or broom; and meeting a teacher or guide are typically seen by the Shaman. The lower world consists of images including entering into the earth through a cave, hollow tree stump, water hole, tunnel, or tube. By being able to interact with the different worlds while manifesting an altered yet ultra-aware state of consciousness, the Shaman is able to exchange information between the world in which we consider normal and the one considered blessed or sacred or spirited.

Since the Shaman plays the role of healer and expert mystic within Shamanic societies, much of what they retrieve is specific to the patient. They may be instructed on which plants to use for treatment, or which person is secretly placing a curse upon a patient. But they also may bring back information on whether to reduce or increase hunting and fishing and whether to seek new gaming grounds. They may be told it is time to appeal to the spirits to bring rain because a drought is coming. They may even find that they must sacrifice themselves so that their tribe can be saved, as sometimes the entities in other worlds exact a heavy price for their treasures. Often the Shaman has, or acquires, one or more familiar helping entities in the spirit worlds; these are often spirits in animal form, spirits of healing plants, or sometimes those of departed Shaman. In many Shamanic societies, magic, magical force, and knowledge are all denoted by one word. Shaman usually enjoy great power and prestige in the community, and are renowned for their spiritual and healing knowledge. But they may also be suspected of harming others and, thus, may be feared as much as they are loved and appreciated.

Overall, Shaman are people who are experts in manipulating the multiple codes through which their tribes' complex belief systems appear. They know the intricacies and personal inter-relations of their culture and hold an integrative bird's-eye view of these in their minds at all times. The Shaman uses the symbols and codes that his tribal family understands and reacts to in predictable ways. They express their meanings verbally, musically, artistically, in dance, and through trance. Meanings are manifested in objects, such as amulets; and also on wings and prayers. Because the tribe understands historical symbology of these manifestations, the placebo effect can be used at its highest level. Even skeptics of Shamanism who have mimicked Shamanic rites without belief in them have become convinced that they, too, are powerful Shaman due to such a high success rate of healing.

In some societies, the Shaman exhibits a two-spirit identity, assuming the dress, attributes, role, or function of the opposite sex, bisexual gender fluidity, and/or same-sex sexual orientation. This practice is common and found among many tribes around the globe. Such two-spirit Shaman are thought to be especially powerful, probably because these Shaman are androgynous exemplars of Shiva/Shakti, Adam/Eve, and Yin/Yang—the omnipotent might of all dualities, including both genders. They are highly respected and sought out in their tribes, as they will also bring high status to their mates.

Although Shaman are still in existence today, their population is surely declining as Western economic hegemony gradually unites the planet. One current trend is similar to that which has occurred in the transformation in the United States of traditional spiritual Raja Yoga to postmodern secular "yog-ercise." While Yoga has been commercialized and co-opted in the West, the spiritual focus has been mostly lost and one part (asana) has been excised to represent the whole. In the case of Shamanism, the so-called New Age movement has attempted to treat Shamanism as one agreed upon method worldwide.

This is claimed even though New Age Shamanism is as patchwork a system as is the eclectic, superficial New Age worldview as a whole. Although there are "Shamanic certifications" available from a smattering of organizations that would fall under the New Age umbrella, they appear to offer such a diluted or syncretic version of original Shamanism that we decided to refrain from giving Shamanism its own entry in this reference guide. Instead, it can be argued that today's Shaman (the psychologists and psychiatrists) dress much differently than their predecessors but share more in common with yesterday's Shaman than today's New Age Shamanic groups out of step with our mainstream Western culture. Remember, Shaman are the guardians and experts of the intricacies of their tribes. Today our current national tribe is mostly, like it or not, a hodgepodge of popular, mainstream culture. Thus, our Shaman must be able to relate to Midwestern suburbanites as well as left coast sweat lodge enthusiasts.

Entering our own literary axis mundi, we now emerge into our more recent history. Myriad twists and turns have occurred as cultures clashed and cooperated for millennia, leaving old dogmas in their wake and creating new ones in our midst. Even as we created what we thought was a dogma-destroying unreligion called "science," the materialistic dogma behind the centuries-old scientific paradigm has mocked its creators. Also, animistic religions have become pantheistic, polytheistic, monotheistic, atheistic, and secularly humanistic. In our newest millennium, we are approaching a spiritual melting pot labeled "anything goes." Are you a strict orthodox Jew? A Buddhist monk fighting Chinese imperialism? A Christian with a Muslim name running for president? A rock starlet yogini? A New Age polyglot? Everything goes in postmodern contemporary spiritual life.

Yet our current paradigm is hardly a random free-for-all, with cavalier acceptance of all beliefs equilaterally. This is because, despite Kant's *Critique of Pure Reason*, we have reasoned our way out of some massive human ills and misconceptions. We now know the Earth is round and spins on its axis just as we know a once elusive force called gravity keeps us from wobbling as we walk. We know how to conquer scourges such as bubonic plague, smallpox, and polio. And we know how to encode so many bits of information within a concentrated space that we can produce functioning telephones that can only be seen with a microscope. The list goes on and on, and clearly we're getting many details right, even as our stubborn cultural blind spots became more widely known and resistant to change.

THE BIRTH OF SCIENTIFIC PSYCHOLOGY

One of the main victories of logic and science in the West has been its contribution to psychology (the study of the soul and/or mind). By many other names, this has been performed ever since humans began ruminating about spiritual topics anywhere from 10,000 to a million years ago. All spiritual practices and religions are thus psychologies, by definition. But scientific psychology did not arrive as such until around 1,100, when the Iraqi Muslim and "father of science" Ibn-al-Haytham (known as Alhazen in the West) presented the scientific method for the first time and invented the word for "experiment." Alhazen's scientific method was similar to our modern scientific method and consisted of the following procedures:

1. Observation

2. Statement of problem

3. Formulation of hypothesis

4. Testing of hypothesis using experimentation

5. Analysis of experimental results

6. Interpretation of data and formulation of conclusion

7. Publication of findings

This system became the basis for the world's first science-based psychiatric hospitals in Iraq, long before Europeans ever rediscovered North America. Early psychology was only one of many interests to Alhazen, and it was many centuries more before psychology as an independent experimental field was founded by William Wundt, MD, at Leipzig University in Germany. Wundt began the first clinical psychology studies upon patients, asking them to introspect about previous and present experiences, feelings, ideas, and fantasies so that he and they might be able to understand and control them in the future. He hypothesized that there was a constant connection between the physical brain and the mind, and therefore, the potential was there for the mind to be studied with the same scientific rigor as the brain. Ergo, psychology and psychiatry are cut from the same cloth.

Wundt sought to understand the human mind by identifying the constituent "parts" of human consciousness in the same way that a chemical compound is broken into various elements. He imagined psychology as a science, much like physics or chemistry, in which consciousness is a collection of identifiable parts. Elements of Wundt's system were developed and championed by his one-time student, Edward Titchener, who described his system as structuralism. In this paradigm, structure is what determines the position of each element making up a larger whole. Every system has a structure, and structuralists are interested in structural laws that deal with coexistence rather than changes. Structures are believed to be the "real" that lies beneath the surface or appearance of things and meanings.

Later structuralism would appear as an aspect of behaviorism, but at first it could not compete with the system elucidated by the other father of modern psychology: philosopher, mystic, and pragmatist William James, MD. James's system was termed functionalism, which views a person's psychological life and general behavior in terms of the person's active adaptation to his or her nonclinical environments. This allowed for the development of psychological theories not easily tested in scientifically controlled experiments. Most of what we know and experience as applied psychology in the present day, and especially those holistic psychologies mentioned throughout this book, emanate from James's pioneering work.

James expressed his mystical side by also penning a seminal book of 1902, *The Varieties of Religious Experience*, in which he boldly states that psychologists should study the mind by entering intense altered states themselves so that they might better understand the pathological altered states of their patients. This voluntary altering of consciousness could come via prayer and meditation, entheogenic medicines (nitrous oxide and peyote were two of his favorites), psychic trance channeling, or any other method. What was important to James was the exploration itself, rather than hypothesizing about what happens when others (psychiatric patients) involuntarily explore similar changes of consciousness (John Dewey, American educational pioneer, also applied this to experiential education). This harkens back to the days of "original psychology," as first chanted and written by ancient Shaman, Yogis, and Taoists. These practitioners sought conscious alteration of consciousness, first and foremost, and subsequent study of the soul and mind came primarily after one's normal waking state was left behind. Perhaps not surprisingly, James's godfather was Ralph Waldo Emerson, who brought Yogic and Vedantic philosophy to Americans for the first time in the form of trancendentalism.

James's penchant for the use of mind-altering medicines was also a conspicuous bridge to the Shamanic psychologists and their cultures that had been so demonized and oppressed by colonizing Western nations such as James's America. Add to this James's love for the paranormal, and his cofounding of the scientific Society for Psychical Research in order to objectively determine whether psychic powers were bona fide, and this particular father of psychology could almost have stepped out of prehistoric Amazonia with Shaman feather and rattle in hand.

Even Wundt's focus on introspection for psychological transformation has within it the beginnings of the Shamanic and Yogic credo: purposefully alter one's state of conscious for the good of one's self, seeming others, and one's environment. By doing so, one will at least gain greater peace, wisdom, and interrelational harmony; at best one will come to fully know one's source. Introspection, contemplation, and meditation have been used by most psychologists from Shaman to present time, as they combine trance and insight within a mild to radical altered state. What Wundt determined analytically others had discovered via rapid drumming; slow, deep breaths in the dark; and maybe a puff of diviner's sage.

From Wundt's German school of psychology lineage came Sigmund Freud, MD, a neurologist with no formal training in experimental psychology. His brilliant, concise descriptions of taboo subjects in the Victorian Age—sexuality, repression, the unconscious mind—led to the highly influential psychoanalysis patient treatment process. In psychoanalysis, Freud instructed patients to "free associate," to lay supine on a couch as he sat behind them silently taking notes. Freud had also studied hypnotherapy early in his training and expertly understood its potential within the backdrop of a ritualized therapy session. Even without a trained hypnotherapist present, try expressing every thought and feeling that arises while lying down at home with a stranger listening behind you and see how long it takes you to enter a trance state. Once entranced, patients' normally unconscious material would surface in patterns, which became more and more patterned and predictable once Freud, Wilhelm Reich, Carl Jung, and many others began to categorize pathological character types and the solutions toward manifesting at least a neutrally healthy temperament instead. For the first time in the modern Western world, the Shamanic induction of freeing a patient's Pandora's box of subconscious processes within a structured healing ceremony was being offered again.

Wilhelm Reich, MD, one of Freud's top students, took the psychoanalytical altered state to a new level, directly inducing his clients to enter into purposeful, long-lasting, extreme emotional expression. Weaving psychoanalytical theory with Laban movement analysis and the observations of German bodyworker extraordinaire, Elsa Gindler, Reich introduced his radical orgonomy to his somewhat shocked colleagues. With patients in an entranced "fight or flight" state, Reich could observe whether their previous sexual and emotional repressions had led to the chronic, unconscious muscular contractions he was observing when they re-enacted earlier emotional scenes on his treatment table. By assisting patients to display optimally healthful physical expression of emotions in this Shamanic-like atmosphere, more healthful emotional well-being could be expressed in the waking state, or any other state, of consciousness.

Reich found that free association could only randomly relieve a patient of chronic neurosis and correlating "body armor." By taking emotions and physical armoring head-on, he believed, one was affecting

change closer to the root source of psychopathology. Distrusting mysticism, Reich yet propounded that every human had an unconditionally loving core that would automatically express itself once the onion-like layers of armor that covered it were dissolved. And though he mocked meditation and prayer to invisible entities, Reich still duplicated the mystics' approach to holistic health via therapeutic altered states. He even invented a "cloud-buster" for creating rain clouds, insisting on its success even as ancient Shaman claimed responsibility for drawing their rain gods' favor.

Western psychologists quickly propagated the efficient and ancient practice of working within a variety of consciousness states in order to manifest greater well-being in every state—including the waking one. Freud accomplished this with patients by way of free association, Reich through orgonomy, and Carl Jung via dream work, but a huge sector of modern psychology has always appreciated the importance of understanding and working within altered states. Many have also directly included the mystical amidst their science, with Jung one of the elders leading directly to the transpersonal, New Age, and integrative psychologies we have with us today. Jung even introduced the concept of archetypes, subconscious imagery that all humans share.

Synchronicity (a concept Jung coined), archetypes include a vast amount of Shamanic content, from power animals to nature deities to geometric yantras and mandalas. Jung insisted that the only route to optimal well-being was to acknowledge our ancient oneness with all of ancestral humanity and learn to embrace and manipulate our shared collective consciousness for the well-being of ourselves, others, and our environments. This included a heavy focus on dream cultivation and interpretation, used in a slightly different form for millennia by Shaman using "dreamtime" healing and divination within aboriginal cultures.

But structuralists, functionalists, and psychoanalysts all met their match with the coming of Pavlov's dogs and behaviorism in the early decades of the twentieth century. Joining the reductionist, materialistic trends visible in medicine, biology, art, and commerce, behaviorists opted for the minimalist approach of "life is a programmable set of behaviors." Behaviorists denied, or claimed irrelevant, that life forms included any Shamanic spiritual force, Reichian orgone, Jungian collective unconscious, or even a mind or internal physiology. Instead, they simply reported on behavior and taught others how to change it. Although this somewhat lifeless approach to life softened around the edges considerably over the next hundred years, behaviorism ruled the psychology roost through the 1950s until beatniks, humanists, hippies, and transpersonalists arrived on the counterculture scene.

Just as Western societal upheaval in the 1960s included the questioning of ethnocentric superiority in general, so did the "third force" of psychology reject the Western materialistic tendencies of "second force" behaviorism and, to a lesser extent, "first force" psychoanalysis. Inherently optimistic, humanistic psychology was developed in the 1950s in reaction to both previous forces and, ironically, arose largely from pessimistic authors of existential philosophy. By emphasizing the subjective experience of individuals and the value of meaning, creativity, and interpersonal relationships, the humanistic approach affirmed a holistic view of human life. It focused on fundamental issues of life, such as self-identity, death, aloneness, freedom, and meaning. First force practitioners focused on the depth of the unconscious human psyche, which they believed must be combined with the awareness of the conscious mind in order to produce a healthy human personality. Second force practitioners barely acknowledged the human psyche but agreed that one could get a human machine functioning more smoothly. Humanists, meanwhile, proclaimed that health was a collective verb since the individual is always part of one or more groups that greatly define him or her.

The five postulates of humanistic psychology became:

1. Human beings cannot be reduced to components.

2. Human beings have in them a uniquely human context.

3. Human consciousness includes an awareness of oneself in the context of other people.

4. Human beings have choices and nondesired responsibilities.

5. Human beings are intentional—they seek meaning, value, and creativity.

Three of the founding theorists behind this school of psychotherapy were Abraham Maslow, PhD; Carl Rogers, PhD; and Fritz Perls, MD; all of whom emphasized the potential for healthy human functioning rather than the pathological focus of Freud and the behaviorists. Connected with Freud via Alfred Adler (Freud's student and Maslow's teacher), Maslow introduced his "hierarchy of needs" back in 1943, illustrating that all people unconsciously or consciously aspire, stepwise, toward fulfilling their human potential all the way to Vedanta-style enlightenment.

Maslow's Hierarchy of Needs

6. Self-realization

5. Self-actualization

4. Self-esteem

3. Ability to give and receive love

2. Safety

1. Food, shelter, clothing

In Maslow's opinion, deficiencies must be met first. Once they are, seeking to satisfy natural human desires automatically drives personal growth. The higher needs in this hierarchy only come into focus when the lower needs in the pyramid are satisfied. Once an individual has moved upwards to the next level, needs in the lower level will no longer be prioritized. If a lower set of needs is no longer being met, the individual will temporarily reprioritize those needs by focusing attention on his or her unfulfilled needs, but will not permanently regress to a lower level. For instance, a businessman at the esteem level who is diagnosed with cancer will spend a great deal of time concentrating on his health (physiological needs), but will continue to value his work performance (esteem needs) and will likely return to work during periods of cancer remission. The main exception to this rule is the self-realized individual who has, by definition, transcended the pyramid as a whole and can no longer be dragged down because all of his or her needs have been permanently met.

Instead, the self-realized naturally help others up and off the pyramid.

Carl Rogers was connected with Freud via Otto Rank (Freud's student and Rogers's teacher). Rogers's person-centered and client-centered therapy was a soothing affair with open-ended questions, occasional compassionate touch (Reich had initiated Western psychotherapeutic touch within orgonomy), and "unconditional positive regard."

To Rogers, optimal human development resulted in a certain process he described as *the good life*, during which a person continually aims to fulfill his or her maximum potential. He listed these characteristics of fully functioning people:

- A growing openness to experience—they move away from defensiveness and negativity.

- An increasingly existential lifestyle—they live each moment fully. This results in excitement, daring, adaptability, tolerance, spontaneity, and a lack of rigidity and suggests a foundation of trust.

- Increasing organismic trust—they trust their own judgment and their ability to choose behavior that is appropriate for each moment. They do not rely on existing codes and social norms.

- Freedom of choice—they are not being shackled by the restrictions that influence an incongruent individual. They are able to make a wider range of choices more freely.

- Creativity—it follows that they will feel more able to be creative. They will also be more creative in the way they adapt to their own circumstances without feeling a need to conform.

- Reliability and constructiveness—they can be trusted to act constructively. Individuals who are open to all their needs will be able to maintain a balance between those needs.

- A rich full life—Rogers describes the life of the fully functioning individual as rich, full, and exciting. He suggests that such individuals experience the stream of life more intensely, including joy and pain, love and heartbreak, fear and courage.

While the ghost of William James may have been tempted to correct Rogers's "stream of life" by including a phrase he coined—stream of consciousness—the unbroken thread between the Shaman's out-of-body journeys and the new psychologist's peak experiences continued to manifest in more and more overt fashion.

Fritz Perls was connected with Freud via Wilhelm Reich, Freud's student and Perls's teacher. His Gestalt therapy was an existential and experiential psychotherapy that focused on the individual's experience in the present moment, the therapist-client relationship, the environmental and social contexts in which these things take place, and the self-regulating adjustments people make as a result of the overall situation. It emphasizes personal responsibility and is built around the central idea that it is only possible to know ourselves against the background of our relationships to other things.

In contrast to the psychoanalytic stance in which patients accept the (hopefully) more healthful attitudes and interpretations of their analyst, in Gestalt therapy clients are encouraged to accept or reject as they continue to progress. Hence, the emphasis here is on avoiding interpretation and encouraging self-discovery, since personal growth is believed to occur through gradual assimilation of experience in a natural way rather than by accepting the interpretations of the analyst. The therapist should not interpret, but rather lead clients to discovery of themselves for themselves.

The Gestalt therapist contrives experiments that lead the client to greater awareness and fuller experience of his or her possibilities. Experiments are often focused on undoing projections and unfinished Gestalts (or "unfinished business" such as unexpressed emotions toward a perceived antagonist). There are many kinds of experiments that might be considered therapeutic within Gestalt, but the essence of the work is that it is experiential rather than interpretive. In honor of their mastery in humanistic patient care, the styles and insights of Perls, neo-Shaman/hypnotherapist Milton Erickson, MD, and family systems humanist Virginia Satir were blended together into a new interpersonal communication model known as neuro-linguistic programming. Neo-Shaman now had yet another system of understanding and manipulating—hopefully for well and not ill—their patients' attitudes, perceptions, and holistic well-being.

Wilhelm Reich reappeared on the humanistic psychology scene via the work of his one time student, Fritz Perls, as well as via Reich's own body-centered orgonomy: character analysis and uninhibited emotional expression and sexuality were elevated nearly to scripture status during the "free love" era of the 1960s. Reichian body-centered therapy, via Alexander Lowen and John Pierrakos' bio-energetics and core energetics, was updated and spiritualized. Other body-oriented psychotherapies, such as Hakomi, polarity therapy, sensory awareness, and rolfing, merged body-mind-spirit and altered states of consciousness in ways unimaginable to the hunter-gatherer Shaman yet approximating the same goal. A unified perspective emerged using an in-depth knowledge of cultural symbols, mores, physical medicine, and psycho-spiritual expertise, in a positive, life-affirming healing environment. Self-help, a form of solo humanistic therapy popular today, joined other progressive psychotherapeutic shifts as the pre-1960s acceptance of external authority began to be questioned while the "me" culture was conceived as the love child of unparalleled cultural wealth and the ever-optimistic, individualistic, naïve American spirit.

Combined with the increased interest in cross-cultural perspectives, especially those of Asian and other developing continents, baby boom era psychology also budded transpersonal psychology off of the humanistic branch. Coined by who else but William James, "transpersonal" alludes to the inherently spiritual aspect of every human being and the importance of focusing on this facet if optimal healing is to occur. Jung, with his discovery of archetypes and appreciation of Raja Yoga and lucid dreamwork, carried the transpersonal torch to Maslow, with his appreciation of peak experiences and ultimate self-realization.

Maslow's colleague from Czechoslavalia, Stanislav Grof, MD, then brought things full circle with his updating and melding of Otto Rank's original work regarding "birth trauma" and that of innumerable Shaman tripping in the forest. Grof agreed with Reich that the root of psychological trauma lay mostly in a person's preverbal years. Reich stopped at infancy, however, where Rank and Grof tread unafraid into the womb. Using what was originally intended to be a reductionist pharmaceutical for stimulating the nervous, respiratory, and circulatory systems, LSD-25 was the perfect tool for helping Grof and his patients access, or at least believe to their cores that they had accessed, memories of their conception through their birth.

Synchronized with Maslow's hierarchy of needs, synthetic LSD was also first introduced in 1943—in this case by Swiss chemist Albert Hofmann, who relived the Shamanic, LSD-amide-laced morning glory seed excursions of a million psychonauts before him. By the time Carl Rogers had published his major work, *Client Centered Therapy*, in 1951, LSD and "psychoactive" psychotherapy had become an essential subject within the field of psychology. Soon Hofmann isolated the active compounds within Shamanic psilocybin mushrooms, which had been introduced to the Western world via a 1957 *Life* magazine article by ethnobotanist Gorgon Watson. Accompanying the article were watercolor renderings of the mushrooms by Dr. Hofmann himself.

Experimentation with the ancient, and now renewed, field of "psychedelic" medicine (coined by psychiatrist Humphrey Osmond in, surprisingly, 1957) was now rife within the professional realms of psychotherapeutics. All psychedelics were legal for private and professional use, and making use of, or at least theorizing about, these potent "mind-manifestors" was nearly automatic for especially the youngest generation of therapists. Not only was there no stigma attached to psychedelic therapy, it was generally believed that a new era of understanding the shocking depths and variations of the human mind had appeared in the form of the strongest psychotropic known to humankind (LSD, psychoactive at the *microgram* level) and its slightly less potent psychedelic plant peers.

Stranger than fiction, an odd couple of Harvard PhD psychologists, Irish American prankster Timothy Leary and Jewish American Richard Alpert (soon to be Baba Ram Dass), were drawn not just to treating patients with the rediscovered medicine of Shaman but of influencing the tumultuous and transformative political times of their day. In true Shamanic style, Leary and Alpert wanted to trip, too. And they did trip—not just tens of times, but thousands of times, using every psychedelic they could find. Unlike Aldous Huxley, the prophetic and refined writer of the 1954 classic psychedelic memoir, *The Doors of Perception*, Leary and Alpert didn't want to reserve the psychedelic experience for the cultural elite. Huxley wrote his book after his first mescaline excursion thanks to a gift from psychedelic therapist, Humphrey Osmond. Holding a rather pessimistic view of human nature (especially capitalistic American), as seen in his anti-utopian *Brave New World* and his wistfully utopian *Island*, Huxley warned of the negative societal consequences of psychedelics going mainstream.

Leary, Alpert, and their long list of colleagues—included poet Allen Ginsberg (a subject of CIA observation); dharma bum beatnik Jack Kerouac; scholar Marshall McLuhen, who inspired Leary to coin the zealous psychedelic motto "tune in, turn on, drop out"; and John Lilly, MD, isolation tank inventor and pioneering dolphin communicator—politely disagreed. Leary reported that he had "learned more about . . . [his] brain and its possibilities . . . [and] more about psychology in the five hours after taking . . . mushrooms than . . . [he] had in the preceding fifteen years of doing research in psychology." That in itself may be hard to swallow for some.

But for the converted, this was nothing to keep to oneself and one's cronies. The good news had to be spread around the world, and Leary grabbed the role of psychedelic prophet with full gusto. After Leary and Alpert were fired from Harvard for passing out psychedelics to students and skipping their own classes, for the first time professionals within the field of psychology began turning a jaundiced eye toward psychedelics. After Alpert returned from India as his alter ego, a full-fledged Yogi-Shaman named Ram Dass, complete with flowing robes, Sanskrit chants, dreamy eyes, and a circle of disciples, more professional eyebrows were raised.

Finally, bus-toting merry prankster, Ken Kesey, author of *One Flew Over the Cuckoo's Nest*, brought matters to a head as his troupe of revelers randomly spiked individuals' drinks with LSD and videotaped the resultant chaos and psychological trauma. Kesey, like Ginsberg, was another volunteer subject of CIA operations. His experience with the government clandestine service was so impactful and bizarre that he turned the story into his best-selling and Oscar-winning novel-movie mentioned above. Yet he replicated the CIA's abuse of psychedelics by dosing many unwitting subjects, seemingly just to see what would happen (the CIA thought the class of drugs might be helpful as a truth serum). Not long afterwards, Western governments began to place psychedelics in the category of Schedule I drugs. This carried the highest incarceration penalties for possession and sale, but also the inherent definition of being drugs with no known potential medical benefits

This irrational drug scheduling did not occur merely because of the excesses of Leary, Kesey, and the millions of recreational psychedelic users around the world. Less obviously, the hammer being applied to the '60s counterculture's chemical catalysts seemed to be a historical repeat of the same hammer that had been applied by Western colonizing governments upon Shamanic societies discovered over and over again in what were to become North and South America, Australia, Africa, and Asia from the fifteenth through the nineteenth centuries. Monotheistic Europe had long ago crushed its own druid/Shamanic cultures, believing them to be devil worshipping conjurers in need of Christian salvation.

This was especially true of female herbalists, often intimately familiar with psychotropic salves and tinctures, who were burned at the stake as black witchcraft practitioners in Europe and the American colonies. The same violent theme song played repeatedly each time European conquerors discovered peoples content with their own spiritual practices, the latter usually fueled one way or another by trance, dance, and the belief that each person could at least communicate with (if not fully unite with) his or her god of choice given the right state of consciousness. But the Western world had already come to the point at which only certain states of consciousness were allowed without penalty. Waking, sleeping, dreaming, and (secret) sex were the major states of consciousness okayed by the authorities; alcohol was the main tolerated drug for achieving a temporary high; and becoming addicted to lethal tobacco was acceptable, since that didn't "do anything at all" (as warbled in a Jefferson Airplane song of the day).

Meantime, wild dancing, communal orgies, frenetic drumming, and day-long psychedelic sessions—the major bonding activities of many Shamanic cultures—were vilified as being tools either of the devil or its incarnation in the form of Leary and the radical left. Leary and others clearly discerned the historical trend of challenging authoritarian rule and consensus belief systems. He and Alpert wrote a groundbreaking article in *The Harvard Review* in 1963, called aptly "The Politics of Consciousness Expansion." In it they write: "The nervous system can be changed, integrated, recircuited, expanded in its function. These possibilities naturally threaten every branch of the Establishment. The dangers of external change appear to frighten us less than the peril of external change. LSD is more frightening than the Bomb!"

One reason mass ingestion of psychedelic drugs, which produce startling, minute-long-to-permanent, internal changes in perception, is feared by political establishments is that if enough people "recircuit" their nervous systems in a manner contrary to the mainstream, societal mutiny is near certain. Beholding the marching protests, love-ins, be-ins, communes, Woodstocks, Kennedys, and Kings of the '60s, Western governments boiled in anger and trembled in fear. Sensing a sea change that threatened the creaky pillars of global politics, governments did the only thing they felt they could do: stop the party. In the midst of the hysteria, the establishment could neither believe nor accept that altered mind-body states could have any therapeutic value, or that at least they should be tested like everything else in science.

Spanning several years, but in retrospect seemingly happening overnight, all major psychedelics were outlawed by the United States Drug Enforcement Agency. The legal definition is "Schedule I" and includes those drugs not available for research or prescription, and deemed not to have medicinal use. Despite the thousands of patients successfully treated and the reams of data supporting their safe and effective use compared with other pharmaceutical treatments of the era, governments had arbitrarily decided that psychedelics had no medical benefit.

Hundreds of researchers, like Stan Grof and Humphrey Osmond, were stopped in their tracks. Most left their psychedelic specialization far behind, pretending they'd never been involved in the first place. Others stood by their principles but had to replace psychedelic therapy with less potent technologies of transformation—such as Grof's LSD replacement:

holotropic breathwork. Still others played rebel until the end, like the "secret chief," Jungian psychologist and U.S. army lieutenant colonel Leo Zeff, PhD. Zeff continued to treat individuals and groups with psychedelics until the end of his life, delineating protocols for safe and effective therapy using medicines such as LSD, psilocybin, MDMA (ecstasy), harmaline, and ibogaine. So afraid was he of prosecution that he only allowed his biography to be posthumously released.

Even some allopaths were miffed at the injustice to science passed off as "national security" long before the neo-cons: Andrew Weil, MD, Harvard medical school graduate and ethnobotanist, began writing about the subject in popular books and arguing with an impressive degree of elegance and reason that altering one's consciousness is as human a need as is sleeping or having sex. *The Natural Mind, The Marriage of the Sun and Moon*, and *From Chocolate to Morphine* were all written with the hope that reason would prevail and psychedelic consciousness-changing would soon be absorbed into the American cultural melting pot. Although Weil has chosen to hide his counterculture beliefs from the mainstream masses that ironically revere him, Weil as Shaman still marches in the annual Telluride Mushroom Festival along with his fellow psilocybin (and chanterelle) enthusiasts. You can take the wild out of the Shaman but not the Shaman out of the Weil.

For twenty years, the anti-Shamanic forces had their way, and as a psychiatrist or psychologist, you were left to study psychoanalysis, functionalism, behaviorism, humanism, transpersonalism, or, increasingly, allopathic medicine—but all without the mind-manifesting catalysts that were as groundbreaking to earlier psychologists as decoding the human genome is for allopaths today. Instead, psychedelic medicine was forgotten, trivialized, or demonized—until 1986. A year earlier, one of the minor counterculture drugs, MDMA, had been placed on Schedule I. This occurred despite a judge's in-depth recommendation that it be placed on Schedule III due to its medical benefits in psychotherapy combined with its low level of toxicity.

MDMA had been resynthesized by rebel chemist, Alexander Shulgin, when he still worked for Dow Corporation as an insecticide inventor. Shulgin passed it on to Leo Zeff, who promptly trained hundreds of therapists around the country as to its proper usage, especially in couples therapy, but also for individual post-traumatic stress disorder and garden variety neuroses such as social anxiety and irritable depression. By the time 1985 rolled around, tens of thousands of Americans were using MDMA regularly for recreation and improved interpersonal communication, with only eight ingestors seeking emergency room assistance over a period of eight years. Once again "the politics of consciousness expansion" reared its head, and MDMA enjoyment was perceived as threatening to society by the reactionary powers that be.

Enter stage left Rick Doblin, toting only some family money, an undergraduate psychology degree from a little known university, and the will of Spartacus. He decided to take on the United States Government on its own legal terms. Although in '85 MDMA had its day in court and eventually lost, Doblin believed that the way to reinstate the legal use of the drug ecstasy was to follow the exact FDA and DEA regulations required of any experimental pharmaceutical drug. His new company, the Multidisciplinary Association for Psychedelic Studies (MAPS), was created for the sole purpose of relegalizing MDMA. But Doblin had been an original student of Grof's holotropic breathwork and knew the great medical potential of all psychedelics. He began studying for a PhD in public policy at the Harvard School of Government and, in the process, began facilitating communication between research universities and various federal governments. MAPS' stated mission is to develop a variety of psychedelic drugs into FDA-approved prescription medicines and to educate the public honestly about their risks and benefits. Although it has taken far longer than Doblin thought to realize a world of legal, medicinal-only use of MDMA, Shamanic psychologists now have a powerful ally.

Since 1995, MAPS has disbursed more than $3 million to research and educational projects including:

- Facilitating FDA and IRB approval to study MDMA-assisted psychotherapy in the treatment of post-traumatic stress disorder in Charleston, South Carolina, with similar research projects now underway in Switzerland and Israel.

- Sponsoring efforts by Professor Lyle Craker, Medicinal Plant Program, University of Massachusetts–Amherst Department of Plant and Soil Sciences, to obtain a license from the Drug Enforcement Administration for a marijuana production facility.

- Pioneering analytical research into the effects of the marijuana vaporizer, leading to the first human study of marijuana vaporizers conducted by Dr. Donald Abrams, University of California–San Francisco.

- Opening an FDA Drug Master File for MDMA. This is required before any drug can be researched in FDA-approved human studies.

- Assisting Charles Grob, MD, to obtain approval for the first FDA-approved study in the U.S. to administer MDMA in trial subjects.

- Assisting in the design and is funding the world's first government-approved scientific study of the therapeutic use of MDMA in Spain.

- Sponsoring studies to analyze the purity and potency of street samples of "ecstasy" and medical marijuana.

- Funding the successful efforts of Donald Abrams, MD, to obtain approval for the first human study in fifteen years into the therapeutic use of marijuana, along with a $1 million grant from the National Institute on Drug Abuse.

- Obtaining Orphan Drug designation from the FDA for smoked marijuana in the treatment of AIDS Wasting Syndrome.

- Funding the synthesis of psilocybin for the first FDA-approved study in twenty-five years to evaluate psilocybin in a patient population.

- Supporting long-term follow-up studies of pioneering research with LSD and psilocybin originally conducted in the 1950s and 1960s.

Currently, MAPS has been given a Schedule I license to conduct research with MDMA on war veterans and survivors of physical or sexual assault who are suffering from post-traumatic stress disorder, as well as with advanced-stage cancer patients who are experiencing anxiety associated with this diagnosis. These are the first licenses the DEA has ever granted for MDMA psychotherapy research. A clinical study of the treatment of cluster headaches using low doses of psilocybin is also being developed by researchers at Harvard Medical School in conjunction with MAPS. And, as we go to print, the first legal dose of LSD has been given to a research subject for the first time in almost forty years; this in Switzerland, home to LSD's recently deceased discoverer.

At long last, psychology students and practitioners who prefer access to all available tools for researching the psyche (the mind and the soul) are on the cusp of having returned to them those medicines that have been part of our psychotherapeutic treatment history from the dawn of humankind. It appears that these medicines never go away. They are too awe-inspiring, terrifying, educative, transformative, and sometimes just plain fun to remain unused by the most curious species on the planet. Governments that try to legislate them away create underground markets with seemingly endless numbers of buyers and sellers. This results in organized criminal elements taking advantage of the high profit margins of officially taboo, but unofficially ubiquitous, products and their accoutrements. The specious "War on Drugs" has cost the American taxpayer billions of dollars per year, partly by incarcerating millions of able-bodied, tax-paying, nonviolent drug users labeled as delinquent by the "politicians of consciousness." Even the politicians are coming around, however, with Bill Clinton admitting to having held some Cannabis in his hand, and Barack Obama nonchalantly stating that he'd done the usual thing and inhaled. Both politicians still claim that they did the wrong thing by using drugs at all. But, of course, politicians like anyone else often use them, too. They simply know that until their drugs of choice are legalized, full honesty from them would result in a fate similar to those academic psychedelic therapists of the '50s and '60s after their drugs were made illegal: vilification, ignominy, or both.

Prospective students may lean toward the field of psychology but wonder where within it they can find their true calling amidst the current pill-pushing of allopathic psychiatry and the "human as computer" cognitive behaviorism that took over the psychol-ogy field in the '60s as it evolved out of behaviorism. In fact, modern psychiatrists may have taken the unkindest cut of all, changing almost against their will from the hypnotic, dreamy, orgone-filled days of Freud, Jung, and Reich to little more than textbook diagnosticians with prosaic prescription drugs that even kids won't steal. Not to belittle the miracles of Prozac and Adderal, especially as they edge closer to a Huxley-esque "soma" quality, but San Pedro mescaline they ain't. On the other hand, those more traditional yet cutting-edge students and practitioners leaning toward alternative psychology—"integrative psychologists," perhaps—can take heart with the recent trend toward reconsidering psychedelics and other cross-cultural techniques as bona fide treatment modalities.

East-West Psychology

Ancient Yogic, Taoist, and Buddhist psychologies are also coming into fuller flower in a different type of Shamanic uprising. Decades ago, humanist/transpersonalist Werner Erhard, also a friend and student of Alan Watts and his Westernized Zen approach, brought mini-satoris and the promise of self-actualization to the masses with his est approach to Large Group Awareness Trainings. More recently, the inception of positive psychology at the American Psychological Association in 1998 is presenting East-West psychology in a more professional manner. Martin Seligman, PhD, introduced this integrative psychology as he began his term as APA president, combining spiritual psychologies based on virtue and transcendence with humanistic/transpersonal psychologies emphasizing the importance of intrinsic human worth, close human relationships, mastering crafts, and learned optimism. The first degree program in positive psychology begins in the fall of 2008 at the University of Pennsylvania and is an excellent example of how archaic practices can be combined with modern updating for the creation of a psychospiritual science appropriate for our time.

The central aim of positive psychology, discovering how humans can attain the highest, most consistent levels of happiness possible, might seem like hopeless fluff for Westerners raised with Freud's *Civilization and Its Discontents* roaming somewhere within their subconscious minds. But most ancient cultures believed that humans were designed for nearly godlike happiness, even though only a few were willing to put in the work required ("the harvest is plenteous, but the laborers are few"). In this regard, times haven't changed much, but what has changed is that some Westerners are waking up to the fact that we have short-changed ourselves into believing that life is troublesome at best and nasty and brutish at worst. Easterners' psychological charts start where Western psychological charts end: at a well-balanced, highly functional life free from chronic worries, with the general acceptable mood from mildly irked to mildly pleased. From this point the Easterner begins the road to more and more enjoyable states of consciousness until a time comes when one's mood varies from mildly pleased to overwhelmingly ecstatic. And whether or not you believe this in entirety, surely we can learn from the East and at least study our own Western potential for stable, ever-new happiness. This is what positive psychology intends to do, and already much numerical data has resulted from their sociological studies. This attention to research has answered some of the critics of humanistic/transpersonal psychology, who correctly pointed out the lack of research data behind many earlier practitioners' claims.

To spoil the positive psychology punchline, practitioners' initial findings are that if you desire consistent contentment then focus on two things above all else: conscious practice of those virtues agreed on by all cultures, and regular cultivation and mastery of the benevolent crafts, skills, or hobbies of your choice. The latter will also help you to regularly enter the "flow" state of consciousness so common to mystic adepts and rigorously studied by positive psychology cofounder, Mihály Csíkszentmihályi , PhD. Five minor focal points toward this same "happy ending" are:

1. Cultivate a rich social network.

2. Share life with a mate.

3. Practice the spiritual path of your choice.

4. Avoid negative thoughts and environments.

5. Live in a wealthy democracy versus an impoverished dictatorship.

Some of these factors are clearly more difficult to accomplish than others, but everyone can make a greater effort to cultivate the cross-cultural virtues of knowledge, courage, humanity, justice, temperance, and transcendence, as well as their many agreed upon derivatives. Positive psychology stresses that the individual should determine his or her already strong virtues and then make sure to live and work these virtues on a daily basis as the individual shores up his or her major virtue deficiencies. This is an example of how updating ancient formulas can be made more effective for our culture. If successful, Western individuals and societies will move from their obsessive focus on the "pleasant life" of material enjoyment. To this will be added the (non-Rogerian) "good life" of flow and immersion in our life's work while using our virtuous strengths and the "meaningful life" Socrates talked about at the original Academy, filled with consistent well-being from being of service to something more important than our individual selves. Unlike the Yogis, positive psychologists aren't yet talking about the attainment of unending bliss. But it's a start.

As a prospective student, you are also poised to help bring about one of the next waves in psychological research by teaming up with psychiatrists such as UCLA professor Charles Grob, MD, who conducted the first U.S. Government-approved tests upon MDMA and who is currently studying the use of psilocybin to help reduce anxiety in end-stage cancer patients. You might perform research, teach, and write regarding the use of cannabis or ketamine for depression, or form a team of scientists who insist that Salvia divinorum must be completely studied from all cultural angles before it is reflexively classified as Schedule I by intelligent but ignorant politicians. Or you can help to create the most accurate, informative database on psychedelic drugs ever compiled, starting where erowid.org leaves off. You might even form a sort of integrative psychology community in order to keep pushing the envelope regarding our understanding of consciousness, as has pundit Ken Wilber.

You might, of course, practice none of the above as you focus on the vast realm of psychology (as Shamanism) that has nothing to do with using medicines to achieve altered states. But unless you devote yourself to the most prosaic examples of cognitive/behavioral talk therapy or institutional research, you no doubt will work with altered states. From structural introspection and hypnosis through psychoanalysis and humanistic/transpersonal psychology, whether working with individuals and groups, you will find persons around you entering altered states, whether you like it or not. As Andrew Weil opined, this is a part of our "natural mind," and all mammalian bodies seek to accomplish it in one way or another and on a regular basis. The more comfortable you can become with the entire range of states yourself, from psychopathological feelings and complete out-of-body dissociation to ecstatic spiritual revelry and seeming oneness with all of creation, the more ease you will have with your patients and their multitude of subtle psychological shape-shiftings.

Like Shaman from previous centuries, as well as those presently offering their services to eco-tourists in the Amazon and elsewhere, you may find that what you thought you knew about the human psyche was a mere atom at the edge of a galactic, experiential, organic database available to us for all the millennia that humans have interacted with psychotropic molecules and other routes toward altered states. At the very least you will understand how Shaman throughout time have used conscious changes in perception to help themselves and others answer for themselves the riddle of meaning, existence, and integrative, holistic health. Our earliest psychologists were humble enough to realize that they could think a trillion thoughts of their own and never become wise enough to fully help their tribes. Instead, they surrendered their mundane consciousness to the consciousness-altering rhythms, body movements, and psychedelic elixirs that automatically opened their hearts and minds to a fuller, less ego-based source of information.

What is this source? Some say gods, spirits, angels, and demons; some say God alone; some say our unconscious or superconscious minds; and some say it's just our brains, stupid! It might take awhile before our science and our suspicions agree on the answer, but perhaps the answer isn't the important thing. Perhaps most important is simply to try to know the source no matter how you conceive of it at present. Clues regarding how to approach and meet the source or fountainhead of existence have existed within every human culture, so there's no need to reinvent this wheel. Prayer, chanting, meditation, self-hypnosis, fasting, all-night vigils, orgies, absorbing music, intense exercise, gathering in mobs, and eating certain "foods of the gods" are the main routes developed over prehistory. Western efforts have added many other psychological modalities, such as orgonomy and holotropic breathwork, which simply work better for some individuals, especially in a modern clinical setting. Future decades will bring ever more routes to those deeper, higher, paradoxical states of consciousness far from our normal "consensus trance," but closer than your next breath or heartbeat.

If psychologists and psychiatrists are not willing to explore these realms and bring them to the less educated in safe and effective forms, who will? If we leave it to governments, recreationalists, or the ever-present counterculture "monkey wrenches," there will be no true Shaman to guide us. Remember, the Shaman knows the cutting-edge intricacies of all major aspects of his society so that he can guide the majority of his tribespeople in a healthful direction. If a Shaman can't live within and relate with our mainstream, then he is basically a Shaman for another tribe. So if you're ready to lead our American and global consciousness into its next cycle of practical knowledge: welcome. You may be who the world has been waiting for.

Western Psychology Movements

Following is a brief overview of the five paradigms of modern Western psychology:

First force: Psychoanalysis (psychodynamic theory), as devised by Sigmund Freud, has as its basis a somewhat Manichean conception of the human psyche. There are two main forces ever working upon us all: the "thanatos" death instinct that craves nonaction and nonexistence and eventually results in violence to self and/or others; and the "eros" creative principle or life instinct. Eros then manifests as the id thesis of usually unconscious, unadulterated biological desires, balanced by the superego antithesis of absorbed authoritarian societal expectations, resulting in the synthesis of the typically discontented, conscious human ego.

Psychic energy has to regulate certain biological

drives in order for civilization to exist, and usually there is conflict. Anxiety occurs when the libido (sexual energy) and other rudimentary emotions cannot express themselves fully. This results in the catalog of human neuroses and psychoses appearing in patients due to their uncontrollable pressures of bottled up emotive energy. Certain behaviors called "defense mechanisms" help to diffuse this tension, but defense mechanisms often themselves cause problems and disrupt daily life for everyone in the sphere of a patient's influence. Freud thought that this inner conflict was the inevitable result of civilization: since we have to cooperate with others and delay physical gratification, we must gain control of our ids. Authoritarian pressure becomes internalized as the necessarily controlling superego. The ego has to find a way to satisfy id drives without breaking the superego rules of society. If the id overpowers the rest of the personality, the individual is generally considered not sane enough to be worked with in therapy.

The type of patient best suited for psychoanalysis is someone with an overdeveloped superego and underdeveloped ego strength. Psychoanalysis typically starts off with free association, or saying the first thing that pops into your awareness. The therapist has to pay careful attention to both what the patient does and doesn't say in order for proper diagnosis and treatment. The patient's dreams also provide material for analysis. In subsequent sessions, the therapist can gain a clear sense of what issues the patient is avoiding consciously but simmering unconsciously. Usually, the therapist will find that the patient recounts past traumas with parents or adult authority figures in childhood (real or imagined). If there is a problem at any stage of psycho-sexual development, the person becomes fixated at that stage and replays those issues. Of course, such patients are unaware of the source of their anxieties and, thus, have no idea why they react the way they do to features in their environment that disturb them. One common defense mechanism is "regression," in which the person reacts to a stressful situation by returning to a mental state prior to inner conflicts. This can be observed in a child-like effect or in childish behavior. A crucial task of the therapist is the analysis of "transference," remaining aloof as the patient eventually directs hostility toward the therapist, treating him or her like a parent figure.

Then, the therapist interprets this behavior, and the patient gains insight.

Traditionally, during sessions the analyst would remain out of the patient's view while the patient lies on a couch. This was done primarily because Freud, who had studied hypnosis thoroughly, knew that relaxation and trance were key parts of the process. Secondarily, he believed transference couldn't occur unless the personality of the therapist faded into the background.

Therapy is rarely done like this today. Although Freud came from a medical background, his "talking cure" was not like the other procedures doctors normally engaged in. Initially the province of psychiatrists, medical training was eventually dropped as a prerequisite to psychoanalytic training. In addition to learning the method in the textbook sense, training requires the therapist to undergo the treatment himself or herself. This is done to prevent "counter-transference," which is when the therapist interprets the patient's situation in light of his or her own issues, interfering with the patient's ability to relive past events.

Psychoanalysis is not a cut-and-dry process, and it lacks a definite timetable because all therapy is directed to experience major psychotherapeutic insights that show no signs of appearing until they occur years into the therapy process. This can deplete one's financial, physical, and emotional resources, so the patient must be really dedicated regarding this route toward possible transformation. Furthermore, the problems addressed in psychoanalysis usually affect the upper classes, from which Freud hailed. In psychodynamic theory, only the well socialized can develop these defense mechanisms fully, so this therapy often only benefits the "worried-well." Coincidentally, since this therapy can be quite expensive, only the well-to-do can usually afford it anyway.

Besides its high costs and inefficient use of therapy time, another thing about psychodynamic theory that turns people off is its generally darker, "Darwinian" view of human nature. Because the id seeks survival first and pleasure a close second, while the superego is almost constantly pulling on id's leash, there is little hope for humankind other than an uneasy truce between two internal factions that have been warring for millennia. If you're not having major life-altering psychological difficulties interfering with your love life or work life, be content with your lot. Things could be much worse.

Second force: Behaviorism appeared on the scene out of questioning the psychoanalytical premise that human nature is automatically at the mercy of biological forces. Some theorists believed that human behavior could be radically altered given the right changes in tactics and environment. Viewing humans as mechanical "black boxes," behaviorists simply wanted to determine the quickest, most effective means toward accomplishing the stated end goal of human behavioral change—including those behaviors such as thoughts and feelings. These practitioners attempted to eliminate all the imprecise methods they saw in previous approaches to psychology, and to this day, their theories are the easiest to test in animal experiments and single-case studies. In scientific procedure, behaviorism is elegantly simple and effective. Techniques from classical conditioning have been shown to be effective in therapies targeting phobias, and operant conditioning is usefully applied in a wide variety of settings, such as in schools, juvenile detention centers, sports teams, companies, and those struggling with developmental disorders. As a theory of psychology, however, behaviorism is severely limited because there is no understanding of underlying cognitive, emotional, and spiritual processes governing the functions of the "black boxes" of humanity.

Behaviorism and its techniques proved inadequate for describing many human activities. Even in some primate and mouse studies, there have been found certain behaviors that are seemingly independent of external reinforcers in their environment. This would indicate the existence of intrinsic motivation in animals (and, by extrapolation, humans), thereby ruining a central premise of behaviorism. Studies like this led to a subschool of cognitive science that is devoted toward understanding memory processes and internal learning systems. This research has cross-pollinated with the field of artificial intelligence and has applications within the field of computer technology. Hardcore behaviorists argue that if researchers kept pursuing traditional methods, it would eventually yield more information. Currently, most theorists combine both approaches into a cognitive-behavioral

system for a more complete picture of learning and memory.

Third force: By the 1940s, these developments led researchers such as Abraham Maslow to conclude that not only does human nature exist, but also the good in human nature may be even more influential than the seeming bad. As within psychodynamic theory, human intentionality was again emphasized. But instead of giving primary importance to our pathological and irrational qualities, a much larger role was given to generosity, creativity, and love. A related philosophy called existential psychology was focusing on human freedom (oxymoron?) and our ability to create meaning in our lives—major proponents of this philosophy included Jean-Paul Sartre, Søren Kierkegaard, and Friedrich Nietzsche. Whereas Freudian techniques are focused on the past, and neo-Freudians, who expanded the role of the conscious ego, concentrate on the present, this approach helps clients look forward to a fuller life in their future. Because of its acknowledgment of the high potential of nearly every human being, this school became known as humanistic psychology.

Despite significant hurdles, psychologists have managed to find creative ways of investigating the subjective aspects of the mind. Carl Jung, who was early on one of Freud's biggest supporters, eventually broke away from his inner circle. Based on his clinical observations and his study of world mythology, Jung hypothesized that the unconscious, which Freud considered private and chaotic, is collectively inherited across all cultures. This collective unconscious forms certain patterns he called "archetypes," symbols found in dreams, myths, stories, and religion. Wilhelm Reich broke away even earlier than Jung and decided that listening to clients talk was near worthless if one wanted to free them from the pressures of id versus superego.

Instead, Reich developed the science of eliminating neuroses and psychoses by directly releasing them from the patient's physical body, in which the patient's unexpressed sexual and otherwise emotive energy had become trapped. Another psychologist who broke from Freud was Alfred Adler, who theorized that humans have a social drive for superiority. He coined the terms "superiority complex" and "inferiority complex" and found that our birth order plays a large role in the development of our personalities. Eric Berne, the founder of transactional analysis, looked at the three parts of the personality: id, ego, and superego and renamed them as the "child," "adult," and "parent." Each aspect of the personality carries with it a script, like continuously playing tapes, which influences our emotional responses to situations. There have been many other important founders of humanistic psychological paradigms, such as Fritz Perls, Carl Rogers, Karen Horney, and Jean Piaget, to name but a few of the most well known.

Abraham Maslow was primarily interested in motivation. He found that everyone has the same essential needs, but differing life conditions demand different priorities from differing individuals. There are deficiency needs and being needs (or "meta-" needs), conceptualized as a hierarchy from purely physical, to psychological/social, to spiritual needs. At the bottom are basic physiological needs: hunger, thirst, air, shelter, etc. The second level constitutes safety needs: structure, order, routine, etc. The third level constitutes affection and belongingness. The fourth level constitutes self-esteem needs and the desire to be needed, respected, and valued by others. The last level was originally self-actualization—the need to understand the world and oneself. This high-level self-development leads to a craving for spiritual evolution, however, and Maslow realized that he needed to create another category for research. This became force number four.

Fourth force: Transpersonal psychology is designed for helping individuals maximize their human potential by acknowledging and working with the divine aspirations (usually hidden) in everyone. One phenomenon introduced by transpersonal psychology, although originally written about in the West by William James in his *Varieties of Religious Experience*, is what Maslow termed "peak experiences." These are transcendent experiences of oneness—with nature, spirit, or the universe—that are non-egoic, non-psychotic, and have been highly encouraged in Eastern traditions from the beginning of history.

Transpersonal psychology has gained many insights in the last thirty years that have changed how many people view religion and spirituality. Especially important is the work of psychiatrist Stanislav Grof, who did pioneering research on chemically induced states of consciousness and later, for legal reasons, psychosomatic responses through breathwork. The more recent appearance of positive psychology has updated transpersonal psychology by not merely having an occasional peak experience or ultimate self-realization as the only goals. Instead, any person can learn a step-by-step approach to so tuning into one's unique divinity on a daily basis that regular, increasing happiness (seemingly unknown to Freud) is the likely result. One need not wait for peak experiences or nirvana, however. Positive psychology says that the route to both is totally fulfilling in its own right.

Fifth force: Whichever psychological system arrives to replace the reductionist approaches of cognitive behaviorism, used to treat the majority of Americans via the HMO/managed care/insurance conglomeration, will probably be given the title of being the fifth and latest psychological force. We have already invoked the presence of a new integral psychology, similar to the integral medicine that is now merging allopathy with CAM modalities in more progressive medical institutions. However, the name integral psychology has already been claimed by Ken Wilber, and other psychologists occasionally state that Wilber's four-quadrant approach to psychology is good enough to claim the fifth force mantle. Wilber himself does not want this title for his system, however, since he thinks psychology as we've known it is dead. Whatever replaces it will be so much more all-encompassing than the first four forces, blending them but adding in the importance of simultaneous focus on the four quadrants that make up human existence as well as the enlightenment experience that transcends them all.

Wilber's four quadrants are:

- the interior, deep, symbolic, emotive lives of both (1) the individual and (2) society (culture), as studied by depth psychology and humanistic/transpersonal psychologists

- (3) the individual's and (4) society's solely exterior lives, as studied by cognitive behaviorism for the individual and evolutionary psychology for society

Evolutionary psychology focuses on the objective organism and how its interaction with the objective environment has resulted, via variation and natural selection, in certain behaviors of the individual organism, most of which originated to serve survival until reproduction. Thus, you tend to behave in the way that you do because a million years of natural selection has left you with stubborn genetic tendencies. Evolutionary theory has a lot of insightful things to say about human behavior and social organization in general, but it is not clinically useful.

The psychospirituality of neurochemistry (as popularized by Candice Pert, PhD) also fits into the vogue "exterior" focus of today's therapies, despite its transpersonal acknowledgments, as this psychological definition of exterior means objective and reductionist. This is as opposed to the interior, difficult-to-measure, subjective worlds of the humanists and transpersonalists.

The main reason that Wilber believes his version of integrative psychology is so outside the psychology box is that he agrees with the mystic perennial philosophy and its dogma of relative realities. His four quadrants make up the phenomenal world, so covering only these quadrants with any sort of integrative psychology at all would keep this hypothetical system well within the psychology box. Wilber, however, believes the only final answer to human psychological needs is spiritual transcendence, at which time the four quadrants no longer apply. If you are consciously and contentedly one with the universe, there aren't four of anything anymore—except in a much more trivial, relative sense. Because Wilber places such importance on end goal enlightenment, he does outdo most transpersonalists who simply include a patient's general spiritual nature within their treatment philosophy and protocols. Whether this is enough to have his theories outdo psychology itself is a question open to debate, especially since ancient Asian spiritual psychologies very much insisted on the importance of this goal: complete liberation from all psychophysiological causes and effects and birth into a spiritual realm with different laws and perspectives. Looked at from this angle, Wilber's "new" system is hardly more than a return to the distant past with some updated language and graphics. Looked at more sympathetically, Wilber's disgust with the current reductionist

state of mass psychology has led him to a place at which he wants to let all present psychologies die a slow death so that the topic can be broached afresh.

Integration is coming to all systems of healing, as well as to all other systems period. Barring cataclysm and apocalypse, integration toward more and more complex and efficient systems is the way that most living organisms and their colonies proceed over time—in their physical structures, psychological development, and cultural expressions. Our current generation is one of the most fascinating times to observe this process, since in the course of a century we have gone from horse drawn carriages to Hybrid Priuses and iPhones. It can be difficult to imagine a time in the future when we will again have such an order of magnitude change in our technological innovations. And though it can be argued that psychology has not kept pace with material technologies, to move from Freud to fifth force in one century is no small leap. Future researchers may look upon the present time as quaintly ignorant, but enough information already exists for each of us to be holistically healthier in body-mind-spirit than any people in any previous era. Since this isn't the case in actuality, perhaps we don't need another "force" but merely application of those forces that lie unused within us already.

Modern Psychology

Psychology is both an academic and applied discipline. It involves the scientific study of mental and emotional processes and behavior, as well as observational study of these same processes using methodology that is from difficult to impossible to test scientifically. There is some tension between scientific psychology, with its program of empirical research at universities, and applied psychology, dealing with practical methods for helping humans and their environments to benefit from the variety of existing psychological hypotheses, as practiced by a master's level counselor or PhD-academic trained or PsyD-clinically trained psychologist.

Psychologists, even behaviorists, attempt to explain the mind and brain in the context of a poignant personal life inevitably full of emotional challenges. In contrast, neurologists utilize a purely physiological approach toward the brain and mind more useful for the treatment of brain injuries. Psychologists study such phenomena as perception, cognition, emotion, personality, behavior, and interpersonal and spiritual relationships. Psychology also refers to the application of such knowledge to various spheres of human activity such as family life, education, work, and the treatment of mental health problems. Cutting-edge psychology is beginning to study psychology in terms of wellness, optimal functioning, and human potential, versus the older psychological focus on labeling and treating specific psychopathologies.

Psychology includes many subfields of study and application concerned with such areas as human development, sports, health, industry, media, law, and transpersonal. So if you a prospective student interested in general psychology, there are a vast number of areas which can be studied both academically and in an applied manner. The field of psychology is generally split into two major categories, each with their own degree acronyms associated with them:

- **Academic psychology:** in which the sharing of intellectual information is the goal rather than direct treatment of patients. Students wishing to put energy in this direction will usually focus on earning a PhD in psychology and, in the process, determine exactly how they would like to focus on their research and scholarship. A systematic, mathematical, objective, test-driven approach can be expected here, and many psychology students find this drier focus upon the human psyche to be unpalatable.

- **Clinical psychology:** which most readers of this book will assume nearly synonymous with the practice of psychology itself, despite the many behind-the-scenes academic psychologists in our midst. It is clinical psychology that can be said to have begun in the first Shamanic "clinics" of our species, perhaps 100,000 years ago, and branched and morphed into the four or five "forces" of applied psychology over the last 150 years. If pursuing a doctorate, the PsyD degree is correlated with clinical expertise as a psychologist, while the MD degree is earned by those preferring psychiatry.

Although there are many clinical techniques used within the four forces which describe the evolution of the discipline, each one utilizes the general form of one expert in psychology guiding one or more individual patients toward a subjective and objective experience of greater peace of mind. This is in regard to internal psychological processes as well as interpersonal and intra-environmental dynamics. More important than specific techniques used within each force is to understand how the forces differ from one another. Once that is known, the prospective student will have a head start regarding the choice of one specific training route over another. All forms of applied psychology "work"—one seminal study found the efficacy of a treatment had more to do with the relationship and trust between client and therapist—so choose an area that is aligned with your intuitive, intellectual, and gut feelings about how the human psyche came to be and how it is best treated for optimal functioning.

It is tempting to construct a historical hierarchy of psychotherapeutic superiority, with the most modern approaches clearly trumping the beliefs and technologies of the Shamanic through the twentieth centuries. Remember, though, that in the world of applied psychology whatever most helps to heal an individual patient is in that moment the best treatment ever devised for them. There will always be a wide variety of approaches to take for practitioners and their patients desiring healing of body, mind, and spirit. It will be the approach you and your patients most believe in that will have the greatest likelihood of success, as Shaman discovered long ago. This is the use of the placebo effect in a conscious way, encouraging its presence so that patients will be much more likely to accept the healing that their bodies, minds, and souls are always working successfully toward if the right resources are there and the worst impediments removed.

PSYCHIATRY

Though psychiatry, like psychology, is a medical specialty that serves the healthy development of the mind, its focus, history, and philosophy is notably different than psychology's origins. Psychiatry is believed to have its earliest roots in the fifth century B.C. At that time, mental disorders, especially patients with outward psychotic symptoms, were considered by the Greeks and Romans to be victims of supernatural manifestations. Elsewhere in Europe and Asia, religious leaders and monarchs used exorcisms and spiritual ceremonies to treat mental disorders. These primitive methods were often harsh, painful, and sadly completely ineffective, frequently resulting in the death of the patient they intended to treat. In the fourth century, Hippocrates, one of the earliest physicians and the most famous Western one, hypothesized that abnormal psychological dispositions may be caused by physiological problems. After noticing that victims of war-related traumas came back from battle with symptoms of madness, he concluded that the physical injuries somehow contributed to unstable psychological states. In this regard, Hippocrates may have treated patients with post-traumatic stress disorder, although there is no evidence to support this claim.

During the medieval era, the earliest psychiatric hospitals were built by Muslims in Baghdad, Fes, and Cairo during the golden age of Islamic rule in the eighth century. Christians, during this time, still relied on earlier demonological explanations for mental illness, and treatment methods for psychosis did not change for nearly a thousand years. The Islamic culture, however, relied on clinical observations done by educated physicians. Purportedly, Islamic doctors are the first group in human history to provide psychotherapy and moral treatment—far more humane healing methods—for the mentally ill. However, no formal method of diagnosis and treatment was formulated.

It was not until the work of French physician Philippe Pinel, often referred to as the father of modern psychiatry, in 1792 that psychiatry emerged as a legitimate faction of medicine. Pinel, after receiving a degree from a medical school in Toulouse, went on to investigate the habits and psychological properties of mental illness after a close friend committed suicide. He subsequently moved to Paris and began working for the most esteemed private sanitarium in the world. During his time there, he developed a system of humane "moral" treatment for the mentally ill. After spending a significant amount of time working with and around the mentally sick, Pinel posited that there were many different types of mental illness and hence no one method could work for all types of diseases. After noticing a motley mix of symptoms—

some patients had a propensity to mania, while others seemed to hallucinate, and others tended to depression—Pinel challenged the prevailing medical paradigm that madness was a single inexplicable disease. On the contrary, Pinel was suggesting that each individual instance of madness, despite common disassociated and inane symptoms, might actually be an altogether different disease with respect to the individual. By treating an individual's condition, on a case-by-case basis, Pinel was able to make far more progress and have more clinical success than other psychiatric methods of the time. Humane or moral treatment may thus be thought of as one of the early forms of holistic psychiatry because Pinel focused on treating the patient rather than the illness. Other notable contemporaries of Pinel include William Tuke, who started a retreat in England for the mentally ill based on Pinel's methods, and Eli Todd, the first director of a retreat for mental patients in the United States.

Psychiatry continued to grow, along with the number of patients in mental asylums throughout the nineteenth century. By the end of the 1880s, the average number of patients in asylums had increased by 927 percent in the United States, with similar numbers in England and Germany. It was clear, both to political officials and scientific practitioners, that the then current method of psychiatric care was unsuccessful. As a result, the reputation of psychiatry in the medical world had hit an extreme low.

During the twentieth century, psychiatry experienced tremendous growth and a type of ideological rebirth with the advent of chemical treatment and prescribed medicine. German psychiatrist and scientist Emil Kraepelin is considered to be the father of modern *scientific* psychiatry and psychopharmacology after his research and discoveries in the early twentieth century. Dr. Kraepelin directly opposed the approach of Sigmund Freud, who regarded and treated mental disorders as the result of psychological factors; instead, Kraepelin argued that mental illness was actually a result of a chemical imbalance in the brain. Ostensibly pioneering the field of biological psychiatry, Kraepelin was the first researcher or practitioner to suggest that mental disorders were all biological in nature. This paradigmatic thinking would later evolve into neurology, neurochemistry, and neuropsychiatry. The goal of the psychiatric community had therefore changed significantly; after Kraepelin's proposed theory of psychopharmacology (the notion that emotive response are results of chemical processes in the brain), psychiatry's new mission became a search for the appropriate combination of chemicals that would correct the imbalance. Effectively, psychiatry gained its infamous "diagnose and treat" formula, treating mental illness at its biologically proposed source.

Kraepelin's ideas had tremendous momentum. The nature of the psychiatric community had fundamentally changed by the middle of the twentieth century and so had the public's response. In 1963, President John F. Kennedy introduced legislation delegating the National Institute of Mental Health to administer Community Mental Health Centers for those being discharged from state psychiatric hospitals. As pharmaceutical and drug companies began to grow in the United States, psychiatrists—as the only mental health doctors who can legally prescribe medicine—gained notoriety. The profession, both economically and scientifically, grew exponentially.

In 1972, esteemed psychologist David Rosenhan published the *Rosenhan Experiment*, a comparative study of validity of psychiatric diagnosis. Rosenhan's controversial study concluded that professional psychiatrists could not distinguish the difference between individuals suffering from serious mental disorders (schizophrenia, bipolar disorder, clinical depression, etc.) and those not suffering from mental illness at all. Though Rosenhan's methodology and conclusions have been critically questioned by members of the psychiatric community, his study sent a serious blow to the profession of psychiatry. It has been clear since Rosenhan's experiment that there are significant inconsistencies and unknowns in psychiatric research and treatment. Critics of psychiatry claim that there is no standardized method for consistent diagnoses, nor is there a correct, fully functional method for choosing the appropriate form of treatment. Modern psychiatry has been accused of fancy and expensive guesswork, with unpredictable efficacy.

Historically speaking, the practice of psychiatry grew out of a community of doctors and scientists, while psychology grew out of a community of philosophers and sociologists. While the two professions are closely related—in some respects their ultimate goal is the same—their competitive growth has incited professional antagonism between the two. For the past fifty years, the rift between the psychiatric and psychological communities has been a point of conflict in the legal and practical applications of medicine. There is currently a great deal of debate in both communities whether it is pragmatically necessary for psychiatrists to attend four years of medical school if they are exclusively prescribing medication in their practice and not using many of the practical skills learned in medical school. Additionally, members of the psychology community are pushing for legislation that would allow them to prescribe medicine without the necessity of attending a four-year medical college, which is unnecessary.

Of course, these debates reflect a larger problem within the greater scientific community—the relative uncertainty of the human brain. When dealing with mental illness and human emotion, there is still a tremendous degree of ambiguity as to how chemicals in our brain dictate human emotions. Additionally, the long-term side effects and social implications of medication (and in some cases overmedication) are still largely undetermined. Until modern science better understands how chemicals in the brain dictate introverted and extroverted relationships, we are still in the dark with regard to mental illness and treatment. The good news is that the science is getting better and genetics look promising—but the ultimate goal of effective treatment and cure for those afflicted with mental illness could be centuries away. Integration of the best treatment modalities from today's CAM and allopathy, as well as the future's unseen medical genius, will likely play a highly significant role.

CAREER INFORMATION

Psychology

This is not the most ideal time to enter the world of graduate level psychology training if you are interested in clinical practice. Most patients do not want to pay for treatment beyond their insurance deductible, and most insurance companies prefer quicker, cheaper, goal-oriented, reductionist, cognitive/behavioral therapy and, of course, pharmaceutical drugs. If anything related to depth psychology is your goal, you will be putting a lot of time, effort, and money into your training yet entering into an economy that often will not fully respect your knowledge and abilities. There will always be some clinical psychologists who will thrive no matter what the social climate, but many will find their hands tied from truly practicing the psychology of their choice while still earning a solid living.

There are other ways to apply psychology versus clinical work alone, however. Applied psychology encompasses both psychological research that is designed to help individuals overcome practical problems as well as the application of this research in a variety of settings. Much of applied psychology research is utilized within other fields, such as business management, product design, ergonomics, nutrition, law, and clinical medicine. Applied psychology also includes the areas of clinical psychology, industrial and organizational psychology, psychology and law, health psychology, school psychology, community psychology, and others. If pursuing a doctorate is your intention, the PhD degree is usually sought by those wanting to follow an academic research career track, while the PsyD or MD-psychiatry degrees are reserved for those wanting to practice clinical applications for the psychology of their choice.

For those with an academic bent, there is also the possible career choice of pure research psychology. Research psychology encompasses the study of behavior for use in academic settings and contains numerous areas: abnormal psychology, biological psychology, cognitive/behavioral psychology, comparative psychology, developmental psychology, health psychology, personality psychology, social psychology, and others. Since this is a guide to emerging degree programs, however, few readers will be likely to prefer the pure reductionist research route alone.

One recent career report suggested that psychology majors earn among the lowest salaries after graduation. However, several recent surveys have suggested that psychology is still one of the most popular college majors. While a study by the National Association of Colleges and Employers found that psychology graduates had the lowest starting pay of any field ($30,000), earnings and salaries of psychologists vary widely depending on education level, experience,

and specialization. The U.S. Department of Labor reports that the middle 50 percent of psychologists earn between $41,850 and $71,880.

Clinical psychology is by far the single largest specialty area for psychologists, with related counseling and developmental psychology as the next major areas of employment. More than 40 percent of psychologists work in the private, for-profit sector or are self-employed. According to the *Occupational Outlook Handbook*, more than four out of ten psychologists were self-employed in 2004, compared to the one in ten in the general population. Educational settings also employ a large number of psychologists with doctoral degrees.

Based on statistics from the U.S. Department of Education, the number of women majoring in psychology has grown tremendously over the last thirty years. While women made up 46 percent of those earning a bachelor's degree in psychology in 1971, this number had grown to a whopping 77.5 percent by 2002.

While minority students made up less than 12 percent of undergraduates in 1976, that number had grown to nearly 25 percent by 2002. There has also been growth in the number of women and minorities earning doctorates in psychology. In 2001, 71 percent of doctoral graduates were women, while 16 percent were minorities.

Employment of psychologists is expected to grow faster than average for all occupations in the field at least through 2014, because of increased demand for psychological services in schools, hospitals, social service agencies, mental health centers, substance abuse treatment clinics, consulting firms, and private companies. Among the specialties in this field, school psychologists—especially those with a specialist degree or higher—may enjoy the best job opportunities. Growing awareness of how students' mental health and behavioral problems, such as bullying, affect learning is increasing demand for school psychologists to offer student counseling and mental health services.

Industrial-organizational psychologists will be in demand to help boost worker productivity and retention rates in a wide range of businesses. Industrial-organizational psychologists will help companies deal with issues such as workplace diversity and antidiscrimination policies. Companies also will use psychologists' expertise in survey design, analysis, and research to develop tools for marketing evaluation and statistical analysis.

Demand should be particularly strong for individuals holding doctorates from leading universities in applied specialties such as counseling, health, and school psychology. Psychologists with extensive training in quantitative research methods and computer science may have a competitive edge over applicants without these backgrounds.

Master's degree holders in fields other than industrial-organizational psychology will face keen competition for jobs because of the limited number of positions that require only a master's degree. Master's degree holders may find jobs as psychological assistants or counselors, providing mental health services under the direct supervision of a licensed psychologist. Still others may find jobs involving research and data collection and analysis in universities, government, or private companies.

Opportunities directly related to psychology will be limited for bachelor's degree holders. Some may find jobs as assistants in rehabilitation centers or in other jobs involving data collection and analysis. Those who meet state certification requirements may become high school psychology teachers. The above statistics will be encouraging for a few, but those desiring to be one of the continuers of the Shamanic psychological offerings from the distant past may understandably wonder where they will put their good intentions into practice. This chapter has given you some historical clues; the rest is up to you.

Marriage and Family Therapy (MFT)

There are other alternatives to traditional psychology or psychiatry for those who want to pursue a career in counseling. Marriage and family therapy (MFT) is a specific branch of psychotherapy that deals with families and intimate relationships. Because familial ties are often among the most problematic yet crucial relationships in an individual's life, this form of counseling practice—in some states called marriage, family, and child counseling (MFCC)—is a separate profession from general psychotherapy. MFTs and MFCCs (there is a slight technical difference between the two) therefore have different, less rigorous edu-

cational and practical licensure requirements. MFTs and MFCCs work in private practice or in clinical settings in hospitals, integrated healing institutions, or counseling organizations.

Licensed MFCCs have formally earned their master of science (MS) degree in counseling with a specialization in marriage, family, and child issues. MFCCs are specifically trained to understand problems systemically, from both individual and familial perspectives. As counselors, they develop strong intervention skills while maintaining a relative understanding of age- and gender-related conflict. The MFCC's practice is similar to an MFT's; the largest difference is in the practitioner's individual choice of educational program and sometimes the title given to the profession in the state practiced. For the most part, the professions' scopes, theories, and execution are similar.

Licensed MFTs earn their master's degree in social work (MSW) with an emphasis on relationships. In this respect, MFTs are social workers, but their practice is limited to family-related therapy. Because MFTs go through a nearly similar education and certification process as MFCCs, it will suffice to discuss the certification and licensing process of the two as one profession. As mentioned before, some states will license MFTs and others will license MFCCs—if it does not specifically refer to the type of master's degree earned, the lexicons are interchangeable.

After completing a bachelor of arts or a bachelor of sciences (BA, BS) degree, potential MFTs can either choose to pursue a conventional master's degree program through an accredited social work institution or they may choose a more rigorous doctoral degree program. A master's program in family therapy usually takes two to three years and provides students with broad foundational knowledge about the various paradigms of understanding relationships. These programs are designed to begin students in marriage and family therapy careers by providing basic clinical and pragmatic skills, as well as theoretical knowledge about socialization and personal growth. Doctoral programs typically take three to five years, preparing students for an academic career in sociological and psychological research or advanced clinical practice and supervision. Doctoral programs also include all of the practical skills offered in a traditional master's program. As there are far too many accredited educational institutions with master's and doctoral programs in family therapy to list, consult the resources later on in this chapter to help you in finding an accredited program in your area.

Students may also pursue their MFT license by earning a graduate degree in another mental heath field. Candidates who graduate from psychiatry, psychology, clinical social work, or psychiatric nursing programs may decide to study MFT in depth in a postgraduate degree clinical training program. This course of action is usually for students who initially think they want to focus in a particular area of psychology and realize that they want to shift their focus to family therapy before they begin their supervised clinical experience. Once students have graduated from an accredited program, they begin the second phase of their professional training: internships and supervised training.

Before gaining a license to begin private practice, graduates must participate in postdegree supervised clinical experience. As always, the requirements for this prerequisite vary from state to state; generally speaking, 3,000 hours of supervised work as an intern or an assistant therapist suffice. However, you should always check with the licensure board in your state for its specific certification requirements. When graduate students have completed their internships—in some respects, the equivalent of a medical residency—they are eligible to apply to their state boards for independent licensure, formally earning the title MFT.

Currently, forty-six states license or certify MFTs. The only remaining requirement, after clinical supervision has been completed, is passing a state licensing exam conducted by the Association of Marital and Family Therapy Regulator Boards (AMFTRB). This comprehensive test assesses students' knowledge, diligence, and experience with traditional terminology and everyday practice associated with the MFT. Once students pass this test, they officially become marriage and family therapists and are legally allowed to open their own practice or work as a full-time social worker at an established firm. It is important to realize that MFTs have different legal rights in different states, as defined by the state licensure boards. In Ohio, for instance, MFTs are *not* allowed to diagnose and treat mental and emotional disorders, practice independently, or bill insurance as psychotherapists.

Psychiatry

A degree in psychiatry is the ultimate long-haul: undergrad, medical school, and residency. Psychiatrists are among the highest paid medical professionals in the United States. According to Salary.com, their average yearly salary is about $168,000, while the top 25 percent of earners make more than $189,000. The Bureau of Labor Statistics predicts that professional psychiatry will grow faster than other industries through 2014, reflecting the overall expansion of the medical industry.

ORGANIZATIONS FOR PSYCHOLOGY AND PSYCHIATRY

The American Psychiatric Association
www.psych.org

The APA is a medical specialty society recognized worldwide. More than 38,000 U.S. and international member physicians work together to ensure humane care and effective treatment for all persons with mental disorders, including mental retardation and substance-related disorders. It is the voice and conscience of modern psychiatry as both an advocacy group and lobbyist organization. Its larger vision is a society that has available, accessible quality psychiatric diagnosis and treatment. The membership of the APA is composed primarily of medical specialists who are legally qualified as psychiatrists.

The American Psychological Association
www.apa.org

Based in Washington, DC, the APA (not to be confused with the American Psychiatric Association) is a scientific and professional organization that represents psychology in the United States. With 148,000 members, APA is the largest association of psychologists worldwide. Its stated goals are to encourage excellence in the practice of modern psychology; promote and improve the methodology of scientific psychological research; improve the qualifications and usefulness of psychology via high standards of ethics, conduct, and education; and increase the diffusion of psychological knowledge to the public through reports, discussions, conferences, and publications.

The American Psychiatric Foundation

www.psychfoundation.org

The APF's mission is to advance public understanding of mental illnesses. It promotes awareness of mental illnesses and the effectiveness of treatment, the importance of early intervention, access to care, and the need for high quality services and treatment through a combination of grants, programs, research funding, and awards. As the philanthropic and educational arm of the American Psychiatric Association (APA), APF combines the knowledge and credibility of the world's largest psychiatric organization with a patient- and family-centered mission. The APF's affiliation with the APA provides it with direct access to the most credible and up-to-date information on mental illness.

The World Psychiatric Association

www.wpanet.org

The WPA was founded in 1950 as the Association for the Organization of World Congresses of Psychiatry. Since then, the organization has changed its focus to strictly create a moral expectation for practicing psychiatrists worldwide. With a manual of procedures, statutes, bylaws, and ethical declarations, the WPA is at the forefront of psychiatric philosophy. It has members in many different countries who adhere to the organization's ethical guidelines when practicing psychiatry. The goal of these documents, along with all their relevant publications and institutional documents, is to promote excellence and raise the standard of practice within the worldwide psychiatric community.

The American Academy of Child and Adolescent Psychiatry

www.aacap.org

AACAP, a 501(c)(3) nonprofit established in 1953, is a membership-based organization, composed of more than 7,500 child and adolescent psychiatrists and other interested physicians. Its members actively research, evaluate, diagnose, and treat psychiatric disorders and pride themselves on giving direction to and responding quickly to new developments in addressing the health care needs of children and their families. AACAP widely distributes information on its Web site, in an effort to promote an understanding of mental illnesses and remove the stigma associated with them. By advancing efforts in prevention of mental illnesses, and assuring proper treatment and access to services for children and adolescents, AACAP hopes to change the face of child and adolescent psychology in the United States.

The Mental Health Activist

www.dearshrink.com/active.htm

MHA, a division of DearShrink.com, is an online mental health center hosted by Dr. Ron Sterling—a geriatric psychiatrist who also specializes in psychotherapy and family therapy. Its Web site provides alerts and links to news articles, reports on legislation, and budding organizations or individuals seeking to improve the state of mental health care in the United States. Currently in the process of updating its archives for the 2008 Washington state legislative session, MHA is a good resource to discover new, relevant networks in the field of psychiatry.

ORGANIZATIONS FOR MFT

The American Association for Marriage and Family Therapy

www.aamft.org

Founded in 1942, the AAMFT is the largest professional association for marriage and family therapists in the United States. It represents the professional interests of more than 24,000 MFTs throughout the world, though its primary focus is on promoting academic and practical excellence in the United States. It publishes the *Journal of Marital and Family Therapy* and newsletters, and has a variety of other public resources to disseminate information about the growing industry of marriage and family therapy. The organization's Web site is the best resource to find legal information about licensure requirements on the Internet. The Virginia Association for Marriage and Family Therapy (www.vamft.org) is the largest chapter of the AAMFT.

Commission on Accreditation for the Marriage and Family Therapy Education

www.aamft.org/about/COAMFTE/AboutCOAMFTE.asp

COAMFTE is a subdivision of the AAMFT. It is responsible for accrediting master's, doctoral, and postgraduate clinical training programs in the United States. Students thinking about pursuing a particular program in family therapy should consult COAMFTE's Web site to make sure that it is part of an accredited institution.

Association of Marital and Family Therapy Regulator Boards

www.amftrb.org

The AMFTRB is legally responsible for regulating the MFT profession by issuing a national exam to candidates applying for state licensure. This organization also serves as a middleman between state boards and national associations. Its Web site is an excellent resource to find state-specific information on the legal and practical concerns of massage and family therapy.

American Family Therapy Academy

www.afta.org

Since its inception in 1977, AFTA has been a nonprofit organization representing family therapy instructors, clinicians, researchers, program directors, policy makers, and practitioners. Its vast and diverse membership promotes dialogue and a collaborative exchange of ideas through the community of family therapy. As a general advocacy group, AFTA seeks to advance theories, therapy, research, and standards of professional education for family therapists. It publishes a newsletter.

California Association of Marriage and Family Therapists

www.camft.org

CAMFT is an independent professional organization that represents the interests of licensed marriage and family therapists. It is dedicated to advancing the profession as an art and a science while maintaining high standards of professional ethics. CAMFT grants honors and awards annually to practitioners and helps MFT students find certified supervisors and internships to meet their licensure requirement.

MENTAL HEALTH PROFESSIONAL ORGANIZATIONS

The Foundation for Shamanic Studies

www.Shamanism.org

FSS is dedicated to the preservation, study, and teaching of Shamanic knowledge for the welfare of the planet and its inhabitants. Internationally renowned anthropologist Michael Harner founded FSS in 1985, creating an international Shamanic community. Now people can benefit from his groundbreaking work in Shamanic journeying through courses in core Shamanism and other spiritual principles that are not bound to a specific cultural group or perspective.

American Association for Humanistic Psychology

www.ahpweb.org

Founded in 1962, AHP is a worldwide network for the development and application of human sciences that recognize the distinctively human qualities and innate potentialities of each individual. AHP links, supports, and stimulates those who support this humanistic vision of the person. It publishes the newsletter *Perspective* and the *Journal of Humanistic Psychology.*

Association for Transpersonal Psychology

www.atpweb.org

Created in 1970 by Anthony Sutich and Abraham Maslow (who with Stanislav Grof named the field "transpersonal" in psychology), ATP is a major voice for the transpersonal movement. It publishes a journal directed by long-time editor Miles Vich and holds an annual conference. It also publishes a national listing of professional members and education programs in transpersonal psychology and a professional journal, *Journal of Transpersonal Psychology.*

National Institute for the Clinical Application of Behavioral Medicine

www.nicabm.com

The NICABM was founded in Connecticut in 1987 to establish practitioner-oriented conferences and seminars for mind-body health care providers focusing specifically on issues at the threshold between physical and emotional health. The institute holds an annual conference with speakers from all areas of integrative medicine, as well as workshops in the northeastern United States.

Dance of the Deer Foundation

www.Shamanism.com

DDF's mission is to preserve the Huichol culture and its Shamanic practices and traditions. The foundation, established in 1979 by Brant Secunda to carry on the vision of his grandfather and teacher, Don José Matsuwa, is a modern center for Shamanic studies. It offers seminars and retreats, consumer consultations, classes in Huichol Shamanism. It has compiled an extensive library about the historical and spiritual practice of Shamanism.

Society for Shamanic Practitioners

www.shamanociety.org

SSP is an alliance of people deeply committed to the re-emergence of Shamanic practices that promote healthy individuals and viable communities. The goal of this not-for-profit public benefit corporation is to support the re-emergence of Shamanism into modern, Western culture. While many other Shamanic organizations seek to document and learn from what has been done in the past, the society is focused on the here and now and is interested in documenting how Shamanism is changing and how it is being used as it interfaces with the twenty-first century world. Currently, the society has approximately 700 members in sixteen countries and continues to grow. Many of members are degreed and licensed health care practitioners, psychologists, and/or social workers who help people by using Shamanic interventions in their practices along with conventional Western therapies.

Erowid

www.erowid.com

Erowid is the best source for information on Schedule I drugs and their effect on the brain, the individual, and society. The Drug Enforcement Agency uses it to keep abreast of the latest trends and substances. Its archives include information on the chemical composition of nearly every psychoactive imaginable, including molecular structures and photographs of substances. Bravo to its two committed and smart founders.

Multidisciplinary Association for Psychedelic Studies

www.maps.org

MAPS is a membership-based, nonprofit research and educational organization. It assists scientists in the design, approval, funding, and reporting on research into the healing and spiritual potential of psychedelics and marijuana. Its newsletter is packed with smart and relevant discussion and research updates. Founded by drug policy pioneer Rick Doblin, PhD, Harvard School of Government.

PERIODICALS—PSYCHOLOGY

Biofeedback and Self-Regulation

http://journalseek.net/cgi-bin/journalseek/
journalsearch.cgi?field=issn&query=0363-3586

A journal dedicated to self-therapies, behavioral therapy, biofeedback training, and psychophysiology

The Humanistic Psychologist

http://journalseek.net/cgi-bin/journalseek/
journalsearch.cgi?field=issn&query=0887-3267

The latest peer-reviewed information and research on humanistic psychology and development

Journal of Humanistic Psychology

www.ahpweb.org/pub/journal/menu.html

Published by the Association for Humanistic Psychology, the JHP is a quarterly publication began in 1961. Topics of special interest are authenticity, identity, personal growth, self-actualization, self-transcendence, I-Thou, encounters, existential and humanistic psychotherapy, community building, and humanistic politics.

The Journal of Transpersonal Psychology

http://atpweb.org/journal.asp

Founded in 1969, this scholarly journal addresses the research, theory, and application of altered states of consciousness, mystical states, and Eastern spiritual practices. It is the official journal of the Association for Transpersonal Psychology.

Psychotherapy Theory, Research, Practice, and Training

www.apa.org/journals/pst/

This journal publishes a wide variety of articles relevant to the field of psychotherapy. Distributed quarterly, the journal strives to create interactions among individuals involved with training, practice, theory, and research since all areas are essential to psychotherapy. Edited by University of Maryland psychology professor Charles J Gelso PhD.

PERIODICALS—MARRIAGE AND FAMILY THERAPY

American Journal of Family Therapy

www.ingentaconnect.com/content/routledg/uaft

Contemporary Family Therapy

www.springerlink.com/content/104691

Published internationally on subjects of behavioral science, psychology, clinical psychology, social sciences, psychiatry, and sociology

The Family Psychotherapist
www.apa.org/divisions/div43/mag.html

Published by Division 43, a subset of the American Psychological Association, on the topic of contemporary family values and issues facing familial relationships

Journal of Family Therapy
www.blackwellpublishing.com/journal.
asp?ref=0163-4445&site=1

This journal advances the understanding and treatment of human relationships constituted in systems such as couples, families, professional networks, and wider groups by publishing articles on theory, research, clinical practice, and training.

Journal of Feminist Family Therapy
www.haworthpressinc.com/store/product.
asp?sku=J086

The JFFT provides an international forum to further explore the relationship between feminist theory and family therapy theory and practice. The journal presents thought-provoking and insightful articles of a theoretical nature, as well as articles focusing on empirical research and clinical application.

Journal of Marriage and Family Therapy
www.jmft.net

The official journal of the American Association for Marriage and Family Therapy

Journal of Sex and Marital Therapy
www.informaworld.
com/smpp/title~content=t713723519~db=all

Published by the Taylor & Francis Group, the JSMT includes articles on impotence and sexual dysfunction, marriage and couples therapy, sex therapy, and general sexuality.

PERIODICALS—PSYCHIATRY

The Multidisciplinary Association for Psychedelic Studies Newsletter
http://www.maps.org

Packed with smart and relevant discussion and research updates

Shaman's Drum
http://shamandrum.org

The American Journal of Psychiatry
http://ajp.psychiatryonline.org

A popular peer-reviewed journal committed to keeping the field of psychiatry vibrant and relevant

Psychiatric News
http://pn.psychiatryonline.org/current.dtl

Current news on advancements, research, and funding opportunities for practicing psychiatrists and other mental health professionals. Printed by American Psychiatric Publishing, Inc.

Clinical Psychiatry News
www.eclinicalpsychiatrynews.com

CPN is an independent newspaper that provides the practicing psychiatrist with timely and relevant news and commentary about clinical developments in the field and about the impact of health care policy on the specialty and the physician's practice. On the CPN Web site, you can subscribe to CPN's newspaper, search old archives, and view current issues.

American Psychiatric Publishing
http://journals.psychiatryonline.org

APPI is the world's premier publisher of books, journals, and other multimedia on psychiatry, mental health, and behavioral science. It offers authoritative, up-to-date, and affordable information geared toward psychiatrists, other mental health professionals, psychiatric residents, medical students, and the general public. Its Web site features nearly every relevant journal or prestigious publication in the field of psychiatry.

GENERAL ONLINE RESOURCES

Allyn & Bacon Family Therapy Web Site
www.abacon.com/famtherapy/index.html

An independent Web site with a comprehensive history and timeline of family therapy. This site also includes therapists' profiles and links to other MFT sites on the Internet.

Georgetown Family Center: Bowen Theory
www.thebowencenter.org/pages/theory.html

A detailed articulation of the Bowen theory of family systems. The Bowen paradigm predicts the consequences of casual relations given the system nature of a family where people are so intensely emotional connected.

Green Lotus Healing Center

www.drpentz.com

The home page of Dr. Judith Penz, a holistic and integrative psychiatrist with board certification in child, adolescent, and adult psychiatry. Dr. Penz is an archetype of an integrative approach that attempts to fuse traditional Western medicine with alternative approaches to personality and psychotherapy.

Traditional and Holistic Healing

www.drjudithorloff.com

The home page of Dr. Judith Orloff, author of *Second Sight* and *Intuitive Healing*. An assistant clinical professor of psychiatric at UCLA, Dr. Orloff asserts that intuitive intelligence is the key to understanding deeper implications of our emotional and physical health. Using a holistic approach to psychiatry, she teaches her patients to use their intuition when dealing with difficult emotional issues.

Psychiatry.com

www.psychiatry.com

A general online forum, for patients and practitioners, dedicated to the practice and philosophy of psychiatric medicine

PsychiatricOnline

www.psychiatryonline.com

Links to various books, journals, and esteemed scholarly papers in the psychiatric community. Its new *DSM-IV-TR®* tool allows members to search journals, textbooks, clinician studies, and medication information handouts all from one Web site.

The Psychotherapy Networker

www.psychotherapynetworker.org

A nonpeer-reviewed magazine for psychotherapists and social workers

BOOKS

Psychology

On Being a Therapist by Jeffrey Kottler

Toward a Psychology of Being by Abraham Maslow

Re-Visioning Psychology by James Hillman

The Adventure of Self-Discovery: Dimensions of Consciousness and New Perspectives in Psychotherapy and

Inner Exploration by Stanislav Grof

The Center of the Cyclone: An Autobiography of Inner Space by John Lilly

Character Analysis by Wilhelm Reich

The Atman Project: A Transpersonal View of Human Development by Ken Wilber

The Master Game by Robert de Ropp

Existential Psychotherapy by Irvin Yalom

The Varieties of Religious Experience by William James

From Chocolate to Morphine: Everything You Need to Know About Mind-Altering Drugs by Winifred Rosen and Andrew Weil

Marriage and Family Therapy

On Being a Therapist by Jeffrey Kottler

An Introduction to Marriage and Family Therapy by Norman L. Winegar, Lorna L. Hecker, and Joseph L. Wetchler

The Practical Practice of Marriage and Family Therapy: Things My Training Supervisor Never Told Me by Mark Odell and Charles F. Campbell

Psychiatry

On Being a Therapist by Jeffrey Kottler

Individual Psychology Psychiatry and Holistic Medicine by Young

Humanizing Madness: Psychiatry and the Cognitive Neurosciences by Niall McLaren MD

Holism and Beyond: The Essence of Holistic Medicine by John Diamond

Essentials of Psychiatry by Jerald Kay and Allan Tasman

Handbook of Complementary and Alternative Therapies in Mental Health by Scott Shannon

Philosophy and Psychiatry by Thomas Schramme and Johannes Thome

EDUCATIONAL INSTITUTIONS

Psychology

Many of the following programs offer both doctorate and master's degrees.

Antioch University Santa Barbara

Santa Barbara, California

www.antiochsb.edu

Programs include MA and PsyD in psychology with a focus in counseling psychology, dance/movement therapy, substance abuse/addiction, marriage and family therapy, and clinical psychology.

California Institute for Human Sciences

Encinitas, California

www.cihs.edu

An integrative and cutting-edge institution, CIHS offers master's and doctorate programs in clinical psychology, comparative religion and philosophy, and several online residency programs from doctoral students. CIHS's doctoral program features classes in the psychology of Shamanism, transpersonal psychology, eco-psychology, expressive arts modalities, and bio-energetic psychological therapy. Master's programs are typically two years, while doctoral programs range from four to six years.

California Institute of Integral Studies

San Francisco, California

www.ciis.edu

CIIS is an accredited institution of higher education that strives to embody spirit, intellect, and wisdom in service to individuals, communities, and the Earth. The institute expands the boundaries of traditional degree programs with interdisciplinary, cross-cultural, and applied studies in psychology, philosophy, religion, cultural anthropology, transformative learning and leadership, integrative health, and the arts. Offering a personal learning environment and supportive community, CIIS provides an extraordinary education for people committed to transforming themselves and the world.

Fielding Graduate University

Santa Barbara, California

www.fielding.edu

Fielding is an institution focused on the role of the media in psychological development. It offers several programs in clinical psychology including a concentration in health psychology and PhD programs in media psychology and social change.

Holy Names University

Oakland, California

www.hnu.edu/academics/counselingpsychology.html

Holy Names University offers four master's and two graduate certificate programs in counseling psychology for students who want to work professionally in the field of counseling. Each program is unique in integrating spirituality with sound theoretical and field-based learning in the area of counseling psychology. MAs are available in forensic psychology and pastoral counseling.

Institute of Transpersonal Psychology

Palo Alto, California

www.itp.edu

ITP is a private, nonsectarian graduate school accredited by the Western Association of Schools and Colleges. Founded in 1975, the institute began as a groundbreaking center of integrative, whole-person learning and training. Today, ITP is a leader in transpersonal research and education of clinicians, spiritual guides, wellness caregivers, and consultants who apply transpersonal principles and values in a variety of settings. The institute's stimulating and transformative educational paradigm, valuing the mind body spirit connection, attracts students from all over the world to both residential and distance-learning programs.

John F. Kennedy University

Orinda, California

www.jfku.edu

JFKU is a learning environment of choice for those seeking a transformative and life-enhancing educational experience. Its stated mission is "to provide access to high-quality, innovative educational opportunities that integrate theory and life experience." JFKU inspires personal, professional, and academic growth and advances the well-being of diverse local and global communities.

Naropa University
Boulder, Colorado
www.naropa.edu

Naropa, a private, nonprofit, nonsectarian liberal arts institution, is dedicated to advancing contemplative education by combing the best of traditional Western education with the spirituality and understanding promoting by Eastern methods. A truly integrated institution, it helps students know themselves more deeply and engage constructively with others. By combining these two storied pedagogies, East and West are indeed meeting every day at Naropa, and the resulting sparks of inspiration are flying. Naropa comprises a four-year undergraduate college and graduate programs in the arts, education, environmental leadership, psychology, and religious studies. It offers BA, BFA, MA, MFA and MDiv degrees, as well as professional development training and classes for the community.

New College of California
San Francisco, California
www.newcollege.edu

New College is an alternative educational institution focusing on living in a just, sacred, and sustainable world. It has graduate programs in psychology on a range of contemporary issues including feminist psychology, humanistic psychology, and social/clinical psychology.

Michigan School for Professional Psychology
Farmington Hills, Michigan
www.mispp.edu

MiSSP's mission "is to educate and train individuals to become reflective scholar-practitioners with the competencies necessary to serve diverse populations as professional humanistic psychologists and psychotherapists." It offers professional programs in clinical psychology as well as a special doctoral degree in humanistic psychology. Dedicated to an environment of collaborative studies, MiSSP is a unique institution founded upon humanistic principles. It is accredited by the Higher Learning Commission, a group that works predominately with schools in the northern-central United States.

Pacifica Graduate Institute
Carpinteria, California
www.pacifica.edu

PGI offers rigorous doctoral and master's graduate programs in alternative psychology. Topics of notable interest include personal/existential thought, depth psychology, psychoanalytic philosophy, Jungian studies, and topics in behavioral perspectives. Graduates of PGI are prepared to apply for the California Clinical Psychology License and/or the California Marriage, Family, and Child Counseling License after completing a two-year master's program. Its PhD program in clinical psychology recently gained APA accreditation.

Saybrook Graduate School and Research Center
San Francisco, California
www.saybrook.edu

Founded in 1971, Saybrook was initially the Humanistic Psychology Institute as part of Sonoma State University. Several years later, it was incorporated and designated as a nonprofit corporation 501(c)(3) organization. Today, Saybrook has become a product of the nationwide wave of innovation in higher education. Founded on the basic humanistic belief that "human consciousness at individual and societal level is a work in progress," Saybrook has become an institutional leader of this ideological movement. Saybrook currently offers a five-year doctoral program for psychology (PsyD). It also offers specializations in Jungian studies, leadership of sustainable systems, marriage and family therapy, and transformative social change.

Seattle University, College of Arts and Sciences
Seattle, Washington
www.seattleu.edu/artsci/gradpsy

Seattle University's College of Arts and Sciences offers a unique master's graduate program in existential and phenomenological psychology. This particular program, founded in 1980, has had an excellent reputation in the mental health community. By looking at how people create meaning out of cognitive experience and drawing upon other psychological paradigm, Seattle University's unique two-year program in alternative psychology allows students to obtain a license as a mental health counselor in the state of Washington and serves as a perquisite for doctoral studies.

Sonoma State University
Rohnert Park, California
www.sonoma.edu/psychology/cdpp

Sonoma State is one of nineteen colleges in the California state university system. The psychology program is humanistically oriented. Most of the Tamalpa Institute's curriculum in dance therapy can now be used to meet the requirements for an MA degree in psychology. Also, Sonoma State offers an external master's degree in person centered expressive therapy and the Institute of Transpersonal Psychology.

Southwestern College
Santa Fe, New Mexico
www.swc.edu/programs/MA_counseling.htm

Southwestern College offers several MA degrees in counseling, art therapy, and counseling with concentrations in grief, loss, and trauma. All master's programs are two years in length.

University of California–Santa Cruz
Santa Cruz, California
http://psych.ucsc.edu

The Psychological Department at UC Santa Cruz prides itself on creative and unique research. Its departmental programs are divided into three major research areas: cognitive, developmental, and social psychology. It provides both graduate and undergraduate programs in clinical psychology, as well as specialized focuses (for graduate students) in areas such as sex and gender, the evolution of cognition, childhood psychopathology, and the psychological impacts of aging.

University of Pennsylvania
Philadelphia, Pennsylvania
http://ppc.sas.upenn.edu

Fall of 2008 is the scheduled date of the first class of students pursuing a master's degree in positive psychology. As alluded to in these pages, "Positive psychology is the scientific study of the strengths and virtues that enable individuals and communities to thrive. The Positive Psychology Center promotes research, training, education, and the dissemination of positive psychology. This field is founded on the belief that people want to lead meaningful and fulfilling lives, cultivate what is best within themselves, and enhance their experiences of love, work, and play." Positive psychology represents the latest link between ancient Asian "perennial philosophy" and modern Western psychotherapy: how to attain and retain happiness at will. A doctoral program is planned for the near future.

University of Santa Monica
Santa Monica, California
http://universityofsantamonica.edu

The psychology program for USM integrates thirty-six counseling skills and approaches them from various alternative paradigms of psychological thought, including person-centered therapy, Jungian psychoanalysis, Gestalt psychology, rational-emotive psychology, neuro-linguistic programming, and psychosynthesis. Classes are offered in weekend format to allow easy access to the university. Additionally, the university offers a unique two- or four-year program in spiritual psychology.

West Georgia College
Carrollton, Georgia
www.westga.edu

West Georgia College, a college within the University of West Georgia network, is an alternative psychology school, which offers doctoral psychology (PsyD) programs in humanistic, transpersonal, existential, critical, psychological, and neuroscientific psychology. Its doctoral programs invite students to pursue their own interests with global understanding and local sensitivity. Most doctoral programs follow the four-year departmental tradition of rigorous and creative scholarly inquiry alongside personal growth.

MFT Programs

For accredited MFT programs only, consult the American Association for Marriage and Family Therapy (www.aamft.org); look for "Online Directories" at the bottom of AAMFT's home page.

Psychiatry

For more information on choosing a medical graduate program with a holistic appreciation, consult chapter 4 on allopathic medicine. Once you have finished four years of medical school, you will have four more years of an applied clinical residency program in psychiatry. From there, it's on to your boards and state licensure. For the official list of allopathic institutions' residency programs, consult the Accreditation Council for Graduate Medical Education at www.acgme.org. During medical school, you will have the time and connections to seek out like-minded researchers and practitioners within residency programs you wish to apply to.

CHAPTER 6

SOCIAL WORK (MSW)

Social work is a cross between society and the individual, between sociology and psychology. The goal of social work is to improve the lives of individuals, groups, and entire societies through direct assistance, awareness, and emotional development. By applying theoretical concepts found in anthropology, economics, sociology, literary theory, and philosophy, social workers incorporate a diverse body of ideas and traditions to serve individuals, families, organizations, and communities. According to the International Federation of Social Workers, the practice draws upon "evidence-based knowledge" from empirical research and practice. By recognizing the "complexity of interactions between humans," social workers play an instrumental role in helping people make smooth, enlightened transitions during difficult periods of their lives. This may take the form of larger social issues, such as case management or community organizing, or more focused, small-scale counseling work, such as individual counseling and small group therapy.

Social workers must therefore use professional lexicons to distinguish between the field's different types. "Macro" social work, for example, refers to big picture professional intervention, serving an entire society, collective group, or country. "Mezzo" social work refers to the practice that serves smaller groups, such as organizations, agencies, or associations. Lastly, "micro" level intervention refers to therapy that is individual or family based. The role of the professional social worker is to recognize inequality, injustice, and social disease in all of its various forms, and treat it with a sophisticated understanding of humanity's social, instinctual, and personal needs.

Social work is a large and far-reaching profession. Clinical practices, which usually take the form of counseling and therapy sessions, may address a multitude of issues from crisis intervention to relationship education. Though the profession is federally regulated (social workers must receive a degree and a state licensure), there is no limit to the scope of the social worker's work. That said, professional social work tends to manifest in two different directions. Currently, there is a great deal of university-based psychological research where scientists, sociologists, and psychologists are trying to understand the chemical connections between

THE GOAL of social work is to improve the lives of individuals, groups, and entire societies through direct assistance, awareness, and emotional development. By recognizing the "complexity of interactions between humans," social workers play an instrumental role in helping people make smooth, enlightened transitions during difficult periods of their lives.

impulses in our brain and how they manifest in social behavior. The other side of the profession includes practitioners who work in a social context, revising their methods not from chemical analyses but from empirical experience with patients, operating under the assumption that similar human beings have comparable needs. The latter types of practitioners tend to be well versed in human emotions and clinical psychology, social conditions, and relationships. In either venue, social work is a practice for the dedicated, curious individual who is uncomfortable with the current state of human interactions.

HISTORY

Social work as a recognized form of therapy originates in the nineteenth century as a religious reaction to poverty in the United States. As America ushered in the technological growth and economic development of the industrial revolution, the poor classes (a significant remnant from the feudal system) became larger and increasingly neglected. The Christian church, at the time a significant moral force in the country, began to organize nonprofit charity groups to feed, house, and cloth the emerging homeless. Social work is historically linked to charity, surfacing mostly from Christian roots, although mainstream social work today is secular.

As the church became more involved in helping the poor class, it became evident that it was not simply a lack of basic sustenance which plagued the poverty stricken but also rampant instances of crime, prostitution, mental illness, and depression. Other secular groups began to see the same problems permeating into the lower and middle classes, and called for a new nonreligious charity, which would promote social welfare without any denominational allegiance to particular dogma or religious sentiment. In the late 1880s, a new so-called "scientific-charity" emerged as one possible answer to the growing ills of an industrialized and socialized society. This has since been historically referred to as the *settlement movement*, a group of secular humanists dedicated to understanding the forces behind and creating treatment for abject poverty without the perspective of religion. Using the "three Rs"—research, reform, and residence—these groups advocated for changes

in social policy through a wide variety of social institutions: education, law, health services, and government. Those concerned and active citizens would later become integrated with the scientific interest in psychology, fusing into a socially conscious and intellectually curious contingent of professional psychotherapists. These individuals laid the foundation for a sociological paradigm and the discipline known today as social work.

CAREER INFORMATION

Social workers may work in many different contexts. As part of a humanitarian group, social workers can work with the sick, homeless, or poor. In a private practice, social workers can specialize in familial intervention, child/adolescent therapy, or relationship counseling. Techniques employed by social workers vary with the practitioner's style, but generally there are three focused areas for professional social workers in the United States: child/family/school, medical/public health, and mental health/substance abuse. Regardless of their focus, most social workers spend their time either seeing clients in an office environment or traveling to see their clients in their life environments.

As of 2006, social workers held 595,000 jobs in the United States. Five out of every ten were in health care and social assistance industries, while three out of ten were employed by state and local government agencies. The Bureau of Labor Statistics expects employment of social workers to increase by "22 percent during the 2006–16 decade," which is a rate of growth faster than other area in health care. The growing elderly population, a legacy from the baby boom generation, will undoubtedly create a need for increased health and social services. All current statistics indicate that social work, and other socially conscious health-related industries, will experience unprecedented periods of economic growth in the next ten to twenty years. The median earnings of social workers were $37,500 as of May 2006, with the middle 50 percent earning between $29,600 and $49,000. The top 10 percent of professionals earn a yearly salary of more than $62,000. Workers unions, advocacy groups, and a plethora of professional organizations employ social workers. Like nursing, it enjoys being a well-networked profession. For information regarding associations and organizations dedicated to social work, consult the resource section.

Every state offers licensure. Standards vary slightly. A growing number of educational programs are placing increased emphasis on communications skills, professional ethics, and sensitivity to cultural diversity issues. To become a licensed, social worker, you must have a bachelor's degree (BSW or BASW), a master's degree (MSW), or a doctoral degree (PhD or DSW) from a program accredited by the Council on Social Work Education. Depending on the particular program or university, a four-year undergraduate degree will generally draw upon the whole gamut of social work practice, including social theory, human development, anthropology, sociology, social policy, research methods, and social planning. Upon completing an accredited program, students are prepared to sit for the Association of Social Work Boards' licensing examination, a comprehensive test that requires students to demonstrate their knowledge of social theory and therapeutic practice. Additionally, students must then have supervised clinical experience through an internship or residency program, which they may begin (in some states) in the final year of school. Most states require two years and 3,000 hours of supervised experience before granted licensure (LSW). For more information on the specific prerequisites to licensure in your state, consult your local chapter of the National Association of Social Workers.

TRAINING PROGRAMS

The Council on Social Work Education (www.cswe.org) accredits social work undergraduate and graduate education programs. It offers a directory of some 300 accredited programs on its Web site. When exploring the community of social work, you may notice that some programs and groups are run through churches and other religious institutions. Because social work originated from the Christian charity movement, there are many professional social workers who are members of the clergy. Pastoral counseling, a branch of counseling in which ordained ministers, rabbis, priests, and other religious officials provide dogmatically inspired therapy services, is a significant pro-

fessional faction within the social work community. While these professionals primarily pursue their education at a seminary or religious institution, counseling can often be a significant part of their religious practice.

ORGANIZATIONS

The National Association of Social Workers
www.socialworkers.org

NASW is the largest membership organization of professional social workers in the world. Boasting more than 150,000 members, NASW is the leading organization for the social work community, representing the profession through research projects, ethical codes, educational standards, legal regulations, and public outreach. Its Web site is a portal to nearly every social work resources on the Internet.

Council on Social Work Education
www.cswe.org

Founded in 1952, the CSWE is a nonprofit national association that represents and accredits undergraduate and graduate programs in social work.

The Association of Social Work Boards
www.aswb.org

AWSB regulates the practice of social work. By maintaining and developing the national licensing examination, it is a central resource for information on the legal regulation and policy regarding social work.

The School Social Work Association of America
www.sswaa.org

SSWAA is a lobbying organization focused on strengthening the social work profession. It assists social workers by creating membership networks locally and online. Based in Washington DC, its legislative advocacy is targeted toward the U.S. Department of Education, Congress, the National Association of Pupil Service, and the Committee for Education Funding.

The Clinical Social Work Association

www.cswf.org

The CSWA is a national profession membership organization for Clinical Social Workers. It represents individual practitioners who provide treatment in agencies, clinics, hospitals, and in private practice. Formerly the Clinical Social Work Federation, the CSWA passionately promotes ethics, professionalism, and networking.

The International Association of Schools of Social Work

www.iassw-aiets.org

IASSW is a global association of social work schools and educators dedicated to the development and standardization of social work education throughout the world. The IASSW holds consultative status in the United Nations and participates as an NGO in Geneva, Vienna, and New York. Using the United Nations as a venue, the IASSW represents social work education at an international level. Members from all fields of social work in all countries are welcome to join the association in its global mission.

The National Organization of Forensic Social Work

www.nofsw.org

The NOFSW is a membership group established to advance education in the field of forensic social work. It facilitates training programs, forums, lectures, group panels, annual conferences, and newsletter publications. It also prints a quarterly journal, *The Journal of Forensic Social Work.*

Association of Oncology Social Work

www.aosw.org

AOSW is a nonprofit international organization dedicated to providing psychosocial services to cancer patients and their families. Since its inception in 1984, AOSW has been working with existing national cancer organizations, currently boasting more than 1,000 of its own members with numerous connections to larger organizations. It publishes a journal for cancer survivors, the *Journal of Psychosocial Oncology.*

The Institute for the Advancement of Social Work Research

www.iaswresearch.org

Founded in 1993 by five national professional organizations that represent social work practice and education communities, IASWR is a nonprofit organization that serves the research needs of the growing social work community. IASWR promotes social work research conducted under the auspices of academic and professional organizations; it does not fund research directly. Its vision is to create an infrastructure for social work research that enhances the professional development of the field. Its Web site also includes a comprehensive listing of all social work organizations on the Internet.

Society for Social Work and Research

www.sswr.org

The SSWR is a nonprofit professional society dedicated to the advancement of social work research. Founded in 1994, the SSWR has more than 1,300 members in forty-five states. It hosts annual conferences, publishes a newsletter, and issues awards for excellence in social worker research. The SSWR also publishes a quarterly journal, *Qualitative Social Work.*

The International Federation of Social Workers

www.ifsw.org

IFSW is a worldwide membership group that represents many social workers in all areas and philosophies of social work. It is dedicated to developing resources, including various publications, seminars, and conferences, as well as increasing solidarity in the social work movement and enhancing social justice globally.

National Association of Deans and Directors Schools of Social Work

www.naddssw.org

NADD represents more than 180 graduate schools of social work in the United States and Canada. It organizes events for leaders in the social work educational community to meet and share ideas, effectively connecting social work educational methodologies in North America.

PERIODICALS

The National Association of Social Work Online Journals

www.naswpressonline.org

The NASW press publishes several online peer-reviewed journals in the field of social work. It publishes four journals: *Social Work,* a journal established in 1956 for all forms of social work; *Health and Social Work,* dedicated to health care professionals; *Social Work Research,* one of the "chief outlets" for primary research in the field; and *Children and Schools* (formerly *Social Work in Education*), a publication established in 1978 that deals with the latest theories and issues faced by social workers employed in schools and community agencies.

Journal of Social Work

http://jsw.sagepub.com

This publication focuses on the theoretical understanding of social work as well as policy, practice, and the promotion of research. The journal welcomes submissions from all fields of social work.

Journal of Social Work Values & Ethics

www.socialworker.com/jswve/

This journal examines the ethical and moral values associated with social work as well as their implications for the practice. JSWVE seeks to raise the standard of excellence in practice and in ethicality by creating a forum for the development of social models, particularly in regard to ethical conflicts. Because ethics and morality play a large part in the practice of social work, the content of this journal is relevant in both social work practice and theory.

Clinical Social Work Journal

www.springerlink.com/content/104850/

The CSWJ, founded in 1973, publishes peer-reviewed articles relevant to the contemporary clinical practice of social work. All of its articles present evidence-based clinical trial for all theories posited by the authors. Devoted to the advancement of clinical knowledge and the betterment of the social work community, CSWJ is one of the elite journals in the social work community.

Social Service Review

www.journals.uchicago.edu/toc/ssr/current

Founded in 1927, SSR is one of the oldest social science journals in the United States. Originally developed to advance the publication of thought provoking original research on social welfare policy, this journal has evolved into a leading voice in the social science and social work community. Articles in the SSR analyze issues from various sociological, economic, and philosophical issues, viewing problems critically in their own context while considering long-range solutions. The journal is distributed quarterly.

ONLINE RESOURCES

The New Social Worker Online

www.socialworker.com

TNSW is a magazine for social workers with a strong online component. On the Web site, practitioners can network with one another, view a list of continuing education programs, post to forums, and look up general information about social work practice. It publishes the *Journal of Social Work Values & Ethics*.

About.com: Mental Health

http://mentalhealth.about.com

Bonnie Burton, a trauma survivor, writes about therapy as a self-healing method. She also details why trauma survivors do not necessarily make the best trauma therapists. This article poses some interesting insights about empathy and its role in a practitioner-client relationship.

Social Work Help

www.socialworkhelp.com

General consumer information on social work. Includes news, links, forums, books, job postings, and a membership program

Disaster Mental Health

www.eyeofthestorminc.com

The personal Web site of John Weaver, LCSW, author of the *Eye of the Storm*, contains practical solutions and programs for workers in a "chaotic" world.

BOOKS

General Systems Approach: Contributions Toward a Holistic Conception of Social Work by Gordon Hearn

Spiritual Diversity in Social Work Practice: The Heart of Helping by Edward Canda and Leola Furman

Handbook of Health Social Work by Sarah Gehlert and Teri Arthur Browne

CHAPTER 7

MASSAGE THERAPY (MT)

Massage therapy is probably the oldest, simplest, most pleasurable medical modality in the world. It is even prehuman—one of our closest ancestor primates, bonobos, regularly massage each other for pleasure and reconciliation. And some claim it is divine, as Hindus tell the story of God as Vishnu being given a foot massage by God as Lakshmi, his wife, in order that Vishnu stay awake almost eternally and keep creation extant. On the human front, all of our earliest civilizations show signs of the practice of massage therapy, either pictorially or in writing. This includes cultures in ancient Egypt, India, China, Japan, Greece, and Rome. In 460 B.C.E., Hippocrates wrote that "the physician must be experienced in many things, but assuredly in rubbing," while the "Yellow Emperor's" Chinese medicine text of 100 B.C.E. recommended "massage of skin and flesh." And bas reliefs at Angkor Wat temple in Cambodia, circa 1150 A.C.E., illustrate the radical technique of "massage abortion," which is little-used today.

Because formalized massage originated in systems of medicine that were inseparable from the religions of Africa and Asia, it was initially part of holistic healing systems that incorporated it as part of a complete body-mind-spirit treatment protocol. An excellent example lies within the massage techniques used in the oldest continuous medical system on our globe: ayurveda. No matter what ailment a patient presents to an ayurvedic doctor, the patient will almost always receive dietary advice, herbal medicines, and meditation suggestions, with a reminder to practice the basics of ayurvedic daily health care. One of the most important of these guidelines is a head-to-toe self-massage using an oil combination specific for one's constitutional type. Another health tonic is to receive regular invigorating and soothing ayurvedic massages from a professional. However, these massages are not merely to assist with aches, pains, and inflammation. They are also to appropriately balance a patient's elemental (earth, water, fire, air, ether) composition in an invisible, energetic, vitalistic way, so that the result is an elemental composition closer to the patient's constitution at birth. If performed

> **MASSAGE THERAPY is probably the oldest, simplest, most pleasurable medical modality in the world. It is even prehuman—one of our closest ancestor primates, bonobos, regularly massage each other for pleasure and reconciliation.**

in a soothing enough way by self or professional, massages can also alter aspects of a patient even more spiritual than the invisible five elements.

These malleable aspects are the gunas: the sattvic (spiritual); rajasic (activating); and tamasic (inhibiting) forces in every person and every atom that far precede the elements within the creation story of Yogic cosmology. If a patient can alter his or her gunas successfully, first toward both the sattvic and rajasic directions and then toward the sattvic alone, then all illnesses can potentially be cured and prevented by treating them at this root-cause guna level. Ayurveda is geared toward healthfully altering the balance of the elements and gunas so that all-around spirit-mind-body health is manifested. This includes the effect of ayurvedic massage. Massage is thus inherently a spiritually evolving modality when viewed within our civilizations' earliest medical systems such as ayurveda and Chinese medicine. Only when the Age of Mysticism had long since given way to the Age of Reason in the West did massage become utterly separated from the comprehensive, holistic medical systems of our archaic past. Countries such as India still retain some of the psychospiritual overtones of massage, since they continue to use ayurveda, or their own ancient medicine, to at least some extent. Other countries began to unravel their medical systems and political systems from the spiritual world a thousand or more years ago. And while this was helpful for ridding especially Western social systems from dogma and superstition, the baby thrown out with the bathwater was deep human connectivity to united body-mind-spirit well-being, which is still greatly lacking in our high-tech world. Reductionism began to overthrow primeval holism, and this splintering continues to resonate in massage therapy offices today.

As the centuries progressed, practitioners continued to use more and more subtle variations within their physical massage arts. Doctors such as Ambroise Pare, a sixteenth-century physician to the French court, touted massage as a treatment for a wide variety of measurable ailments of body and mind—each viewed as quite separate from the other. The Victorian Age added a dose of shame and ignorance regarding the importance of the body and its functions, yet in the midst of it all came an unlikely pairing to reproclaim the importance of conscious touch.

Modern Western massage came to fruition in the nineteenth century via a traveling Swedish theologian who learned some hands-on techniques from a Chinese martial arts and "tuina" massage expert named "Ming." These compiled techniques later became known as "Swedish massage," and the theologian who organized them was Per Henrik Ling. Ling and Ming became fencing and exercise partners in Copenhagen, and Ling apprenticed with Ming in order to make use of techniques for healing his frequent athletic injuries. Back in Sweden, Ling began teaching massage and fencing at Lund University and became determined to place Ming's teachings into a system that could benefit the masses. He went to medical school and learned Western anatomy, physiology, and human pathology. He then elaborated a system of gymnastics, exercises, and massage maneuvers, which he divided into four branches: 1) pedagogical, 2) medical, 3) military, and 4) aesthetic.

This Swedish Movement System carried out his hypotheses borrowed from China, India, Egypt, Greece, and Rome, and demonstrated the necessary Western scientific rigor required to be integrated or approved by established medical practitioners. Ling finally obtained the cooperation of the Swedish government in 1813. The Royal Gymnastic Central Institute, created for the training of gymnastic instructors, was opened in Stockholm with Ling as principal. Despite the claims of Dr. Pare two centuries earlier, orthodox medical practitioners were usually opposed to the broader claims made by Ling and his pupils regarding the system's panacea-like action upon a variety of diseases. However, doctors could not ignore the clear benefits it had upon patients' musculoskeletal ailments, moods, and more. The fact that in 1831 Ling was elected a member of the Swedish General Medical Association shows that in his own country his methods were ultimately regarded as medically adequate.

The field of modern Western physical therapy, originating in 1894, is also said by some to have been based on Ling's Swedish Movement System as well. But other physiotherapy sources don't mention his influence at all, and still others claim that Ling had little to do with Swedish massage either! The most common tale, however, is that a Dutch physician, Georg Mezger, MD, coined the term "Swedish massage" in 1839 when he reduced the number of Ling's excessive variety of maneuvers and placed French names upon them as well. To this day, four of the five strokes that comprise Swedish massage have retained these French names in America: effleurage, petrissage, tapotement, and frictions. "Vibration" was added later. Few articles ever mention that all of these massage techniques had been present in ancient Asian massage systems long before Ming or Ling were born, and currently the "Swedish" massage label goes officially unchallenged.

The alternate story regarding the origin of Swedish massage says that, despite Mezger's work, at some point in the late nineteenth century Ling's Swedish Movement System was transposed into the Swedish Massage System via a simple semantic, clerical error. Also, when the first books were written about Ling's original Swedish Movement System, the writers included the French terms used by Mezger and may have confused future writers into thinking that Ling had devised the truncated version developed by Mezger. Either way, Asian massage, as understood by a Swede and as revised by a Dutchman, forms the true core of "Swedish massage."

From the nineteenth century onward, massage continued to be used in both mainstream and CAM medical practices. As the allopaths began using the new pharmaceuticals of the twentieth century, however, massage started to be phased out and by the end of the 1950s remained a mostly alternative modality. Even CAM practitioners adopted the new technologies of the modern age, replacing much of their hands-on contact with electrical stimulation machines and mechanized massage tools. The 1960s counterculture movements affected almost every dimension of human life in the West, however, including medical practices. One overarching theme of the 1960s was tolerance, acceptance, and respect for other cultures' practices as being at least equal to our own. Ethnocentrism was widely villainized by a large cross section of America for the first time, and cross-cultural medicine began to seem commonplace in American urban environments. The general wave of interest in natural healing, brought forth in hippie philosophy and similar in outlook to the paradigms of ayurveda, Chinese medicine, and other similar global CAM systems, also re-energized the realm of hands-on massage. Since that time, massage has gradually reappeared as a popular form of regular preventive stress-reducing medicine as well as a direct curative modality. Massage therapy is now the most common CAM modality in use, helping Americans to control at least a fraction of the increased stress they are feeling from the ever-increasing speed and complexity of life.

By 1997, Americans were spending between $4 billion and $6 billion on massage therapy, according to the American Massage Therapy Association. This claim borders on the unbelievable; however, clearly it's a big number. Massage therapy makes up 30 percent of the total amount of money spent on CAM treatments in the United States. Because insurance companies often do not cover all massage appointments for their clients, Americans have gotten used to paying out of pocket for massage therapy. This runs counter to the direction of out-of-pocket medical expenses in general, as most Americans spend less than ever on medical treatments not covered by insurance. Insurance premiums and deductibles are high enough now that Americans often feel they shouldn't have to spend yet more money on receiving medical treatment. This has made it difficult for CAM practitioners who can't or aren't covered by insurance. But massage therapists have bucked this trend, perhaps because of the immediate pleasure felt by recipients of massage versus the delayed response and less noticeable enjoyment received from appointments with chiropractors, acupuncturists, naturopaths, and most other CAM providers.

The 1960s was the crucible that spawned many other branches of massage therapy that may interest readers with a more psychospiritual bent. Although the fusion of massage and psychospiritual well-being began at least as far back as the origins of Egyptian and ayurvedic medicine, the Western world retained little of the holistic perspective of the East. Holistic nursing, which debuted in the West with Florence Nightingale's service during the Crimean War of the mid-1850s, did acknowledge the importance of treating body, mind, and spirit, but promoted compassionate touching of patients more than massage therapy per se. Physiotherapy, perhaps originally based on Ling's system, was established with the foundation in 1894 of the European Society of

Trained Masseurs. During World War I, patients suffering from nerve injury or shell shock were treated with massage. St. Thomas's Hospital, London, had a department of massage until 1934. However, later breakthroughs in medical technology and pharmacology eclipsed massage as physiotherapists began to increasingly favor electrical instruments over manual methods for tissue healing.

Even Wilhelm Reich, MD, who in the 1930s introduced the concept of combining bodywork and psychotherapy via his groundbreaking method of orgonomy, left out the "spirit" aspect of holistic medicine. Viewing the Nazi uprising as an occult-fueled outburst of sociopathy, Reich mistrusted spirituality and religion until his passing. When the counterculture challenges of the 1960s occurred on both sides of the Atlantic, however, Reich's methods re-emerged and found a ready audience who quickly spiritualized his work to suit themselves. Although Reich had never made any such claims, his version of the life force, termed "orgone," was now equated to ayurveda's "prana" and Taoism's "chi," as well as other similar concepts from distinctly vitalistic traditions. Reich's overtly mechanistic, though body-centered, approach to psychotherapy was not enough for the more ethereal aspirations of the Age of Aquaruis portion of the '60s. Soon holistic offshoots appeared directly from Reich's students, including Alexander Lowen's and John Pierrakos's bio-energetics; Pierrokas's core energetics; and Charles Kelley's radix work. Once patients left the bodywork table as practitioners added movement to Reich's original protocol, and once spirituality overtly entered and balanced the work, any resemblance of neo-Reichian bodywork to massage therapy quickly diminished.

Reich's second wife was a student of Elsa Gindler, who many historians feel is the true founder of Western body-mind therapy. This can be collectively termed, "somatic psychology," and Gindler's vision preceded Reich's and probably greatly influenced him. A gymnast rather than an MD, Gindler and her work did not share Reich's focus on sexual expression that so impressed the free love counterculture. She never earned much status in America, but Gindler's approach to continuous mindfulness of breath and movement for healing psychosomatic ailments and maximizing human experience inspired the founders

of therapies still popular today: Feldenkrais, Gestalt therapy, and Esalen massage. Gindler's direct link to the U.S. was via her student, Charlotte Selver. Selver renamed Gindler's system "sensory awareness" and taught thousands of Americans at the famous Esalen Institute in coastal California starting in 1963. By way of her work at Esalen, Selver strongly inspired the "human potential movement" and the related humanistic psychologies that peaked in influence during the 1970s. Aspects of her work, especially the conscious sensing of the body and the following of physical sensations that she'd learned from Gindler, flowed into many of the methods of physical therapy and psychotherapy that exist today. In the 1930s, Marion Rosen studied with Lucy Heyer, who had been trained by Elsa Gindler. Licensed in physical therapy at the Mayo Clinic, Rosen developed her Rosen Method over the course of many years in private practice as a physical therapist. Her movement training and bodywork style is now more commonly known than sensory awareness, as the popular representatives of somatic psychology change from decade to decade.

Rolfing, Hellerwork, somatic emotional therapy, and somatic experiencing are yet four more psychosomatic bodywork styles that have arisen since the 1960s and are either beholden to Gindler, Reich, or both. Each contain fascinating "twists" that differentiate it from the next, similar style, in a manner alike to the different sects of one overarching religion. In fact, many of these therapies have become cult-like at one time or another, especially when the founders were embodied and teaching their students directly. Therapeutic touch, a mostly noncontact form of "energetic" massage devised by mystic Dora Kunz and Dolores Krieger, an RN, was introduced in the 1970s and returned a strong sense of sacred purpose to bodywork, as did the introduction to the West of Japanese reiki, nearly identical to the chi kung of Chinese medicine.

Yet both left behind the benefits of hands-on touch, so yearned for by traumatized humans acting much like laboratory Rhesus monkey infants left without their affectionate mothers. Somatic experiencing was conceived of by zoologist Peter Levine in the 1980s after observing how animals healthfully process psychosomatic trauma. Yet he began teaching his system in the CAM stronghold of Berkeley, California, and was surely aware of Reich's intent to return his patients back to their free-flowing mammalian motions alike to wild animals and healthy infant humans.

Because the CAM massage so popular today with mainstream Americans is usually either spiritually diluted Asian massage or inherently secular Swedish, sports, or deep tissue massage, the holistic inroads made during the counterculture are utilized by just a small percentage of Americans today. And while there is absolutely nothing amiss with receiving a massage for pleasure, relaxation, and physical healing, could we increase the benefits for massage recipients if as a field we incorporated nondogmatic psychospiritual aspects into our massage sessions? Are we missing our chance to assist psychologically troubled and spiritually bereft individuals by not making use of the many deep psychosomatic insights of bodywork over the last hundred years and the spirituo-somatic insights of the last millennia? These are answers that future massage therapists will have to answer for themselves and for their field as a whole.

Almost every public health measure is a balance between giving the people what they want and giving the people what will likely keep them alive and well. Since current human instinct doesn't provide infallibility in choosing health options, sometimes it is helpful for others to step in and "enrich" those options chosen by many out of simple desires for short-term pleasure and relaxation. This is, perhaps, one challenge for future massage therapists: to reunite massage with its holistic roots while keeping the psychospiritual additions cutting edge, enjoyable, and effective at producing healthful improvements at all levels of the human organism.

One dictionary's definition and description of massage therapy runs: "Massage therapy is the scientific manipulation of the soft tissues of the body for the purpose of normalizing those tissues and consists of manual techniques that include applying fixed or movable pressure, holding, and/or causing movement of or to the body. Generally, massage is known to affect the circulation of blood and the flow of blood and lymph, reduce muscular tension or flaccidity, affect the nervous system through stimulation or sedation, and enhance tissue healing. Massage therapy

. . . can also reduce . . . anxiety and stress." Given the much greater potential of massage and bodywork regarding psychospiritual healing, the increasing psychospiritual distress partially created by our frenetic Western culture, and the already high usage of massage therapy in the general populace, perhaps the time is ripe for a subtle, graceful, vitalistic revolution within the mostly mechanistic world of mass market massage.

TECHNIQUES

The following techniques have been accorded an unofficial top ten status within the popular culture of twenty-first century America:

Swedish massage: uses soothing, tapping, and kneading strokes to work the entire body, relieving muscle tension and loosening sore joints. Swedish massage therapists use five basic strokes, which anyone can learn for use upon themselves and others. These are: effleurage (stroking); petrissage (muscles are lightly grabbed and lifted); friction (thumbs and fingertips work in deep circles into the thickest part of muscles); tapotement (chopping, beating, and tapping strokes); and vibration (fingers are pressed or flattened firmly on a muscle, then the area is shaken rapidly for a few seconds).

Deep tissue massage: targets chronic tension in muscles that lie far below the surface of your body. You have five layers of muscle in your back, for example, and while Swedish massage may help the first couple of layers, it may not do much to directly impact the muscles underneath. Deep tissue techniques usually involve slow strokes, direct pressure, and friction movements that go across the grain of the muscles. Massage therapists use their fingers, thumbs, and occasionally elbows in order to apply needed pressure.

Sports massage: designed to help exercisers train and recover more optimally, whether they're a world champion or an average Joe. Its techniques are similar to those within Swedish and deep tissue massage, but sports massage versions are adapted to meet every athlete's special needs. Pre-event massage can help invigorate muscles and improve circulation before competition, but it can also energize or relax an athlete and help him to focus on competition. Postevent massage can help to detoxify waste products out of the body and improve muscle recovery time. Massage during exercise or competition may do more practical harm than good, according to some players who agree that their muscles seem to fatigue more quickly than normal following massage treatment during match play.

Neuromuscular massage (or therapy) is a form of deep tissue massage that is applied to individual muscles, one thumb-sized portion at a time. It is used to increase blood flow, reduce pain, and release pressure on nerves caused by injuries to, or tension in, muscles and other soft tissue. Neuromuscular massage helps release trigger points: intense knots of tense, often inflamed muscle that many times also "refer" pain to remote muscles elsewhere on the patient's body. Relieving a tense trigger point in your back, for example, could help ease pain in your shoulder or reduce headaches.

Rolfing (also known as structural reintegration) seeks to reeducate patients' body-minds regarding posture. When posture is poor, it can be reflected in a myriad of health problems, such as backaches, headaches, joint pain, and a long list of psychopathologies. Rolfers seek to realign and straighten patients' bodies by working mainly upon their myofascia, the connective tissue that surrounds all muscles and helps to hold musculoskeletal systems together. The initial, ten-session, head-to-toe rolfing program was rather painful initially, but new versions of rolfing techniques employing a therapist's hands and elbows are quite tolerable and just as effective at improving one's posture. Long-stored emotions are frequently released during rolfing sessions, so choosing a rolfer with psychotherapeutic training as well as a history of being a patient of psychotherapy is likely a helpful choice to make. No one likes spontaneously generated emotions to be negatively reacted upon by a supposedly professional therapist. Remember, rolfers are skilled bodyworkers but not necessarily psychologists—or exorcists.

Hellerwork is an offshoot of rolfing that adds both mental and movement reeducation to the physical work. In a series of eleven sessions, instruction is given on how to change poor posture habits. Patients also receive massages that focus on returning their muscles, and other tissues, to their proper positions. As with many body-centered therapies, results can be dramatically beneficial as expert human hands help to release "nearer to the root cause" areas of long-held psychophysical tension. "Sometimes we can greatly increase the spaces in your joints to the point where you may have grown three-fourths of an inch taller before you're done," one Hellerworker has said. Psychological growth and maturation is also connoted by this form of treatment, and many others on this massage list, probably acknowledged by humankind for as long as we have been able to sense the reduction of body-mind stress in others via the power of our own touch.

Craniosacral therapy focuses on the skull and spinal column. Therapists use very gentle hand pressure, no more than the weight of a nickel, to facilitate optimal cerebrospinal fluid flow. The hypothesis is that specific craniosacral manipulations will reduce overall patient tension and counteract any trauma experienced to their bodies (and minds?) over the years. The meditative ambience during treatment often creates a healing environment beyond the techniques themselves. For a lengthier discussion of craniosacral therapy, and its direct link to osteopathy, see section 2.

Feldenkrais treats every body as an individual work of art, with differing postures and movement patterns. Practitioners seek to teach their clients ideal patterns of movement through slow, gentle, exercise-like sessions. It also includes a gentle massage that is designed to teach patients how to expand their ranges of motion. It's often useful for victims of stroke or accidents, and any who have lost movement capabilities overall.

Tragerwork uses gentle, rocking massage to help release the body's harmful "holding patterns." If you injured your left shoulder as a child, for example, you still may unconsciously carry it lower than your right shoulder, throwing your body-mind off balance and robbing you of energy. Therapists employ very light, gentle shaking techniques that are unlike traditional Swedish-style massage. Tragerwork helps people to be more aware of their bodies, especially the way they move and hold themselves. For several reasons, helping to free people from their chronic physical holding patterns also seems to rid them of emotional stress associated with the prior injury.

Despite the popularity of the above massage approaches in America, several others are worth mentioning out of respect for their respective traditions as well as their influence on nearly all present-day bodywork systems. Although every culture has traditions regarding healing with touch, the following styles from India, China, and Kurdistan will be described in order to offer up a slice of our global massage expertise:

Ayurveda: Although Africa likely produced our original massage techniques, due to the cradle of humanity that rests there, references to authentic African massage techniques are obscure and esoteric. The ancient Indian system of ayurvedic medicine placed great importance on massage for long-term health, and there is a historical record that can be traced. In ayurveda, massage therapy is for everyday usage, something even the most luxury-loving American scarcely considers. Ayurvedic massage can be performed by self or another, but the intent is not so much psychophysiological relaxation but rather keeping in balance the five elements (earth, water, fire, air, ether) that are believed to manifest as the human body. By doing so, the overall health of both the individual and group body-mind can be sustained as part of a medical system that developed in ancient India and still is used to treat billions today. Each person has an ideal combination of oils, such as sesame, sunflower, mustard, and coconut, which will best keep his or her elements in balance if it is applied to the skin each day. As with most Eastern practices, regularity and depth of concentrated practice is more important than time spent any given day in practice. This is also true with ayurvedic massage, so if you are feeling pressed for time, the ideal daily full body oil rubdown can be altered to include just face and/or feet. In general, long, brisk, medium-depth strokes are suggested in ayurveda, especially upon the limbs. If you are fortunate enough to have the time to perform thirty minutes of self-massage or massage receiving once or twice a day, that is ideal. However, one minute of complete full-body massage is said to be an excellent, and mostly forgotten, tonic for prevention of almost all body-mind ills.

In rural areas of India, massage is often still done by family members upon each other. And there still exists in many regions a compulsory and ceremonial premarriage massage for husbands and wives-to-be. Giving and receiving love is believed to be enhanced if one is practiced in giving and receiving loving massage. Babies are thus also massaged regularly, often using a small ball of dough dipped in vegetable oil.

The Yoga- and Hindu-based system of ayurveda is believed to have offered to the world the first system of energy point stimulation for improving health. The "marma" points identified by Yogis are quite similar to the chi points familiar to us from traditional Chinese medicine. Marma massage can be applied one at a time, in a manner alike to acupressure, or via the long massage strokes mentioned previously. Within the multi-step, intensive "panchakarma" rejuvenative treatment in ayurvedic medicine, massage is used upon patients to bring imbalanced elements to certain regions (such as stomach and intestines) for later expulsion. Relaxing massage is also performed via oil poured upon the forehead, showing that massage can be accomplished via tools other than hands. Of course, many massage tools have existed throughout time, with oil pouring being uncommon in the West compared with mechanical "thumpers" or hi-tech electrostimluation. The question remains whether the West will ever make optimal use of the body-mind, health-giving properties of daily, lifelong massage. Any approach we take as a culture toward that goal will likely result in greater distance from whatever negative traits Americans received from our more Puritanical ancestors.

Chinese medicine: In this system, greatly related to ayurveda in its spiritual, vitalistic, and element-focused approach, massage may occur at specific chi points in order to affect the human organ systems at their respective meridians. It may also be applied in a specific manner to balance body-mind yin and yang in a more general way. Still another approach is to apply hands-on chi kung (energy transmission) treatment directly through a patient's skin. The five major massage types within Chinese medicine are:

- *Amno, press and rub:* used for rejuvenation and health maintenance. Commonly performed as self-help home care, in martial arts and general sports therapy, and as an adjunct to chi kung.

- *Tuina, push and grasp:* sophisticated medical massage used to treat injuries, joint and muscle problems, and internal disorders as classified by Chinese medicine.

- *Infant Tuina:* one of the primary ways in which the Chinese medically treat babies and young children. The points and channels used can be quite different to the standards ones used, reflecting the evolution and alteration of chi flow within a growing organism.

- *Dian Xue, point press:* familiar to Americans as acupressure. Uses simple, held pressure techniques, especially upon meridian chi points. It is both a home remedy and a replacement for acupuncture for practitioners who are voluntarily or involuntarily without needles.

- *Wai Qi Liao Fa, curing with external Ch'i:* healing by direct transmission from chi kung practitioners, ideally after years of training and discipline.

Breema (Kurdistani) bodywork: Just as Kurdistan is barely known as a nation without a country that stretches throughout northern Afghanistan, Iraq, and Iran, so is the Breema bodywork that hails from Kurdistan little known in the West. It is mentioned here as a segue between the ancient bodywork systems of Asia and the more choreographed processes of orgonomy and rolfing in the West. Breema is a mesmerizing massage style performed upon fully clothed patients lying upon cushiony oriental rugs. The massage strokes of Breema are more like rhythmic heel-of-the-hand pressings along a recipient's marma/chi point meridians. Breema rhythms are so slow and soothing that a majority of patients fall asleep during sessions. They are also so choreographed that expert practitioners perform a variety of intricately memorized massage "dances" around their supine patients

for hour after hour. And while physical benefits are similar to other forms of massage (decreased pain, increased range of motion, better posture, subjective relaxation), Breema practitioners believe it is also a route to greater psychospiritual evolution. It is also a remarkably earthy style of contact, with practitioners encouraged to always be aware of their own calm breath and the felt sense of their body weight upon the floor. It is believed that if these two acts are practiced well enough, nothing else is needed to produce a successful patient treatment session. Perhaps taking a cue from ancient Muslim Breema practitioners and the crusading Europeans who copied their skills, many choreographed bodywork systems appeared in the West following the groundbreaking work of Elsa Gindler and Wilhelm Reich in the earliest twentieth century.

Despite the clear leap forward that their refined and psychologically transformative systems represented versus the more open-ended, slower-paced earlier hands-on approaches to comprehensive well-being, the massage therapy technique that has ended up being the most popular in America is simply the one for pleasure and relaxation. Is it possible to fuse the best of massage with the best of transformative bodywork to offer Americans what they want but also more of what our increasingly depressed and anxious culture needs? Can an ecumenical spiritual benefit be supplied as well, using techniques from ancient medical systems, such as ayurveda and Chinese medicine, which addresses spiritual, psychological, and physical health with equal vigor? In the meantime, integrative massage, integrative bodywork, integrative medicine, as well as an integrative approach to just about every other solution we seek, is likely to the wisest tack to take. As a prospective student, it is up to you to decide what combination of hands-on healing and effect upon your patients' bodies, minds, and souls you are willing to settle for. While everyone appreciates the short-term relaxation benefits and longer-term musculoskeletal, circulation, and immune system benefits from receiving the common forms of Western massage, the technologies of massage have not kept pace with other technological advances of our time. With the health needs of Americans so great, and with so many Americans receiving massage, it is a shame we are not offering more atomic age improvements on top of those gains that muscle-kneading bonobos have offered to their kin for millions of years. Massage is great; our health needs are greater. How can you help?

WHERE PRACTICED

Massage therapists most often work in the following venues:

Self-employed practitioner: Many massage therapists choose to start their own private practice sometimes taking several years to build a loyal sustaining clientele base. Self-employed practitioners set their own hours and fees but are solely responsible for finding their clients, promoting their practice, and providing their service. Private practitioners tend to rent an office space or room, work out of their home, and/or provide outcall services.

Multidisciplinary clinics: Frequently massage therapists and other holistic healers team up in a full-service clinic. The clinic may be restricted to massage therapy, offering a variety of different modalities.

Spas, salons, and holistic centers: Spas are the single largest growing revenue source for massage therapists in the United States. Massage is the number one requested service at spas. High-end spas offer packages that include massage therapy, and, depending on the spa's popularity and notoriety, there might be a demand for technique specific massage modalities rather than the more popularized Swedish or deep tissue massage.

Doctors' or chiropractors' offices: Massage therapy can be a complement to traditional allopathic medicine, as well as chiropractic medicine.

Rehabilitation centers: Massage therapy is often a useful adjunct to physical and mental healing.

Nursing homes or hospitals: Massage is an increasingly common therapy for the elderly or sick. As the baby boom generation gets older, there is an increasing demand for massage therapists in hospitals and nursing home. The greatest challenge of doing massage in a nursing home is getting past the reticence of people who have never experienced massage therapy before.

Health clubs or fitness facilities: These opportunities vary widely because of the variety of different types of facilities. Becoming associated with a high-end club could be a terrific opportunity, while being associated with a budget facility might be a waste of time. Most therapists found in a health club rent a space from the club but are not employees of the club itself. Though it's unlikely that a massage therapist would be hired by a health club full-time, it may be worthwhile fostering reciprocal relationships with a number of fitness clubs in the therapist's area, as well as for growing a client list for personal practice.

Sports teams or sports medicine clinics: This is probably the most lucrative atmosphere for a massage therapist. Professional teams have large budgets, and a lot of them have a sports massage therapist working for them full time. They can pay top dollar, but they will also expect: the best in terms of practice, professionalism, and that therapists perform nontherapy duties such as lugging equipment when not actively in session. Sports medicine clinics are in much the same league. Most of their services are being retained by professional athletes or amateur athletes with promise and good insurance. Financially, working in a sports medicine clinic can be rewarding; however, massaging athletes can notoriously be a more stressful task, and higher rewards almost always bring higher stakes and expectations.

On-site massage in the workplace: Many therapists in private practice find this to be a good way to subsidize their income. Massage is increasingly being offered as a work perk by employers. Some employers foot the whole bill, while others pay a portion. This method requires strong sales techniques when pitching the benefits of massage to corporations; other essential skills include ability to network as well as building a secure relationship with potential employers.

House calls: Some therapists do this kind of work as their sole practice. It takes a particular kind of personality to be able to travel from location to location, constantly cart equipment in and out of locations, all while being able to project relaxed confidence in a client's home. The upshot, however, is that this can be a low-cost way to start an independent and profitable practice. It provides lots of opportunities to claim deductions related to income taxes.

CERTIFICATION AND CAREER INFORMATION

There is little difference between the nomenclatures of accreditation. It is, however, important to distinguish between national certification and local licensure or certification. National certification occurs when a student graduates from an accredited massage school and passes the comprehensive examination given by the National Certification Board for Therapeutic Massage and Bodywork (NCBTMB). To practice massage therapy in most states, graduates must apply for licensure (sometimes called local certification) through their state's board. Additionally, some states require passing a separate examination, often with a practical component before granting candidates licensure. National certification, according to most practitioners, makes the licensure process easier as the NCBTMB test will prepare candidates for local licensure examinations anywhere. When practitioners become licensed in their state, they essentially progress from an amateur or student to a therapist, earning the legal ability to conduct their own practice.

The NCBTMB has been issuing a nationwide test to nationally certify and standardize massage practices across the United States for the past decade. Though nationally licensed massage therapists must still be certified in each state they choose to practice in, it is highly recommended to pursue national certification as soon as you graduate from massage school. Laurie Azzarella, who is nationally certified in therapeutic massage and bodywork, a seminar director of Earthwalk-USA, as well as a career reflexologist, is a strong advocate for national standardization: "National certification in massage therapy is the highest standard

degree in the practice. It allows for personal mobility and general notoriety. Practitioners will find it much easier to get degrees in different states if they are nationally certified."

According to the NCBTMB, there are two ways to become nationally certified in therapeutic massage and bodywork. Individuals who have graduated with at least 500 hours of formal training at an accredited school of massage are eligible to sit for the national exam before pursuing state licensure. The NCBTMB also recognizes apprenticeships and informal training as a legitimate way to learn massage; however, students wishing to waive the 500 credit-hour requirement must submit a personal portfolio and application in order to be approved to sit for the exam.

School doesn't stop after passing the national certification exam. Most states require postgraduate education to maintain a legal license. Though requirements vary from state to state, most states require massage therapists to participate in at least forty-eight credit hours every four years. This precedent was set by the American Massage Therapy Association and has been embraced by many other accrediting organizations and state institutions. Postgraduate education ensures that practitioners are current and fresh in their training and aware of new methods, practices, and research in the field. Azzarella also supports national postgraduate education requirements: "As a massage therapist, your license is really a license to learn. The knowledge you will acquire is a bag of tools that you will synthesize and integrate into your own private practice; this bag must always be open, welcoming new methods, techniques, and modalities." In this sense, even the most advanced practitioners and instructors are always learning.

Relevant Degrees

Though it appears that there are many different types of licensures and certifications for massage therapists, the various acronyms reflect state-by-state differences. For instance, in Florida, practitioners become certified as CMTs (certified massage therapist) after massage school and LMT (licensed massage therapist) upon completion of licensing exam; in Washington, the same career is certified as LMT (licensed massage therapist), and in California, the same degree is called CLMT (certified licensed massage therapist).

- **LMP:** Licensed Massage Practitioner
- **LMT:** Licensed Massage Therapist
- **RMT:** Registered Massage Therapist
- **MT:** Massage Therapist
- **CLMP:** Certified Licensed Massage Practitioner
- **CLMT:** Certified Licensed Massage Therapist
- **CMP:** Certified Massage Practitioner
- **AMT:** Advanced Massage Therapist *(postgraduate)*
- **AOS:** Associate Degree of Occupational Studies in Massage Therapy *(postgraduate)*
- **NCTMB:** Nationally Certified Therapeutic Massage and Bodywork

TRAINING PROGRAMS

Education and training programs in massage therapy are numerous throughout the United States, and growing every day. With more than 1,500 established massage schools in the United States from which to choose, picking a school can be a daunting and overwhelming process. In this section, you'll find resources to make the search a little easier. Depending on the program and the scope of the curriculum, massage schools typically graduate students in six to eighteen months. Some programs are geared toward intense therapeutic theory and practice, while others consist of late-night classes for people who want a less ambitious part-time career. The Commission on Massage Therapy Accreditation (COMTA) has been formally accrediting massage schools throughout the U.S. since 1984. All accredited schools meet a rigorous standard of study and focus and represent the most elite massage therapy training programs. They typically also tend to be the most expensive. Many community college and trade schools have jumped on the bandwagon, leading to lower standards and poorer training. Tuition for a complete program ranges from $5,000 to $12,000, depending on the length of the program.

Commission on Massage Therapy Accreditation
www.comta.org

The COMTA is a nonprofit independent body, which is responsible for accrediting massage schools in the United States. For a list of formally accredited massage schools in the United States, consult the COMTA Web site. The commission is recognized both by the AMTA and NCBTMB as the only formal accrediting agency for massage schools in the United States.

Massage Therapy Web Central
www.qwl.com/mts.html

MTWC is a private Web site that contains listings of massage schools, associations, journals, and practitioner guides to the Internet. The site, designed and run by massage therapists, is a resource for consumers, corporations, and private practitioners.

Massage Schools Guide
www.massageschoolsguide.com

This group offers an organized directory of massage schools, which are cataloged by location, programs offered, difficulty, and user reviews.

Natural Healers
www.naturalhealers.com

Natural Healers is a leading directory of massage schools in the United States and Canada. Hundreds of accredited massage schools advertise on the Natural Healers site. Users can browse by state, degree, or school name.

Massage Therapy Careers
www.massagetherapycareers.com

Written by massage therapists specifically targeting prospective students of the discipline, this independent resource gives students all the practical information they need to start a professional career in massage therapy.

ORGANIZATIONS

The American Massage Therapy Association
www.amtamassage.org

AMTA is the largest massage-related organization in the United States. Representing more than 58,000 massage therapists, AMTA seeks to establish and facilitate the practice of massage therapy as an alternative method of health care in the United States. It oversees many research projects in the United States and serves as the main advocacy group for massage practice in legal, educational, and public venues. Its Web site contains important information for all types of bodyworkers in the United States.

The American Medical Massage Association
www.americanmedicalmassage.com

AMMA was created to represent the image of medical message therapists. It seeks to promote medical massage through publications and education, and increase awareness within the massage community. AMMA has defined a code of ethics, which best represent the practical expectations of medical massage practitioners.

Associated Bodywork and Massage Professionals
www.abmp.com

ABMP is a professional membership organization, which is open to a diverse array of somatic therapists and skin care professionals. Certified memberships enjoy liability coverage up to $2 million, as well as enhanced listings on massagetherapy.com's online referral service. This professional organization is a great way for practitioners to promote their practice and network with similar professionals.

Bureau of Health Education Schools
www.abhes.org

BHES is the only agency recognized by the U.S. Department of Education as an institutional and specialized accrediting body, which focuses on health care education and training. As a result, BHES is responsible for accrediting all heath-related schools in the United States, insofar that they may receive federal funding from the Department of Education.

Commission on Massage Therapy Accreditation
www.comta.org

COMTA is a nonprofit independent body, which his responsible for accrediting massage schools in the United States. Founded in 1982, COMTA seeks to improve the quality of education for students seeking education in massage by maintaining a strict and rigorous standard of professionalism from educational institutions.

Esalen Institute
www.esalen.org

Esalen is a particular type of massage that focuses on some of the unexplored areas of the human body. The institute, based in California, is dedicated to understanding and exploring a new modality of body-oriented therapy. It offers classes, workshops, annual massage events, and conferences, as well as publishes a catalog with interesting information about this new technique.

The International Association of Infant Massage
www.iaim.ws

The IAIM is attempting to bring back the ancient tradition of infant massage. By promoting nurturing therapeutic touch and spreading information about the importance and benefits of infant massage, the IAIM hopes to spread the method of infant massage throughout the global massage community.

International Massage Association
www.imagroup.com

IMA supports massage practitioners globally through advocacy, networking, and general public outreach. It publishes a newsletter and offers many practice-related benefits to its members. IMA appeals to practitioners of more than 150 different massage techniques.

Massage Therapy Foundation
www.massagetherapyfoundation.org

MTF advances the practice and knowledge of massage therapy by supporting evidence-based scientific research. By raising the standard of education and scientific inquiry in massage therapy, MTF hopes to prove the scientific efficacy of massage treatment. It publishes several electronic journals, which document the foundation's research projects, and also hosts educational outreach programs and workshops.

Massage Therapy Research Consortium
www.massagetherapyresearchconsortium.com

MTRC advances massage therapy education and practice through a network of participating schools, practitioners, and organizations. By collaboratively building research capacity in massage institutions, and by fostering partnerships with research scientists in our communities, MTRC seeks to enhance public health, as well as the overall standards in the massage community.

National Certification Board for Therapeutic Massage and Bodywork
www.ncbtmb.com

Established in 1992, NCBTMB currently runs the certification process for all licensed and registered massage practitioners in the United States. This independent, nonprofit organization has certified more than 90,000 therapists since its inception. It defines the standard of education for prospective students of massage therapy. Currently, to become nationally certified by NCBTMB, one must complete a minimum of 500 instruction hours, demonstrate core skills, and pass NCBTMB's comprehensive examination.

United States Association for Body Psychotherapy

www.usabp.org

The USABP is a national professional organization focusing on body-mind practitioners. It is committed to organizing, representing, and shaping the emerging professions related to body psychotherapies. Founded in 1996 and achieving nonprofit status in 1997, the USABP is a resource for information on the expanding and relatively enigmatic field of body psychotherapy. It publishes a journal, hosts conferences, and has a membership network.

The United States Medical Massage Association

www.usmedicalmassage.org

The USMMA's mission is to represent medical massage therapists nationwide by educating massage practitioners in the ethical practice of medical massage. USMMA promotes the standardization and national certification of medical massage, while defending the rights of medical massage therapists as members of the holistic somatic community. In addition, USMMA will endorse, recognize, or accept professional medical massage organizations that abide by the ethics and medical standards and practices recognized by medical authorities.

PERIODICALS

Massage Magazine

www.massagemag.com

Massage Today

www.massagetoday.com

Massage & Bodywork

www.massageandbodywork.com

Massage Therapy Magazine

www.massagetherapypractice.com

JOURNALS

Massage Therapy Journal

www.amtamassage.org/journal/home.html

The official publication of the American Massage Therapy Association

The International Journal of Therapeutic Message and Bodywork

http://journals.sfu.ca/ijtmb/index.php/ijtmb

A peer-reviewed publication concerned with the expanding network of massage therapy and bodywork. The journal addresses research, education, and practice methodology in current paradigms of bodywork.

Journal of Bodywork and Movement Therapies

www.elsevier.com/wps/find/journaldescription. cws_home/623047/description#description

The official journal of the National Association of Myofascial Trigger Point Therapists, the JBMT covers the latest therapeutic techniques and professional debates on topics such as physical therapy, osteopathy, chiropractic, massage therapy, Pilates, and Yoga.

ONLINE RESOURCES

Know Your Source

www.knowyoursource.com

In addition to transparent sourcing of practitioner supplies to integrative health care providers, KYS offers a hip social network at knowyoursource.com and a corresponding progressive consumer directory at knowyourhealer.net.

Massage Therapy Web Central

www.qwl.com/mts.html

Massage Register State Requirements

www.massageregister.com/StateRequirements.asp

This easy-to-use Web site details the different state requirements for massage and bodywork licensure.

Natural Healers

www.naturalhealers.com

Lippincott Williams & Wilkins

www.lww.com/massage

LWW publishes and reviews books, journals, magazines, and articles relevant to massage and holistic psychotherapy. Its archives are a great resources for massage students and teachers. It also has links for upcoming events, conferences, and training in massage therapy.

BOOKS

Massage: A Career at Your Fingertips by Martin Ashley

Business Mastery: 4th Edition by Cherie Sohnen-Moe

Tappan's Handbook of Healing Massage Techniques by Francis M. Tappan

Massage Therapy Career Guide for Hands-On Success by Steve Capellini

The Complete Book of Massage by Clare Maxwell-Hudson

CHAPTER 8

NATUROPATHIC MEDICINE (ND)

Naturopathic medicine is as old as medicine itself. The medicinal use of herbs dates as far back as 13,000 years ago, as depicted by the cave paintings of Lascaux, France. The earliest known civilizations of India and Pakistan utilized the holistic ayurveda system of health care. Ancient Shamanic, Egyptian, Chinese, Babylonian, Persian, Hebrew, Greco-Roman, and all global medicinal systems before the European Renaissance would also have been considered naturopathic medicine by today's standards. This is because naturopathic medicine is defined as much by its holistic principles as by its techniques.

There are Seven Principles of modern naturopathy:

1. **Do no harm** (*Primum non nocere*). Don't make the treatment worse than the disease. Use the gentlest, least invasive therapies first. Move on to more potent, more side-effect ridden therapeutics only if necessary. Let nature take its healing course, avoid symptom suppression and assist it with minimal force.

2. **Respect the healing power of nature** (*Vis medicatrix naturae*). There is an innate healing force within all life that is always attempting to prevent and/or heal every possible illness. Skin abrasions heal, broken bones reconnect, grief fades, so long as this "life force" flows in a balanced, unimpeded way. Naturopaths help their patients to optimize this innate force via positive lifestyle changes and nontoxic therapies.

3. **Treat the cause** (*Tolle causum*). Seek to find and heal the deepest source of any ailment. Don't be satisfied with merely alleviating patient symptoms, which are often only the superficial manifestations of deeper disease patterns.

4. **Doctor as teacher** (*Docere*). Educate patients so that they become their own doctors for most of their illnesses. Empower patients to prevent and treat their own patterns of ill health via ever-increasing self-awareness and self-control. Remove any barriers of

NATUROPATHIC MEDICINE is an integrative and vitalistic medical system that always tends toward the most natural and preventive, least harsh, and most lifestyle altering treatment protocols for the purpose of getting to the root cause of illness. It helps patients manifest not just passive recovery, but optimal health.

inequality between doctor and patient so that ideal communication can occur. Last but not least, "walk your talk" and be a living example of balanced health.

5. **Prevention**. Far better than treating ailments is to prevent them before they arise. Encourage patients to consider their thoughts, words, and deeds as actions that prevent either ill health or well-being. Even when patients are feeling well, annual visits to a doctor are recommended in order to detect subtle changes in direction toward health or illness.

6. **Treat the whole person**. Each human consists of a body-mind-spirit complex within many layers of socialization. Every aspect of a patient's life manifests wellness or disease somewhere along the spectrum of health. A naturopath is aware of the different layers of patient complexity and treats all layers equally.

7. **Wellness**. Health is the radiant, vibrant expression of well-being rather than merely the absence of disease signs and symptoms within any given patient. Physical vitality, psychological peace, spiritual depth, social grace, and compassionate global outreach are all examples of wellness attributes. Actively cultivating these attributes is the responsibility of each individual, for his or her own sake and for the sake of the society in which he or she lives.

Most medical systems in place before the rise of modern Western medicine in Renaissance Europe followed the basic principles above. They were "vitalistic" in nature, meaning that a spiritual "vital force" or "life force" was believed to be both the source of existence and the essential healing force for every person. Ayurveda's "prana," Chinese medicine's "chi," and Hippocrates' "humours" are all versions of the vital force within early naturopathic systems. These systems also focused on treating the causes of disease by treating the whole person—spirit, mind, and body. They all promoted wellness-oriented, preventive medicine as primary in importance. Healing via the least invasive method possible was secondary, as summed up in American colonial times: "An ounce of prevention is worth a pound of cure." *Docere*, or

doctor as teacher, was the most ignored naturopathic principle in earlier times, since many practitioners of yore preferred to retain their elevated status by keeping their knowledge secret.

Experimental, scientific, chemically oriented medicine appeared around 1400 A.C.E. and began to flourish by the 1700s. This was a new medical system to challenge the vitalistic medical practices being used around the globe. Traditional practitioners argued that allopaths (coined as a derogatory term in the 1800s by the first homeopath) were using toxic substances as medicines and ignoring the most important parts of patients' lives when attempting a cure. Allopaths argued that traditionalists were living in a mythical past of unproven and obsolete philosophies and techniques. The battle for medical supremacy was on and is still being fought to this day.

In the midst of this arena came a nineteenth century German monk, Father Sebastian Kneipp. Kneipp spent most of his days and nights treating a steady stream of hundreds of patients with a hydrotherapy "water cure" he had learned in order to treat his own tuberculosis. Benedict Lust (pronounced Loost) was successfully treated by Kneipp in 1896 and was encouraged to promote in the Unites States the nature-based medicine from which he had benefited. This included not only hydrotherapy, but also herbalism, exercise, optimal nutrition, spirituality, a balanced life of work and recreation amidst fresh air, sunshine, and even walking daily with bare feet on the grass. The United States already had a Native American/colonial system of natural medicine; Lust's primary introduction was the European version of natural medicine centered on hydrotherapy.

Lust established the Kneipp Water-Cure Institute, one of the earliest health food stores, and several English and German language periodicals advocating Kneipp's "nature cure." He also graduated from the New York Homeopathic Medical College in 1901 and the Universal College of Osteopathy in 1902. Lust then purchased the term "naturopathy" from John Scheel, a holistic medical doctor. Scheel coined the term in 1895 after being impressed by Kneipp's methods. Lust founded the American Institute of Naturopathy in New York City, the nation's first naturopathic college. He also began calling himself a naturopath when the school received its charter in

1905. The Kneipp Societies were replaced with the Naturopathic Society of America, which later became the American Naturopathic Association. Henry Lindlahr, MD, further systematized naturopathy in America after he visited Kneipp for help in curing his own diabetes. He also opened a health sanitarium and school in Chicago devoted to naturopathic principles.

At the turn of the century, the competition for U.S. medical superiority had reached its zenith, with naturopaths, allopaths, chiropractors, osteopaths, eclectics, and homeopaths all running neck and neck. At the profession's peak, it is estimated that there were more than 10,000 NDs in the United States. However, some naturopathic colleges were seen as little more than diploma mills requiring little coursework and even less patient contact. The Flexner Report of 1910 turned the tide in favor of the allopaths, resulting in the closure of most U.S. medical schools that did not teach an allopathic curriculum. An American Medical Association (AMA) study in 1927 alleged that there were twelve naturopathy schools training fewer than 200 students. These numbers would continue to decline until the 1970s. Yet Lust and other advocates continued to work diligently for state licensure of naturopaths, and, by 1935, approximately half of all states offered legal support for NDs. The 1920s and 1930s are considered the peak years for naturopathy, complete with nationwide conventions, popular journals, and high public awareness.

Soon scientific advances, such as effective antibiotics, corticosteroids, and improved surgical techniques, were impressing upon the public consciousness. The political influence of the AMA continued to grow, as did the power of pharmaceutical and insurance companies. Meanwhile, the death of Lust in 1945 and consistent infighting between schools of natural therapeutics steadily drained interest from the realm of naturopathy. By the 1950s, few naturopaths or ND schools existed, and those that did existed on the medical fringe. In 1956, the National College of Naturopathic Medicine opened in Portland, Oregon. For the first time, scientific philosophy and procedures were used to support traditional naturopathic training based on traditional folklore. Modern naturopathic medicine had arrived to little notice. For more than twenty years, the National

College remained the only training site recognized by the states licensing naturopathic doctors, frequently schooling fewer than ten students per year. Finally, in 1978, John Bastyr College of Naturopathic Medicine opened its doors in Seattle, Washington. The college was named after a naturopath-chiropractor-midwife who was instrumental in keeping interest in licensed naturopathy alive throughout the dormant 1950s and 1960s. John Bastyr College is now known as Bastyr University. The next ten years brought increasing public recognition to naturopathic medicine. Two more colleges of naturopathic medicine were founded: one in Tempe, Arizona, and one in Bridgeport, Connecticut.

The Clinton administration ushered in a new era for NDs. In 1992, the Office of Alternative Medicine of the National Institute of Health (NIH), created by an act of Congress, invited several NDs to serve on federal advisory panels. They helped to define priorities and design protocols for state-of-the-art alternative medical research. In 1994, the NIH selected Bastyr University as the national center for research on alternative treatments for HIV/AIDS. At a $1 million level of funding, this action represented the first formal recognition by the federal government of the legitimacy and significance of naturopathic medicine. In October 1996, the Natural Medicine Clinic opened in Kent, Washington. This was a major development for both public health and integrative medicine, as for the first time both naturopaths and allopaths officially worked together as equal practitioners under the same roof. Funded by the King County Seattle Department of Public Health, the Natural Medicine Clinic was the first medical facility in the nation to offer naturopathic medical treatments paid for by U.S. tax dollars. Bastyr University was selected, over several leading Seattle-area hospitals, to operate this groundbreaking clinic.

Bastyr University was founded with the intent that science would be a cornerstone of naturopathy, not merely a supporting figure. At the current time, six programs/institutions that train naturopathic physicians are recognized in the U.S. The Council on Naturopathic Medical Education is the U.S. Department of Education accrediting body that monitors and maintains the recognized standards to train licensable naturopathic physicians.

Modern naturopathic doctors now often prefer to defend their treatments of choice by pointing to supportive research. It is no longer enough to say that since a natural remedy has been used in the past there is no need for further evidence of its effectiveness. Though vitalistic thinking is still common, NDs appreciate that science can both bolster their validity and eliminate ineffective folk remedies of the past. Modern NDs perform the same medical exams, order the same lab tests and diagnostic imaging, and speak the same biomedical language as MDs. The combination of treating the whole person, supporting the body's healing processes with nature's medicines, and using scientific diagnostics make the modern naturopathic doctor unique.

Today's naturopathic medicine is a modern twist on ancient healing practices. It includes more than it excludes, making it difficult to pinpoint an exact definition. Naturopathic medicine is an integrative and vitalistic medical system that always tends toward the most natural and preventive, least harsh, and most lifestyle altering treatment protocols for the purpose of getting to the root cause of illness. It helps patients manifest not just passive recovery, but optimal health. This is the opposite of allopathy's focus on the symptom-relieving, potent-pill quick fix. Naturopathy includes a broad array of modalities, including nutritional, exercise, stress reduction, and lifestyle counseling; botanical medicine; nutraceuticals (all of the vitamins, minerals, and other food supplements seen on the shelves of health food stores); homeopathy; physical medicine (which includes joint adjustments, hydrotherapy, and massage); preventive medicine; environmental medicine; and drug-minimizing baby delivery or midwifery. Naturopaths' training includes minor office surgical procedures, such as removal of skin lesions and pharmacology, or prescription drug use. Some naturopathic doctors also pursue extra training in ayurvedic medicine or in acupuncture and Oriental medicine which gives them an expanded scope of practice.

So what makes a naturopath a naturopath? It is the principles of their practice and breadth of their training more than anything else. No other practitioner is exposed to learning so many different "alternative" medical modalities within such a concentrated period of time. Yet they also receive comparable training as allopaths in anatomy, physiology, biochemistry, endocrinology, and all of the other -ologies of standard Western medical studies. During their four to six years of medical school, ND students are trained as general practitioners. Specializing in one modality is not encouraged. After graduation, some naturopathic doctors focus on one modality or approach to treatment while others practice a more generalized medicine. Keep in mind that if you stay general you will likely have a hard time differentiating yourself.

NATUROPATHIC DIAGNOSTIC AND TREATMENT MODALITIES

There are a large number of medical systems and treatment modalities that are considered naturopathic. Many of these, such as ayurvedic medicine, homeopathy and acupuncture, are also their own disciplines. The prospective student should be aware that any medical practice that follows the Seven Principles of Naturopathy can be considered naturopathic. This is both its boon and its bane, as unproven methodologies are occasionally placed on equal footing with those proven through the scientific method. Here we focus on those practices taught at naturopathic universities for the specific purpose of acquiring an ND degree.

Preventive medicine: One of the Seven Principles of Naturopathy, it is also an overarching naturopathic modality, since NDs always have in the back of their minds how to help patients prevent future health woes by analyzing current patient lifestyle habits. Specific areas analyzed are diet, exercise, stress reduction, creativity, connection to nature, spirituality and community, work satisfaction, interpersonal relationships, and environmental toxins.

Nutritional medicine: To a great extent, the health of our body and minds are determined by the foods we eat. Every individual requires a certain amount of water, micronutrients (vitamins, minerals, coenzymes), macronutrients (proteins, fats, carbohydrates), fiber, "energetics," and more in order to function at an optimal level. Yet no two people are identical. Every person manifests "biochemical individuality" when it comes to those nutrient sources which are best for them. Although all NDs recommend a whole foods diet, some also use many different nutritional systems (ayurveda, systemized diets, orthomolecular) to assist their patients in preventing and treating every possible ailment as well as to encourage active well-being. Typical of naturopathy is that it is not so important which nutritional system is used. What is important is that patients understand that improving one's diet leads to improved well-being. Specific ailments are also prevented and treated by the use of specific foods and food supplements. These are termed by some "nutraceuticals."

Botanical medicine: Plant medicine has been used by humans for more than 10,000 years. Most of our Western medicines were plant based until the last half century of synthetic pharmaceutical inventions. The majority of the world's population continues to use herbal medicine as their main medical modality. Scientific research has validated some herbal medicines and debunked others. Herbal medicines can be considered concentrated food sources of biochemicals. They can be taken preventively or curatively on a daily or as-needed basis for the treatment of every illness. They can also be considered agents that alter the human vital force in specific energetic ways deduced by practitioners within pre-allopathic systems of traditional medicine. These energetic effects are difficult to study scientifically. Plant preparations may be applied externally, inhaled, ingested, or introduced into the body via any orifice. Modern NDs tend to use processed herbs that have been "standardized" to a known content of one assumed active ingredient.

Homeopathy: This is one of the most controversial systems in all of medicine. The main reason for this is that the most potent remedies in homeopathy are so dilute that nothing can be physically measured other than the sugar pill or water that holds the remedy. Healing effects are presumed to be due to either energetics, placebo, or both. Samuel Hahnemann, MD, was a nineteenth century prodigy who taught as a medical school professor as a teenager. He became disenchanted with allopathy (a derogatory term he coined) and searched for his own panacea. Hahnemann discovered that an extremely small dose of a substance, which in large amounts would cause certain symptoms in a healthy person, would alleviate these same symptoms in a suffering patient. The smaller the prescribed dose, the more potent was the symptom relief. This method was found to be especially effective if the dose was diluted in water and shaken repeatedly. NDs who use homeopathy either perform a lengthy oral interview with a patient to determine that patient's overall constitutional type, or they focus their intake on the patient's current chronic and acute symptoms. They then determine the exact remedy that matches the patient's constitutional type or symptom profile. Generic homeopathic formulas are also available for NDs less familiar with homeopathic interviewing. Homeopathic remedies are extremely safe and nontoxic.

Physical medicine. This is a large treatment area that includes massage, naturopathic manipulation (naturopathy's name for therapeutic joint adjustment similar to chiropractic); hydrotherapy; colonic irrigation; and ultrasound treatment (not lab diagnosis), diathermy, interferential, and other similar machines used to introduce therapeutic heat and/or electricity into a patient's tissues. Normally an ND specializes in physical medicine after graduation in order to focus upon this broad spectrum of physical medicine treatments. NDs must remain well disciplined and not dilute their efforts by trying to master too many specialties simultaneously.

Brief descriptions follow for the physical medicine modalities mentioned above.

- **Massage:** All naturopaths learn basic massage techniques, including Swedish-style and deep tissue work. These are excellent to use for reducing patient stress, forging a stronger doctor-patient bond, helping to heal musculoskeletal injuries, and strengthening the lymphatic portion of the immune system. However, most NDs avoid massage work in their practice other than as preparatory work for joint adjustment. Instead, they refer general massage work on to a licensed massage therapist.

- **Naturopathic manipulation:** By law, the ND profession is not allowed to call their work either chiropractic or osteopathy, even though the techniques used are similar. NDs are usually vitalists, though unlike traditional osteopaths and chiropractors they do not believe that a well-aligned joint structure in a patient by itself equals optimal life force flow and well-being. Naturopathic manipulation is simply one technique used among many and is no more important than any other.

- **Hydrotherapy:** This is the ancient modality used by Father Kneipp to help cure himself and Benedict Lust of their tuberculoses. It can be considered the reason that naturopathy, as we know it, exists in the U.S. today. Hydrotherapy, or water therapy, is the application of water to initiate cure. Because the water is usually very hot or very cold, some have reasoned that it is the temperature and not the water that is initiating the healing process. It is a safe and painless therapy that can be done anywhere for all types of injuries and illness. Some common hydrotherapy treatments are hot foot baths, constitutional hydrotherapy, immersion bath, Russian sauna, warming socks, and the well-known ice pack.

- **Colonic irrigation:** This uncommon treatment is used if a patient is experiencing incomplete bowel evacuation, parasites, hemorrhoids, or is manifesting other intestinal challenges. A flexible plastic tube is inserted into the patient's rectum and low-pressure, body-temperature water is gradually introduced into the colon. When the patient signals the need to evacuate, the practitioner redirects the pressure and the introduced water is flushed out. A viewing area is present so that excreted fecal matter can be assessed for relative healthfulness. Often the ND massages the patient's abdominal area for ease of evacuation. Usually more than one "colonic" is required to restore proper bowel function. Coffee or other herbs can be added to the water solution to maximize colonic effect.

- **Ultrasound/diathermy/interferential:** Electromagnetic waves that penetrate the human skin are known to have therapeutic benefits for healing types of diseased tissue. Decrease of inflammation, pain, and muscle spasm, as well as increase of muscle strength and range of motion are common patient results. NDs learn the use of several machines useful for conducting sound, heat, and electricity into the human body. Most NDs leave the use of these machines to chiropractors and osteopaths.

Laboratory diagnosis: NDs are well instructed in understanding which diagnostic lab tests are appropriate to order for any given patient. Once the lab tests arrive, NDs have been trained to analyze them just as a medical doctor does. Examples of labwork that may be requested by an ND include blood testing, urinalysis, ultrasound, x-ray, MRI, biopsy, saliva analysis, and hair analysis.

Minor office procedures: All naturopathic students are trained to perform minor office procedures such as lesion removal and the suturing of wounds. The authority to incorporate these skills into practice depends on the laws of the jurisdiction in which the graduate practices.

Naturopathic obstetrics: Similar to minor surgery, there are a couple of classes on obstetrics (the science and art of assisting the approximately nine-month birthing process) taught at naturopathic universities. Only NDs who continue on toward midwifery certification are legally allowed to be the primary physician present during labor and birth. This certification entails more university coursework and internships with midwives covering many births. All licensed NDs may legally give advice on how to prepare for pregnancy and how to maintain health for the family system during the changes leading up to, and after, birth itself.

Lifestyle counseling: Compared with other doctors, NDs spend a large amount of time assessing and communicating with patients about their lifestyles. This is because for NDs an excellent health predictor is the sum total of a patient's positive lifestyle traits (such as eating whole foods and performing daily exercise) minus their negative lifestyle habits (such as smoking tobacco and working eighty-hour weeks). Following their "doctor as teacher" principle, NDs educate their patients regarding which habits are positive or negative and why. NDs are also trained in basic psychology skills and use these to encourage patients to discuss areas of their life that are troubling them. They also train patients to improve their methods of thinking, feeling, and behaving, so that their psyches are working on their behalf instead of against them. Few patients in America are craving a change in lifestyle. Most would rather take a pill and continue living as they always have. NDs remind patients that to attain optimal health on a daily basis, one's lifestyle must adhere to basic habits that are excellent predictors of well-being.

Pharmacology: NDs are not usually associated with the recommendation of prescription drugs. However, most states allow NDs to prescribe certain antibiotics, topical corticosteroids, and other substances that require little additional training in allopathy in order to keep patients safe from inappropriate use or negative side effects. Some NDs would prefer to have a much larger "legend list" of allowable prescription drugs, so that patients need not go to two different physicians for basic medications. Many other NDs never recommend a prescription drug, believing that they are "the last refuge of the incompetent." Most NDs leave prescription drugs for life-threatening illnesses, if they use them at all.

Acupuncture: It has now been proven via scientific methodology that penetrating the human skin with thin needles at specific points is helpful for the treatment of a variety of ailments. Traditional Chinese medicine posits that all ailments can be improved by this method. NDs must receive extensive training for years beyond their basic curriculum in order to legally practice acupuncture. In fact, they must earn a licensed acupuncture (LAc) degree before, during, or after their ND schooling in order to gain permission from most states to penetrate a patient's skin with acupuncture needles. Few ND students are willing to attend the extra classes required to earn the LAc simultaneously with an ND degree. Working toward one medical degree alone is usually one of the most difficult assignments that a student completes during his or her lifetime. Two degrees earned at once also tends to mean that short shrift is given to fully understanding all coursework due to sheer lack of time. However, once an ND has an LAc degree, his or her income status increases greatly. All potential ND students should give consideration to earning a

legal means to offering acupuncture to patients for this reason alone.

Environmental medicine: There is the inner environment of the body and mind, and the outer environment that surrounds it. No matter how healthy patients are, put them in a toxic enough arena and their health will fail. NDs assess the toxins in a patient's work, home, and recreation sites and determine whether or not they are cause for concern and can then be reduced or eliminated. Some individuals are especially susceptible to environmental toxins, referred to as "chemical sensitivity." Once a patient is diagnosed as such, special guidance is given so that the patient understands what materials to avoid as well as how to alter his or her body-mind so that decreasing chemical sensitivity is experienced. Blood tests and hair analyses can detect toxic chemical levels in a patient's body, and a variety of substances can be prescribed to remove these toxins. Given the increasing toxicity of our planet at the present time, this specialty may increase in importance for the foreseeable future.

CAREER AND TRAINING

Naturopathic doctors are primary care providers who are trained in conventional medical sciences, diagnosis, and treatment but who choose preventive medicine and "natural" therapeutics as their main focus of patient care. Each prospective student must complete standard premedical coursework, including two college semesters (or three quarters) of general chemistry, organic chemistry, physics, and biology. Mathematics and psychology coursework may also be required. MCAT exams are not required.

Each of the six accredited naturopathic universities offers a four- to six-year program toward the naturopathic doctor degree. This time frame can be extended to five years or longer if the student wishes to attend part time. Assuming a four-year track, ND students' first two years cover basic medical sciences mostly via lecture, group study, and book learning. Cadaver dissection is one notable exception. The second two years are clinic focused, where the student actively participates in the treatment of patients while completing the clinical training. Before graduation, each student must see a minimum of patient contacts before graduation. Hands-on coursework, such as massage and naturopathic joint manipulation, is also incorporated at this stage.

Naturopathic medical schools are accredited by an independent agency, the Council on Naturopathic Medical Education (CNME), which is recognized and regulated by the U.S. Department of Education.. In June 2008, the National Advisory Committee on Institutional Quality and Integrity (NACIQI) at a regularly scheduled hearing on the CNME's application to the U.S. Department of Education for re-recognition as an accrediting agency recommended that CNME be granted a five-year re-recognition, which is the maximum length of time.

Upon graduation, students must pass all of the state board naturopathic exams for those licensed states in which they are choosing to practice. These board exams are provided by the North American Board of Naturopathic Examiners (NABNE). Continuing medical education coursework is required for NDs to retain their licensure. Most states do not require a residency for naturopathic doctors to practice. There are residency positions available, but not enough exist for all graduates to obtain one. Unlike internship and residency requirements for DOs and MDs, however, due to philosophical differences, it is difficult for NDs to find a medical institution that will take them on as an intern or resident. It is considered an honor for an ND to be received as a postgraduate in this manner, as there are few spaces for residents at the six naturopathic universities.

Many medical practitioners rightly say that it is during their internships and residencies that they learn the majority of their practical medical knowledge. So NDs are often criticized for stopping their learning process just when it should be taking off. But NDs will have little choice in this regard until American hospitals open their doors to NDs. In the meantime, most graduates start their own private practice or join an integrated practice that might include MDs, acupuncturists, therapists, or other practitioners. A small number of graduates choose to enter the research field and pursue training in public health and join research teams that investigate alternative medicine.

At least fifteen states, plus Washington, DC; the U.S. Virgin Islands; Puerto Rico; and four Canadian provinces, have formal licensing and educational requirements. Two states outlaw the practice of naturopathic medicine, while other states and provinces generally ignore naturopathic medicine and have no laws relating to practice. In unlicensed states and provinces, naturopaths who have learned their trade via apprenticeship or correspondence schools are not differentiated from clinically trained NDs who have studied at accredited universities. This has created angry legal battles between the two sides: NDs versus "un-Ds," as some NDs put it. Some unlicensed naturopaths may have far greater medical skills than their university-trained colleagues. Clearly a legal resolution is needed, as naturopaths without formal, accredited education and clinical training are often aggressive opponents against naturopathy becoming licensed in their own states. Fighting successfully against licensure allows unlicensed naturopaths to continue practicing without persecution in most states, yet keeps modern naturopathic medicine from being exposed to, and embraced by, the country as a whole.

One solution would be to rename the modern ND degree so that it reflects the integration with allopathy begun with the founding of Bastyr University in 1978 and illustrated at the integrative Natural Medicine Clinic. This would also allow traditional doctors of natural medicine within licensed states to continue using the name of naturopath. And this seems only fair, since the medicine of Kneipp and Lust is more accurately expressed by the traditional naturopath and not by the modern licensed ND. Others disagree. Prospective students of natural medicine may someday be choosing from accredited programs offering IMD (integrative medical doctor) or IND (integrative naturopathic doctor) degrees. Students should be aware that the letters ND will be confusing to most laypeople who don't understand the difference between traditional and modern naturopaths.

The abovementioned legal and philosophical battles within their own medical field have hit NDs hard in one major area: the pocketbook. On average, NDs earn less income than similarly trained doctors in North America. The top-tier ND makes an annual income in the range of $70,000 to $100,000; however, while no actual numbers exist, informal surveys for this book indicate that many struggle financially, earn more like $40,000 per year, and believe that the handful of top-tier ND programs have not been truthful about graduate success rates. Information regarding graduate success is expected in most professional fields, such as law, business, and medicine, from universities themselves as well as publications such as *U.S. News and World Report.* The combination of the high opportunity cost—five years, the $80,000+ tuition, the institutional stronghold of allopathy, and the generally low salary (barring the exceptional doctor often good at self-promotion) means that you must be realistic about your ambitions and drive.

As of 2008, unlike an ND, an MD or DO can pay off their student loans with an average entry salary of $100,000 per year. While no hard numbers exist, informal surveys of ND graduates from the major schools indicate that only 45 percent are in practice five years after graduation. If it's not true, ND career student centers should set the record straight. If it is true, ND programs are misinforming students about realistic career expectations.

Unless there is a major change in the public perception of naturopathic medicine, paying for an ND degree may be one of the poorest returns on investment of any degree undertaken in America. Carefully consider whether naturopathy is your calling and if you are willing to sacrifice income and degree recognition. If not, there are other holistic medical options that may be more appropriate. If you are willing to accept the hardships that have come with being a pioneer, you will be needed for carrying the time-honored thread of naturopathic medical principles into a society much in need of your services—whether it currently acknowledges you or not.

Each year several hundred clinically trained NDs graduate from the seven accredited universities in North America. This number will probably continue to grow at a slow rate until more favorable integrative health care legislation takes effect in the U.S. and Canada. Until that time, many aspiring NDs will choose to attend chiropractic, osteopathic, traditional Chinese medicine, and other schools whose degree programs lead to more reliable economic success. And until that time, success in the field of naturopathic medicine will often be more dependent on

your personal sales and business building skills than on your skill level as a physician. In summary, inspecting modern naturopathic medicine from several viewpoints, including the traditional, the idealistic, the political, and the economical, will allow prospective students to make the wisest choice for their own professional careers.

STATE-SPECIFIC LICENSURE

As of 2008, fifteen states and the District of Columbia license naturopathic physicians: Alaska, Arizona, California, Connecticut, Florida, Hawaii, Idaho, Kansas, Maine, Montana, New Hampshire, Oregon, Utah, Vermont, and Washington. In several states, licensed naturopathic physicians must also qualify for a certificate to practice natural childbirth (midwifery), acupuncture, or to dispense a natural substance or device. For more on state-based licensure requirements and regulations, refer to www.naturopathic.org.

Additional Information

Profile of Profession: Naturopathic Practice
Center for the Health Professions
University of California, San Francisco
www.futurehealth.ucsf.edu/pdf_files/Naturo2.pdf

ORGANIZATIONS

American Association of Naturopathic Physicians
www.naturopathic.org

The AANP is the largest naturopathic advocacy networking group for naturopathic physicians in North America. It is involved in almost all naturopathic legal, regulatory, and research movements, including education, licensing standards, and spreading awareness about the profession.

Association of Accredited Naturopathic Medical Colleges
www.aanmc.org

The AANMC was established in February 2001 to propel and foster the naturopathic medical profession by actively supporting the academic efforts of accredited and recognized schools of naturopathic medicine. Since its birth, the AANMC has represented six accredited colleges in the United States and Canada.

The Council on Naturopathic Medical Education
www.cnme.org

The CNME's mission is quality assurance: serving the public by accrediting naturopathic medical education programs that voluntarily seek recognition so that they meet or exceed its standards. Students and graduates of programs accredited or preaccredited (candidacy) by CNME are eligible to apply for the naturopathic licensing examinations administered by the North American Board of Naturopathic Examiners and are generally eligible for state and provincial licensure in the U.S. and Canada.

Oncology Association of Naturopathic Physicians
www.oncanp.org

The OANP is a membership organization dedicated to the survival and quality of life for people living with cancer through the integration of naturopathic oncology in cancer care. The OANP has its own board certification, continuing education programs, practitioner networking recourses, and research initiatives.

North American Board of Naturopathic Examiners
www.nabne.org

The NPLEX (Naturopathic Physicians Licensing Examinations) is the multi-part examination that graduates of accredited naturopathic medical colleges must pass in order to be licensed in any of the fifteen states, the District of Columbia, or five Canadian provinces that license/register naturopathic physicians. NABNE is responsible for approving applicants to take the NPLEX and for administering the examinations.

STATE-BASED ASSOCIATIONS

Arizona Naturopathic Medical Association
www.aznma.com

California Naturopathic Doctors Association
www.calnd.org

Colorado Association of Naturopathic Physicians
www.coanp.org

Connecticut Naturopathic Association
www.cnpaonline.org

Florida Naturopathic Physicians Association
www.fnpa.org

Hawaii Association of Naturopathic Physicians
www.hawaiind.org

Illinois Association of Naturopathic Physicians
www.ilanp.org

Indiana Association of Naturopathic Physicians
www.inanp.org

Maine Association of Naturopathic Doctors
www.mand.org

Massachusetts Society of Naturopathic Doctors
www.msnd.org

Michigan Association of Naturopathic Physicians
www.michnd.org

Minnesota Association of Naturopathic Physicians
www.mnanp.org

Missouri Association of Naturopathic Physicians
www.missourinaturopath.org

Montana Association of Naturopathic Physicians
www.mtnd.org

New Hampshire Association of Naturopathic Doctors
www.nhand.org

New York Association of Naturopathic Physicians
www.nyanp.org

North Carolina Association of Naturopathic Physicians
www.ncanp.com

Ohio Chapter of the American Association of Naturopathic Physicians
www.ocaanp.org

Oregon Association of Naturopathic Physicians
www.oanp.org

Pennsylvania Association of Naturopathic Physicians
www.panp.org

Vermont Association of Naturopathic Physicians
www.vanp.org

Virginia Association of Naturopathic Physicians
www.vaanp.org

Washington Association of Naturopathic Physicians
www.wanp.org

Wisconsin Naturopathic Physicians Association
www.wisconsin-nd.org

PERIODICALS

Alternative Medicine Review
www.thorne.com/altmedrev

Alternative Therapies in Health and Medicine
www.alternative-therapies.com

American Family Physician
www.aafp.org
Official publication of the American Academy of Family Physicians

Complementary Therapies in Medicine
www.harcourt-international.com/journals/ctim

Integrative Medicine: A Clinician's Journal
www.imjournal.com

Journal of Alternative and Complementary Medicine
www.liebertpub.com/ACM
Research on paradigm, practice, and policy

Journal of Naturopathic Medicine
Official publication of the American Association of Naturopathic Physicians

BOOKS

Textbook of Natural Medicine by Joseph Pizzorno, ND, and Michael Murray, ND

Total Wellness by Joseph Pizzorno, ND

Complete Botanical Prescriber by John Sherman, ND

Nature Cure by Henry Lindlahr, MD

Planet Medicine by Richard Grossinger

EDUCATIONAL INSTITUTIONS

The following naturopathic schools are the only schools in North America that are accredited by the AANMC. To become a licensed naturopathic physician in states that recognize the licensure, you must graduate from one of the following programs:

Bastyr University
Kenmore, Washington
www.bastyr.edu

Boucher Institute of Naturopathic Medicine
New Westminster, British Columbia, Canada
www.binm.org/

Canadian College of Naturopathic Medicine
Toronto, Canada
www.ccnm.edu

National College of Natural Medicine
Portland, Oregon
www.ncnm.edu

Southwest College of Naturopathic Medicine and Health Sciences
Tempe, Arizona
www.scnm.edu

University of Bridgeport College of Naturopathic Medicine
Bridgeport, Connecticut
www.bridgeport.edu/ub/nm/

National College of Health Sciences
Chicago, Illinois
http://www.nuhs.edu/

CHAPTER 9

HOLISTIC NURSING (RN)

Nursing has been practiced throughout the entirety of human history, since most human beings instinctively care for one another during times of illness and crisis. However, the way nursing is defined and the way in which it is practiced has changed greatly within the last several hundred years. The original nurses who went by that specific title were the "wet" and "dry" nurses of fourteenth century England. They either suckled another woman's baby ("wet") or performed general service to a young child without suckling ("dry"). Within a hundred years, this definition had been expanded to include any human being caring for another.

Between the time of Shakespeare's England and the Crimean War of the 1850s (pitting England and France against Russia), professional nursing was nearly always performed by nuns or military "hangers-on." These latter women were of the poorer classes and hoped to make some wages by cooking and otherwise caring for the troops. Few career choices were viewed as so demeaning for those not living in a convent.

The nursing profession began its great change when a twenty-four-year old named Florence Nightingale followed what she felt was a divine calling by announcing to her horror-struck upper-class family that she was devoting her life to caring for the poor. She started by successfully advocating for improvement in medical conditions at blue-collar London infirmaries and later traveled to Turkey with forty other nurse volunteers to tend the British wounded during the Crimean War. There she began her attempts to lessen client fatalities via improved hygiene, nutrition, medical equipment, statistical analysis, and compassion.

Her nickname of "The Lady of the Lamp" conjures up the idealistic image of the holistic nurse, gliding through the dark, war-torn night and nurturing the bodies, minds, and souls of the afflicted. After the war, Nightingale was said to be the most famous person in England after Queen Victoria. This fame made nursing a respected profession and allowed Nightingale to successfully influence the English Army to overhaul its entire system of medical care. Due to her influence, the English

HOLISTIC NURSES are committed to care that recognizes the inherent physical, psychological, and spiritual integration within each human being. With this in mind, holistic nurses take care to create an environment conducive to client healing and focus their care on interventions that promote client peace, comfort, and a subjective sense of harmony. Nurses are often in key management roles within health services. The coming integration of health care and need to control costs suggests that nurses in positions of influence will likely be holistic.

also established their first army medical school and instituted their first comprehensive system of medical recording.

Other Nightingale accomplishments include: pioneering "medical tourism, by directing the poor to travel to other countries for inexpensive, high-quality treatment; using family money to establish the first Nightingale Training School for Nurses; writing *Notes on Nursing*, the first nursing textbook that was also sold to the public as a popular introduction to nursing; consulting with the Union Army during the American Civil War; pioneering the use of statistics-based illustrations to chart epidemics; and mentoring Linda Richards, the first American-trained nurse. Richards was the first student at the first American nursing school: a skeleton two-year program started in 1872 at the New England Hospital for Women and Children in Boston, Massachusetts. She later founded more nursing schools in both the United States and Japan.

Meanwhile, nurse Clara Barton more than consulted with the Union Army. She was under their full employment and, unlike Nightingale, was given permission to treat soldiers directly on the battlefield. In 1881, she became president of the American branch of the International Red Cross, devoted to bringing emergency assistance to those affected by wars and other calamities. New Zealand was the first country to regulate nurses nationally, with the adoption of the Nurses Registration Act in 1901. North Carolina was the first state in the United States to pass a nursing licensure law in 1903, though it wasn't until 1909 that the University of Minnesota created the first bachelor's degree program in nursing. In 1952, males joined females for the first time under the same registry in the United Kingdom. This followed on the heels of the establishment of the National Health Service, a mostly free "cradle-to-grave" welfare state health care service for all British residents. Shortly thereafter, Columbia University began offering the first master's degree in nursing. Holistic nurses of the present time believe that Florence Nightingale's personal example, writings, and speeches laid the groundwork for modern holistic care.

Much of Nightingale's advice regarding holistic client care has been ignored for the last 150 years, but there have been occasional bursts of interest in her opinions. Most recently, the Civil Rights Movement during the 1960s brought with it new focus on alternative approaches to human relations. This included the relationship between doctors, nurses, clients, and the extended family of health care practitioners. In 1971, the rights of the dying client were addressed by the founding of the hospice movement. At that time, Florence Wald resigned from her post as the dean of the Yale School of Nursing and joined forces with two pediatricians and a chaplain to establish the first hospice in Branford, Connecticut. In 1980, the Roper, Logan, and Tierney model of nursing was published. This model lists the twelve major modes of activity for humans (communicating, walking, sleeping, etc.) and insists that nurses should use this list for initial client assessment through final treatment.

Nurses have often experienced difficulty with the historical medical hierarchy that has tended to state that a nurse's primary purpose is to follow the direction of doctors. This setup was perhaps inevitable during the long centuries of nurses as poor hangers-on, hoping for a pittance in exchange for their nurturance. But in Nightingale's *Notes on Nursing*, doctors are mentioned infrequently, and sometimes critically, particularly relating to their bedside manner. In the author's opinion, nursing was a profession with principles and rules of its own, having little to do with whether or not a doctor was present. Present-day holistic nurses will find this attitude to be helpful, as most doctors today are allopathically, not holistically, inclined. The modern era has seen the development of holistic and certification programs and the introduction of numerous sympathetic journals to broaden the knowledge base of the profession. Nurses are often in key management roles within health services and hold research posts at universities. The coming integration of health care and need to control costs suggests that nurses in positions of influence will likely be holistic.

Holistic nursing is defined by the American Holistic Nurses Association as "all nursing practice that has healing the whole person as its goal." It can be further defined as a practice that draws on nursing knowledge, theories, expertise, and intuition for the purpose of guiding nurses to become therapeutic partners with their clients. Holistic nursing prefers the word "client" to the word "patient," since "patient" assumes the standard allopathic medical relationship of a relatively ignorant ill person being cared for by an impatient expert. Holistic nurses work to strengthen their clients' facilitation of their own healing process and to help them achieve a greater feeling of overall fulfillment within their lives. The practice of holistic nursing is grounded in various theories of nursing theory. While each holistic nurse chooses which nursing theory to apply in any individual case, the nursing theories of Jean Watson (*Theory of Transpersonal Caring*), Helen Erickson (*Modeling and Role-Modeling*), Martha Rogers (*Science of Unitary Human Beings*), Margaret Newman (*Health as Expanding Consciousness*), and Rosemarie Rizzo Parse (*Theory of Human Becoming*) are most frequently used to support holistic nursing practices.

There are two general viewpoints within the nursing profession regarding holism. One view defines an integral vision in terms of its component parts—biology, psychology, social network, spirituality—with the belief that the whole is greater than these parts. The other viewpoint defines the whole as an irreducible unit. While both may be correct when debated from different angles, the more practical of the two viewpoints seems to be the first. This viewpoint allows nurses to guide their clients to focus on improving the various aspects of their lives one by one. Because there are a limited number of major categories of life, clients may feel empowered knowing that a little effort at introspection and self-improvement will go a long way.

Unlike allopathic nursing, holistic nursing requires the nurse to integrate client self-care and self-responsibility into his or her own life. Holistic nurses also help clients to understand the desirability of striving for an awareness of the interconnectedness of individual humans and global ecological community. Perhaps equally important, holistic nursing also shines the spotlight on care for the caregiver. Holistic nurses are taught that they must walk their talk and manifest balanced health in their own lives.

If a caregiver ignores self-care, burn out and ill health are the likely results. Yet within allopathic medical training, little time is spent instructing students on the importance of maintaining their own well-being for the sake of themselves and their clients. Holistic nursing schools embrace the viewpoint, "nurse, heal thyself," in a manner similar to that which all student practitioners receive within their field of holistic medicine.

Holistic nurses are committed to care that recognizes the inherent physical, psychological, and spiritual integration within each human being. With this in mind, holistic nurses take care to create an environment conducive to client healing and focus their care on interventions that promote client peace, comfort, and a subjective sense of harmony. Modalities frequently used include the following interventions listed in the Nursing Interventions Classification (NIC): art therapy, acupressure, animal-assisted therapy, music therapy, therapeutic touch (or other energy-based modalities such as healing touch), guided imagery, massage, and relaxation therapy.

Interventions frequently employed in holistic nursing practice include anxiety reduction, bodywork, emotional support, exercise promotion, forgiveness facilitation, hope installation, journaling, counseling, cognitive therapy, and spiritual support. Holistic nursing also requires the nurse to understand the phenomenon of creating a physical environment conducive to healing, ideally in the form of soothing, colorful surroundings; harmonious music, including that from nature; a clear view of nature at all times; pleasant aromas, including those from optimally healthful meals; nurturing touch sensations, including bedding, clothes, and nurturing touch—in short, a healing boost to all of the client's senses.

In one sense, all nursing practice can be holistic—that is, all nursing practice may have healing the whole person as its goal. What makes holistic nursing practice a specialty is that there is a body of holistic medical knowledge and an advanced set of nursing skills that when applied goes well beyond the client care skills learned at the basic level of nursing training.

The following philosophical principles form the backbone for holistic nursing practice:

- Humans manifest an essential unity of body, mind, and spirit.

- Human experience is contextually and culturally defined.

- Health and illness are basic human experiences.

- The presence of illness does not preclude health, nor does optimal health preclude illness.

- Human experiences are subjectively described, and health and illness are determined by the viewpoint of each individual.

- The relationship between nurse and client involves participation of both during the process of care.

- The interaction between nurse and client occurs within the values and beliefs of the client and the nurse.

- Public policy and the health care delivery system influence the health and well-being of society and professional nursing.

- Holistic nurses emphasize the care of the whole client, not merely the treatment of symptoms and disease.

- A holistic model of nursing focuses on patterns and root causes of illness and views disease and suffering as opportunities for healing and growth.

- Holistic nurses emphasize health promotion, prevention, self-awareness, self-exploration, self-care, and self-responsibility.

- Holistic nursing understands that each client is an interactive system of physical, mental, emotional, social, spiritual, environmental, and other factors.

The American Holistic Nurses Association credits Florence Nightingale as being the first holistic nurse. Nightingale recognized the importance of caring for the whole person and encouraged interventions that enhanced individuals' abilities to draw upon their own healing powers. She considered touch, light, aromatics, empathetic listening, music, quiet reflection, and similar healing measures as essential ingredients to good nursing care. Illustrating her balanced approach to scientific, statistical, and holistic care, she wrote, "Nursing is an art; and if it is to be made an art, it requires an exclusive devotion as hard a preparation as any painter's or sculptor's work; for what is the having to do with dead canvas or dead marble, compared with having to do with the living body,

the temple of God's spirit? It is one of the Fine Arts: I had almost said, the finest of Fine Arts." As such, holistic nursing combines the medical sciences with the universal arts of interpersonal healing and radically compassionate client care.

TECHNIQUES

The origin of holistic nursing occurred over a hundred years ago. But it is only within the last few decades that the nursing field as a whole has manifested enough progressive changes to allow for holistic nursing to grow into a respected subspecialty of its own. Below are some of the main treatment methods learned by holistic nursing students:

Therapeutic touch: Similar to the "hands-off" therapeutic healing energy transmission from doctor to client within Chinese medicine's system of chi kung, therapeutic touch was developed by self-proclaimed psychic Dora Kunz and her apprentice, Dolores Krieger, PhD, RN. In 1972, they began teaching classes in therapeutic touch at the Theosophical Society's Pumpkin Hill Farm spiritual retreat center in rural upstate New York. Students are taught how to sense a client's energy field via moving their hands slowly above the client's body.

Once the relative health of the client's emanating life force is determined, therapeutic touch practitioners use more slow hand movements to manipulate any imbalanced energy flow into a more balanced, healthful pattern by sending the client healing vital force of their own. Treatments usually last no longer than twenty minutes. Patients frequently report pain relief, mood elevation, and increased vitality. Practitioners acknowledge that there is a scarcity of science behind the exact energy field they feel they are sensing and altering. This they attribute to current technological shortcomings.

Because therapeutic touch cofounder Dolores Krieger is a registered nurse, the nursing field was the main initial recipient of therapeutic touch trainings. For this reason, there are thousands of therapeutic touch trained nurses around the world, and therapeutic touch is often thought of synonymously with the nursing profession. However, any layperson with no medical training can also receive therapeutic touch instruction. The Chinese claim that there are multiple scientific studies supporting the claim that chi kung is an effective treatment for almost any ailment. Therapeutic touch practitioners make the same panacea-like claim for their version of energy healing. However, the only studies to-date have repudiated its effectiveness beyond the placebo effect.

Massage: Nurses, unlike doctors, have always had the legal right to touch clients with therapeutic intent. Performing a variety of massage techniques upon clients is therefore an obvious modality for holistic nurses to employ with their clients. All of the common massage techniques, from Swedish to shiatsu, are taught in the various holistic nursing programs across the United States. This allows the holistic nurse to offer the type of touch appropriate for different conditions: reducing stress, healing injuries, or improving lymphatic system function.

Unlike therapeutic touch, which includes no physical touch, massage techniques have been widely proven to offer scientifically significant benefits for a variety of ailments. According to the National Institutes of Health Center for Complementary and Alternative Medicine, massage helps to alleviate joint, muscle, and migraine pain; shorten birth labor; enhance immune system function; decrease depression and anxiety; reduce post-surgery swelling; enhance sleep, energy, circulation, and concentration; decrease blood pressure and premenstrual cramping; improve the air flow of asthmatic children; and even improve the weight gain of children if they are premature. Although elixir claims should be viewed with skepticism, the range of ailments which massage is able to improve at least lends credence to the argument that a panacea is not an impossibility.

Psychoneuroimmunology: More a field of research than a specific therapy, the mouthful psychoneuroimmunology (PNI) was a radical hypothesis for the West in 1974 when it was advanced by Robert Ader, PhD, a psychiatric researcher at the University of Rochester Medical Center. Ader found that experimental rats' immune function changed depending upon the relative stressfulness of their environment. This finding was counter to the prevailing medical belief of the times, which held that the human immune system was unlike other organ systems in that it was not affected by the nervous system.

PNI is therefore the simple statement that there are no exceptions to the fact that every body part is impacted by the mind via the brain and the rest of the nervous system .The communication goes both ways, in that the relative state of health of the body also impacts clients' minds via the same nervous system. Because of the overarching impact of the mind on the body, and vice versa, it would be more accurate to call this field of research, "psychoneurobiology," so that newcomers to the term don't think that the mind only influences the immune system and not all other body systems as well.

Holistic nurses make practical use of PNI by assessing the relative distress of a client's environment as well as a client's tendencies to lean toward optimism or pessimism, hope or despair, forgiveness or hostility. They then offer advice on the environmental changes, stress reduction techniques, counseling, biofeedback training, and the like that support a healthy immune system.

Stress reduction: Technically, there are two types of stress, only one of which is desirable to reduce. *Eustress* is that which challenges, enriches, and strengthens us—such as a strenuous hike through alpine meadows. *Distress* is that which threatens, enervates, and debilitates us, such as being attacked by a grizzly bear. Even distress is harmless, and potentially helpful, if it is short term. Brief releases of the neurochemicals that facilitate our bear-escaping, "fight or flight" response can save our lives in powerful, involuntary fashion. Lingering too long under the sway of distress chemicals, on the other hand, quickly begins to injure multiple systems of the body-mind. High blood pressure; lackluster immunity; chronic, alternating depression/anxiety; and shallow rapid breathing leading to poor oxygenation are just a few of the results of a runaway fight or flight mechanism.

Unfortunately for modern-day urban dwellers, the fast pace, noise, workaholism, anonymity, and concrete environment of our cities are a recipe for keeping individuals in a state of chronic fight or flight. Without using tools to switch our nervous systems from the fight or flight "sympathetic" nervous system to the rest and relax, "parasympathetic" nervous system, most people never realize that they can consciously choose greater calmness over instinctive anxiety. To help clients lower distress levels, holistic nurses offer a range of exercises, from deep breathing to sitting and walking meditation to guided imagery to hypnosis, which clients can immediately begin to use while ill to improve their rate of healing. Clients can then continue such exercises at home on a daily basis so that there is a greater chance for them to prevent future illness.

Holistic nurses also give instruction to clients on how to use indirect stress reduction techniques, such as daily physical exercise and improving family communication skills, so as to reduce the total overall time that a client spends in sympathetic nervous system overdrive. The formula is simple, if not easy, to put into effect: remain in the parasympathetic rest and relax response as much as possible; allow the sympathetic fight or flight response to remain only as long as it helps you to get out of imminent danger. Then return to rest and relax as quickly as possible. Cultivating this skill is one of the most direct routes to improved health and happiness.

Counseling: Holistic nurses are not trained as psychologists, but they do learn the basics of healthy and dysfunctional human psychology as well as a variety of counseling techniques that are usually related to those within the fields of humanistic, cognitive/behavioral, and transpersonal psychology. Unconditional positive regard; encouraging rational, willfully optimistic changes in thoughts and actions; and training clients how to focus in a practical way on their spiritual faith of choice are common attitudes taken by holistic nurses as counselors. As in the area of stress reduction, holistic nurses incorporate counseling tools such as guided imagery and lifestyle introspection. And counseling may be kept informal, so that clients do not feel that they are being considered psychologically unsound. Instead, counseling may be provided under the umbrellas of stress reduction and preventive medicine.

Because allopathic providers are often criticized for the brevity and brusqueness of their bedside manner, counseling in the form of nonjudgmental listening by a holistic nurse can result in greater positive client response than the degree of counseling would seem to warrant. It is a great relief to clients to be counseled by their health providers, the majority of whom are allopathically trained.

Biofeedback: This is the real-time measurement of a client's body processes, such as heart rate, blood pressure, perspiration, skin temperature, muscle tension, and brain wave patterns, so that the client may learn to consciously control these previously involuntary processes. A biofeedback machine emits a sound, or produces an effect on a video screen, to tell the client whether he or she is increasing or decreasing his or her skin temperature, or other physical process being measured. Because each of the above processes is closely related to stress reduction, it would be easy to think that all biofeedback is stress reduction related.

However, ADHD and epileptic clients are trained via biofeedback to increase the speed of their brain waves. This would normally tend to increase a client's perception of distress, but these clients instead feel more focused and less convulsive, respectively. Normally relaxing alpha and theta waves can also be used in therapy by helping clients to remember and resolve previously traumatic events. Although it has been used within medicine since the mid-1960s, the potential of biofeedback to help clients gain healthful control over the functioning of their body-minds has barely been tapped.

Hypnotherapy and guided imagery: Hypnotherapy, or the use of hypnosis for improving health, has been practiced for thousands of years. Ancient Egyptians, East Indians, and Greeks used it in their temples devoted to the healing powers of sleep; premier physicians such as Paracelsus and Avicenna practiced it during the Middle Ages; and Franz Mesmer and Sigmund Freud were two modern Europeans who used hypnotherapy enthusiastically at some point during their careers. The American Medical Association approved the therapeutic use of hypnosis in 1958, and since that time, hypnotherapy has become a common, if misunderstood, treatment for ailments as diverse as phobias, addictions, bedwetting, depression, and post-traumatic stress disorder. The greater the client trust in the hypnotherapist, and the less anxiety the client feels in general, the easier it is for a client to be hypnotized.

This means that a client will be in a semiconscious trance state in which he or she is much more suggestible than normal to statements made by the hypnotist. The client also exhibits paradoxical physiological responses, such as pupil dilation after exposure to bright light. Holistic nurses may use hypnotherapy to treat specific ailments by giving, for example, the entranced client suggestions of improved immunity or improved wound healing. More common is the use of hypnotism for general client stress reduction, including teaching self-hypnotism to clients for daily use at home.

Guided imagery is the use of specific thoughts and suggestions in order to influence the client's imagination toward a state of relaxation, more healthful emotional expression, or the belief that specific healing is occurring within ailing organ systems. It was developed in the 1950s by German psychiatrist, Hanscarl Leuner, MD, who soon added LSD to his protocols and became one of the world's most prominent psychedelic therapists until his retirement in 1986. A client needn't be in a hypnotic trance in order to receive benefits from guided imagery exercises received via an in-person practitioner, an audio recording, or self-induction.

However, the state of consciousness commonly reached during guided imagery is similar enough to the hypnotic state that it likely taps into similar healing powers of the imagining subconscious mind. A common exercise in guided imagery is to soothingly instruct a client to imagine a beautiful walk through nature leading to his or her personal epitome of a relaxing scenic destination. This destination can then be revisited by the imagining client at will in order to help him or her prevent or treat subsequent anxiety by consciously eliciting peace of mind.

Herbology: Holistic nurses can take coursework in herbal medicine that gives them a basic understanding of both the vitalistic/energetic approach of various herbal folk traditions and the more materialistic, phyto-pharmacological postmodern era of current herbal researchers. Holistic nurses rarely rely solely, or even primarily, on herbal medicine for client treatment. Instead, allopathic prescription drugs are usually the main medicines used, with the holistic aspect of holistic nursing coming from the complementary use of various natural medicine modalities to support the actions of the two allopathic staples of synthetic drugs and surgery. Learning even fifty herbal medicines gives the holistic nurse an effective adjunct for treating most client complaints, including infection, inflammation, fatigue, and anxiety/depression.

Advanced holistic assessment: It is more and more common for nurses to participate in a client's primary diagnosis and treatment along with presiding MDs, osteopaths, et al. Holistic nurses assess clients using a broad spectrum approach as regarding those categories of life that are deemed important to health. This includes the spiritual, emotional, intellectual, creative, environmental, sexual, interpersonal, community, global, and, finally, physical aspects of an individual's life. Holistic assessment takes considerable more time than a standard ten-minute allopathic intake typically based on presenting symptoms only. Taking a greater amount of time during a first office call often saves much more time overall, as a practitioner can more easily assess the root cause of an ailment and treat this cause immediately within the initial treatment protocol. Clients also report that experiencing a holistic intake assessment gives them a greater sense of being cared for and understood.

Integral healing modalities: Holistic nursing embraces as wide a spectrum of medical modalities as does naturopathic medicine, since everything considered holistic is usually considered naturopathic as well. This means that holistic nurses can expect to learn the basics of ayurvedic and Chinese medicine, as well as Western herbal medicine, exercise physiology, nutritional science, meditation, reiki, reflexology, and therapeutic touch, either through required coursework, electives, or continuing education. Holistic nurses cannot expect to always have a receptive audience from coworkers and clients regarding some of the alternative modalities that have an obvious lack of scientific backing.

At this point in history, however, most medical personnel and clients appreciate the intelligent combination of allopathic and science-backed complementary and alternative medicine. This is what integrative medicine is all about, and given the somewhat dated connotation of the word, "holistic," integrative nursing is perhaps a more accurate expression for the cutting-edge style of nursing of which Florence Nightingale would be most proud.

CAREER AND TRAINING

Holistic nursing is practiced everywhere that nursing is in general, which means it is practiced in all states and around the world. A holistic nursing degree or certification will allow you to greatly improve your client care by balancing allopathic nursing skills, such as physical examinations and prescription drug administration, with the range of complementary skills described above. Interest in integrative medicine is increasing yearly, and your new skills will be widely accepted within today's nursing field. This is especially true of the clients with whom you come into contact. While there remain individuals skeptical of holistic treatments from their doctors, few clients hesitate when offered similar suggestions from their nursing staff. Although this may be viewed as a double standard, part of the reason behind this phenomenon is that many clients remain convinced that modern allopathy must be the first line of treatment while complementary medicine should remain just that: a complement to our culturally accepted form of Western allopathic medicine. Since nurses are usually viewed as complementary aides to presiding doctors, despite the efforts of Florence Nightingale, accepting therapies from holistic nurses fits well within clients' conception of the age-old hierarchy of both medical providers and medical modalities.

Trends bode well for the field of holistic nursing in the United States. A study in 2003 by the University of Texas School of Nursing found that nursing schools across the country are responding to increasing consumer use of integrative medicine by incorporating holistic modalities into their curricula. Approximately 60 percent of the 585 U.S.-based schools recognize the definition of holistic nursing in their curricula, while 85 percent included integrative modalities within their coursework. In December 2006, holistic nursing was officially recognized by the American Nurses Association. This recognition gives registered nurses (RNs) who practice in this area increased credibility as well as legitimacy.

The first degree program specifically in holistic nursing was at New York University's College of Nursing, where a Holistic Nurse Practitioner (HNP) Master's Degree can be earned within the Advanced Practice Holistic Nursing Graduate Program. Established in 1998, the first graduates entered the workforce in 2001, after the required three years of training. Each student enters the program with BA and RN degrees, and most students already have several years of nursing practice in their résumé. Since that time, a second HNP master's degree program has been initiated at Tennessee State University. This program is completed entirely online and offers RN practitioners nationwide the opportunity to earn an HNP degree without considering a move to New York. Upon graduation, holistic nurses easily integrate into private and group medical practices as well as hospital-based integrative healing centers.

What makes the HNP program unique is that, in combination with advanced instruction in the sciences of pharmacology, pathology, and psychoneuroimmunology, students are taught the equal importance of nutrition, exercise, stress reduction, spirituality, meditation, cross-cultural perspective, emotional balance, and the basis for all "vitalistic" medical systems since the advent of humankind: optimal energy. Graduates learn to make holistic diagnoses that incorporate all factors of the human body-mind-spirit complex and then to offer equally integrative medical treatments.

Income for holistic nurses will be higher than that for the registered nurse profession as a whole, as any further degree earnings beyond that of RN tends to bring about a percentage increase in salary. Because an added master's degree tends to elicit higher earnings than an added certification, students should consider earning a master's degree in holistic nursing. Of course, given the small number of holistic nursing programs currently available, students may choose to earn certifications after nursing school closer to their current homes, jobs, and families.

The average salary for holistic nurses nationwide is $55,000. Although the average salary for RNs without added specialization is only $52,000, remember that this average for holistic nurses includes all of those with certifications only, versus those who have earned the more lucrative HNP master's degree. And, more optimistic than the above numbers, nurses with specializations beyond an RN degree claim to earn $9,000 more per year. This is especially true if you should choose to set up a private practice of your own.

The fields of nursing and CAM are both booming simultaneously. There is an ongoing shortage of nurses nationwide and worldwide. Nurses can usually choose whatever geographic region in which they prefer to work and can often negotiate signing bonuses from $2,000 to $20,000 as well as paid relocation. Integrative practitioners are becoming more and more respected, especially those who combine allopathy and CAM in an integrative form. If you are a prospective student with a holistic mind-set desiring the greatest likelihood of career success and fulfillment in the medical field, strongly consider holistic nursing. There are few careers that offer so many job opportunities and so much appreciation from both your clients, your heart, and your pocketbook.

WHERE PRACTICED

Holistic nurses tend to work as part of a larger integrated clinic, which may be a traditional allopathic institution or a progressive center for integrative and alternative medicine. Refer to the General Resources section of this book for information on cutting-edge centers for integrative health. With proper licensing and certification, some nurses choose to form an independent practice, which must meet the legal standards for private health care practices as defined by states' boards. As most nurses tend to be women, there is a significant contingent of holistic nurses who work primarily in the field of women's health care, in areas such as obstetrics (pregnancy) and gynecology.

EDUCATION REQUIREMENTS

To achieve or be eligible for an RN (registered nurse) title, you must graduate from a state-approved school of nursing; these programs tend to be either four-year university programs, three-year diploma programs, or two-year associate programs. The programs, accredited by the American Nurses' Credentialing Center, range in difficulty and in prerequisite application requirements. Some require experience in the sciences, while others do not require even a high school diploma.

Once students have completed a two- to four-year program, they are eligible to sit for a state-based RN licensing examination administered by the National Council Licensure Examination for Registered Nurses (NCLEX-RN). For more information on testing locations and prerequisites in your state, consult your state's board of nursing.

DEGREES, LICENSURE, ACCREDITATION, AND CERTIFICATION

There are two basic types of certification that students of nursing may pursue. The first type of certification is a standard RN certification, which is a state-regulated modality of health care. RNs are not necessarily holistic in practice, and therefore, the process to become an RN is not unlike pursuing other standardized medical professions. For more information on this licensed certification, consult the American Nurses' Association's Web site: www.nursingworld. org.

The other type of nursing certification is a three-step process done through the American Holistic Nurses' Certification Corporation (AHNCC). Most holistic nurses will gain their RN certification first and then go on to pursue an additional program in holistic nursing. Applicants must write an essay that illustrates their understanding and pass a quantitative examination given by the AHNCC tri-annually. It is important to note that holistic certification is not a federally licensed or endorsed program. It is a private certification program that connotes proficiency in holistic nursing, but it does not in and of itself constitute a license to be a health care provider. For this reason, all applicants for holistic nursing certificate programs must already be licensed.

Certified holistic nurses are able to expand their practice by gaining smaller certifications in specific modalities, such as therapeutic touch, energy medicine, biofeedback, and other areas of mind-body medicine. A certificate in holistic nursing is a license to continue learning and pursuing CAM therapies, which are relevant to practice.

Relevant Licensed Nursing Degrees

- **BSN:** A bachelor of science in nursing degree is one of the highest nursing degrees (save master's or PhD programs) achievable in the medical world. Providing information on nursing theory, sciences, humanities, behavioral science, and professional nursing, these four-year programs widen the scope of nursing practice and allow students to pursue a career as a primary health care provider. As of 2005, more than 570 colleges and universities in the United States offer a BSN or a comparable advanced nursing degree.

- **ADN:** A two-year associate degree in nursing prepares individuals for a defined technical scope of practice. The general education focuses on technical proficiency and nursing theory. Most RNs whose first degree is an ADN return to school to earn their bachelor's degree in nursing. In 2006, associate nursing degrees accounted for about 59 percent of nursing education programs in the United States.

- **Diploma:** Diploma nursing programs are usually associated with a hospital or medical institution as they combine classroom experience with clinical instruction over a three-year period. Although diploma programs were once common in the nursing community, programs have diminished steadily over the past ten years. As of 2006, three-year diploma programs only account for 4 percent of nursing education program in the United States.

CONTINUING EDUCATION

As in most licensed medical professions, RNs must continue their medical education during their practice to maintain their license. Unlike MD continuing education requirements, continuing education in nursing is fairly open: there are many programs, both in the classroom and online, which may count for "contact hour" credit. Credit hours and requirements tend to vary slightly from state to state.

ORGANIZATIONS

American Holistic Nurses Association
www.ahna.org

The largest advocacy group and the current "voice" of holistic nursing in the United States, the AHNA is a membership group that hosts conferences, funds holistic research initiatives, and lobbies for standards of education in the nursing community. It is a nonprofit agency dedicated to promoting excellence for the holistic profession.

American Nurses Association
www.nursingworld.org

This is the largest non-holistic nursing advocacy not-for-profit group in the United States. Its Web site contains many types of useful information about the nursing profession.

American Holistic Nurses' Certification Corporation
www.ahncc.org

AHNCC is responsible for administering the Holistic Nurses Certification Examination (HNCE) and certifying holistic nurses for private practice. The board of directors ensure the validity, reliability, and integrity of the certification process by overseeing all of the organization's directional aims.

American Nurses Credentialing Center
www.nursecredentialing.org

ANCC is the leading nurse credentialing center in the United States. It certifies health care providers, accredits education providers, recognizes excellence in nursing, educates the public about the benefits of nursing, and supports credentialing through research and other consultative services.

American Board of Nursing Specialists
www.nursingcertification.org

ABNS is a not-for-profit organization with two arms: a Membership Assembly and an Accreditation Council. Each is governed by elected representatives. ABNS is an advocate for consumer protection by establishing specialty nursing certification. Member organizations of ABNS represent more than a half million certified registered nurses around the world.

National Council of State Boards of Nursing

www.ncsbn.org/index.htm

The council's membership is comprised of all fifty states' nursing boards including the four territories.

Nightingale Initiative for Global Health

www.nighcommunities.org

The mission of this social outreach organization is to inform and empower nurses to work in local, national, and global communities to build a healthy world.

National Association of Nurse Massage Therapists

www.nanmt.org

This is an advocacy/membership group for holistic nurses who practice massage therapy.

The International Society for the Study of Subtle Energies and Energy Medicine

www.issseem.org

An international nonprofit interdisciplinary organization, ISSSEEM is dedicated to exploring and applying subtle energies as they relate to the experience of consciousness, healing, and human potential.

Nurse Radio

nurseradio.org/nurseradio/Index.shtm

This cool nonprofit Internet radio station is dedicated to nurses and nurse leaders.

The Nursing Organization Alliance

www.nursing-alliance.org

The alliance is a coalition of nursing organizations that unified to create a stronger voice for nurses. It includes membership and newsletters.

PEER-REVIEWED PERIODICALS

Journal of Holistic Nursing

jhn.sagepub.com

Official journal of the American Holistic Nurses Association. Quarterly.

Holistic Nursing Practice

www.hnpjournal.com

This publication takes a whole-person approach to nursing addressing both medical and psychosocial concerns. Each issue provides in-depth coverage of a single topic applicable to daily clinical practice. Emphasis is on health-oriented, biobehavioral research and the controversies inherent in holistic nursing practice.

Nursing Research

www.ovid.com/site/catalog/Journal/572.jsp?top=2&mid=3&bottom=7&subsection=12

Celebrating its fiftieth year of publication in 2001, *Nursing Research* is the most prestigious and sought-after research journal in the field, publishing articles on research techniques, quantitative and qualitative studies, and state-of-the-art methodology, including information not yet found in textbooks.

American Journal of Nursing

www.ajnonline.com

The oldest and largest currently circulating nursing journal in the world, the AJN is a peer-reviewed periodical founded upon the dissemination of evidence-based research and dedicated to promoting excellence in nursing and health care.

BOOKS

Holistic Nursing: A Handbook for Practice (Dossey, Holistic Nursing) by Barbara Montgomery Dossey, Lynn Keegan, and Cathie E. Guzzetta

Complementary/Alternative Therapies in Nursing by Mariah Snyder and Ruth Lindquist

AHNA Standards of Holistic Nursing Practice: Guidelines for Caring and Healing by Barbara Montgomery Dossey, Cathie E. Guzzetta, Johanne A. Quinn, and Noreen Cavan Frisch

Guidelines for Holistic Nursing: A Handbook for Practice by Barbara Montgomery Dossey

Critical Care Nursing: A Holistic Approach by Patricia Gonce Morton, Dorrie Fontaine, Carolyn M Hudak, and Barbara M Gallo

Essential Readings in Holistic Nursing by Cathie E. Guzzetta

EDUCATIONAL INSTITUTIONS

There are a plethora of nursing schools in the country. For a comprehensive list of general nursing schools, arranged geographically and by expertise, consult the All Nursing Schools Organization Web site at www. allnursingschools.com.

The American Holistic Nurses' Certification Corporation endorses a few nursing schools that specialize in holistic nursing. While this list is not absolute, all of the following accredited schools have active programs in integrative therapies and classes in holistic health.

Xavier University Department of Nursing
Cincinnati, Ohio
www.xavier.edu/nursing

Metropolitan State University School of Nursing
St. Paul, Minnesota
www.metrostate.edu/cnhs

Humboldt State University, School of Nursing
Arcata, California
www.humboldt.edu/~nurs

Western Michigan University, Bronson School of Nursing
Kalamazoo, Michigan
www.wmich.edu/hhs/nursing

University of Colorado–Colorado Springs
Colorado Springs, Colorado
www.uccs.edu/~bethel/dnp.htm

New York University, Department of Nursing
New York, New York
www.nyu.edu/nursing

Indiana University School of Nursing
South Bend, Indiana
www.nursing.iupui.edu

West Virginia University School of Nursing
Morgantown, West Virginia
www.hsc.wvu.edu/son

University of Texas Medical Branch at Galveston, School of Nursing
Galveston, Texas
www.son.utmb.edu

Dominican University of California, School of Arts and Science
San Rafael, California
www.dominican.edu/academics/artssciences/natbehealth/nursing.html

University of Colorado–Denver
Denver, Colorado
www.uchsc.edu/ahec/mapp/about

University of Texas–Brownsville and Texas Southmost College
Brownsville, Texas
http://blue.utb.edu/shs

Tennessee State University
Nashville, Tennessee
www.tnstate.edu/interior.asp?ptid=1&mid=288

NONDEGREE PROGRAMS

ALEXANDER TECHNIQUE

Frederick Matthias Alexander was a Shakespearean actor in the early 1900s. Toward the middle of his acting career, he pioneered a simple and effective approach to rebalancing the body through awareness, movement, and touch. Inspired by his own vocal problems, Alexander noticed that his recurring loss of voice was caused by unconscious and imbalanced movements of his neck and throat. Essentially, he believed that his strained neck muscles caused the loss of his voice. He developed a method that used breathing patterns to consciously lessen muscular tension where needed and distribute the "stress" of movement more evenly throughout his body. In a short period of time, Alexander fully recovered his voice. He was able to act again; more importantly, his observations led to the conclusion that correct alignment in regard to one's head, neck, and back are essential for optimal movement and vocal functionality. The Alexander method teaches one how to replace often damaging, unconscious bodily habits with newer, conscious ones that improve general movement and thereby correct physiological problems.

After his career in drama, Alexander went on to formulate his techniques into a scientific therapy. He empirically found that any movement including walking, sitting, standing, and even speaking could be made physically easier by examining a person's movements in multiple mirrors, isolating muscles or ligaments that were stressed by the activity, and rebalancing the strain to the rest of the body. Ostensibly, Alexander's technique focuses on activities that are strenuous to one zone of the body and seeks to distribute appropriate muscle tension to other areas, which are not being used optimally.

The Alexander Technique is a self-therapy that is typically taught by an expert of another specialty. Just like many other CAM therapies, the Alexander Technique involves a sound integration between body and mind, so the therapy achieves its most potent results when participants have faith that they are indeed helping their bodies. The benefits of this therapy are relatively subjective. However, there seems to be no limit to its efficacy in certain individuals. The Alexander Technique has been used to improve the strength and stamina in dancers, actors, musicians, vocal performers, and Olympic and professional athletes. Some research indicates that the Alexander Technique is useful in helping patients cope with Parkinson's disease. Other research suggests that the Alexander Technique may be beneficial for treating chronic back pain when incorporated as part of a multidisciplinary approach including chiropractic medicine, acupuncture, and/or psychological intervention and treatment.

In a typical session, the student will lie upon a table, sit on a stool, or remain standing or walking while the instructor tells the student to move, for example, his or her head forward and up in order to allow the torso to stretch vertically. The instructor encourages kinesthetic awareness by instructing students to visualize a relationship between their back, neck, and head, thus beginning the process of a newly constructed body image. This "new" image allows students (or patients) to become conscious of the otherwise unnoticeable subtleties of their movements, upon which they can find and address more specific physiological problems. It should be noted that the Alexander technique can be a difficult and counterinstinctive process to master. Most teachers consider twenty to forty lessons to be required before self-therapy can be effective. As a result, the learning environment, knowledge of the instructor, and the relationship of the student with the instructor often have a drastic impact on the functionality and efficiency of the technique.

The Alexander Technique can be found as curriculum in performance schools of dance, acting, circus, music, voice, and some athletic training. It is appropriate for those starting at any fitness level and is also used as remedial movement education within the fields of physical therapy and pain management.

Although in the United States the Alexander Technique is considered by those in its field to be primarily educational—taught in a student/teacher relationship as compared to being a treatment regimen between client and practitioner—it is regarded by the United Kingdom National Health Service as an alternative and complementary treatment for many medical complaints. A partial list of ailments include back problems; unlearning and avoiding repetitive strain injury; improving ergonomics; stuttering, speech training, and voice loss; coping with mobility for those with Parkinson's disease; and posture or balance problems.

The Alexander Technique has also been known to help performers with getting past the plateau effect of little improvement with much effort; performance anxiety; getting beyond a supposed "lack of talent"; and sharpening discrimination and descriptive ability. It has also helped individuals control unwanted reactions, phobias, and depression.

In a cross-cultural comparison, the Alexander Technique can be compared with the ancient Asian concept of mindfulness. Typically used by practitioners of spiritual practices such as Raja Yoga, Buddhism, and Taoism, complete mindfulness includes simultaneous awareness of body movements and tension; breath rate and depth; emotional flux, expression, or suppression; the near-constant stream of intellectual or other thoughts; interpersonal dynamics; detailed external environment; and, most importantly, spirit, in whatever way is most inspiring to the individual.

A version of this challenging task is also reflected in the super-precise movements of martial arts masters of the Asian-style fighting forms who, like actors, emphasize material success and physical prowess over spiritual striving. Long ago, members of certain cultures developed to the extreme the philosophy that specific styles of body movements influenced the mind-set of both mover and the one being moved around. The Japanese tea ceremony is yet another example of ancient, moving mindfulness. Practitioners of the tea ceremony and the Alexander Technique share a similar appearance of effortless floating compared with those who have done no movement therapy. F.M. Alexander was able to accomplish through sheer observation, physical need, and a Western cultural slant the same optimal muscular physics that other cultures have determined via different means.

As is the case with many similar CAM therapies, concentrated focus is more important than an exact modality. Increased body awareness in general can increase effectiveness and contentment in all other areas of life. Choose your favorite method and apply with zeal! Any practice is better than no practice at all, and you'll be a better practitioner because of it.

RESOURCES

BOOKS

How You Stand, How You Move, How You Live: Learning the Alexander Technique to Explore Your Mind-Body Connection and Achieve Self-Mastery by Missy Vineyard

Body Learning: An Introduction to the Alexander Technique by Michael J. Gelb

The Alexander Technique Manual: Take Control of Your Posture and Your Life by Richard Brennan

How to Learn the Alexander Technique: A Manual for Students by Barbara Conable

Voice and the Alexander Technique by Jane Heirich

The Use of the Self by F.M. Alexander and Wilfred Barlow

The Alexander Technique: A Complete Course in How to Hold and Use Your Body for Maximum Energy by John Gray

Indirect Procedures: A Musician's Guide to the Alexander Technique by Pedro de Alcantara

PERIODICAL

Direction Journal
www.directionjournal.com

For musicians, performers, and other types of professions with high stress. This journal researches effective means of treatment for people with jobs that put stress on the body.

ONLINE

The Complete Guide to the Alexander Technique
www.alexandertechnique.com

A consumer targeted FAQ

Alexander Technique Center
www.alexandercenter.com

An article written by Marian Goldberg on the history and philosophy of the Alexander Technique; includes applications for musicians as well as stress reduction for other professions

Physical Therapy and Alexander Technique
http://physicaltherapy.org

Dedicated to the intersection of physical therapy and the Alexander Technique used interactively

Alexander Technique for Self-Care
www.alexanderlessons.com

Nonprofessional consumer tricks for promoting mental and physical health in daily life

InteliHealth: Alexander Technique
www.intelihealth.com/IH/ihtIH/WS/8513/34968/360044.html?d=dmtContent

InteliHealth's article on the efficacy of, and research done upon, the Alexander Technique

ORGANIZATIONS

Alexander Technique International
www.ati-net.com

A worldwide organization of teachers, students, and friends of the Alexander Technique created to promote and advance the work begun by F. Matthias Alexander. ATI embraces the diversity of the international Alexander Technique community and is working to promote international dialogue. For a list of articles on the Alexander Technique, consult www.ati-net.com/ati-artl.php.

American Society for the Alexander Technique
www.alexandertech.org

The largest professional organization of AT practitioners in the United States

Association of Theatre Movement Educators
www.atmeweb.org

Promotes the highest possible standards for theater movement training and the application of those standards to educational and professional theater, especially in regard to kinesthetic education and the Alexander Technique

TRAINING

American Center for the Alexander Technique
New York, New York
www.acatnyc.org

Urbana-Champaign Teachers of the Alexander Technique
Urbana, Illinois
www.prairienet.org/alexandertech

The Alexander Educational Center
Berkeley, California
www.alexandertechnique.org

The Alexander Educational Center Virginia
Charlottesville, Virginia
www.alexandertechniquecentre.com

St. Louis Center for the Alexander Technique
St. Louis, Missouri
www.slat.us

The Art of Learning Center
San Francisco and Berkeley, California
www.mtpress.com/graduates.htm

Alexander Technique Center of Washington D.C.
Washington, D.C.
www.alexandercenter.com/atcwdc.html

Alexander Technique School New England
Amherst, Massachusetts
www.atcne.com/training.htm

The Oregon Center for the Alexander Technique
Portland, Oregon
www.oregonalexander.com

APPLIED KINESIOLOGY

Applied kinesiology (AK) was developed by George Goodheart, DC, in 1964, as his interpretation of a book, *Muscles, Testing, and Function*, which was written by two physical therapists. It is a practice of using manual muscle-strength testing, first for medical diagnosis and then for determination of prescribed treatment therapy. It purportedly gives feedback on the moment-to-moment functional status of the body in a quick acting manner, without the use of machines.

AK is a subjective diagnostic method used by approximately 40 percent of chiropractors, as well as other practitioners, for the purpose of diagnosing patients' specific areas of physical, psychological, and chemical imbalance. To accomplish this feat, the practitioner chooses one or more muscle groups to test upon a given patient. For example, a doctor asks a patient to hold up his or her arm and resist when the doctor attempts to pull it down. If the patient resists smoothly and strongly, the nervous system has indicated that it is strong within this muscle group, as well as within any organ system that is believed to be functionally connected to the muscle group being tested. If the patient resists the doctor's downward pull in a spasmodic or weakened manner, then that patient's nervous system has indicated dysfunction within the related muscles and organ systems. After an immediate attempt to treat this condition, the same muscle group is again tested. If the chiropractor feels that the muscle group is now strong, the treatment is considered a success.

Using the same AK technique, some practitioners also believe that the appropriateness of specific medications can be deduced for any given patient. One common method for discovering this information is to first determine a subjective baseline reading for a strong muscle group in a patient's body. For example, the chiropractor feels a smooth, strong response from a patient's muscles when he attempts to push down the patient's arm. Next, a small amount of a medication is placed under the patient's tongue (or sometimes is simply kept in its container and held in the patient's hand) and the same muscle group is tested. A strong response is interpreted to mean that this medication is appropriate for the patient; a staccato or weakened response means that the medication is inappropriate. Similar tests can be performed by way of verbal questioning, with baseline muscle strength assessed before a "yes" or "no" question is asked of the patient. If the muscle remains strong, that is a "yes" answer in the language of the patient's nervous system. If the muscle weakens, that is a "no." This is one basic AK methodology, and many more complex versions are also used.

There is understandable criticism directed at AK by the scientific community because the results of AK testing are solely and subjectively determined by the doctor doing the testing. Although anecdotal evidence exists, a review of peer-reviewed studies concluded that the "evidence to date does not support the use of [AK] for the diagnosis of organic disease or pre/subclinical conditions." AK proponents usu-

ally agree that because the testing is subjective one must choose an AK practitioner with care. And since many CAM diagnostic techniques are subjective in nature (pulse and tongue diagnoses within the more respected systems of ayurvedic and traditional Chinese medicine are some longstanding examples), subjectivity alone is not evidence of fraud or practitioner ignorance.

RESOURCES

BOOKS

Applied Kinesiology: A Training Manual and Reference Book of Basic Principles and Practices by Robert Frost

Your Body Can Talk: How to Use Simple Muscle Testing to Learn What Your Body Knows and Needs: The Art and Application of Clinical Kinesiology by Susan L. Levy and Carol Lehr

Applied Kinesiology by Tom and Carole Valentine

Applied Kinesiology: Basic Procedures and Muscle Testing by David S. Walther

Brumstrom's Clinical Kinesiology by Laura K. Smith, Elizabeth Lawrence Weiss, and L. Don Lehmkuhl

ONLINE

Research in Kinesiologic Medicine
www.kinesiology.net/research.asp

International Journal of Applied Kinesiology and Kinesiologic Medicine
www.kinmed.com

Education in Applied Kinesiology
www.akse.de/eng

This organization provides information on English seminars around the world. This is not a certification program.

ORGANIZATIONS

International College of Applied Kinesiology
www.icak.com

For training, membership, and all international information on the discipline

International College of Applied Kinesiology
www.icakusa.com

Relevant information for American practitioners

Applied Kinesiology
www.appliedkinesiology.com

This organization promotes information and research that supports the efficacy and use of applied kinesiology.

Systems DC
www.systemsdc.com

Systems DC was developed by David S. Walther, DC, DIBAK, in 1974 to promote teaching applied kinesiology to primary care physicians.

AROMATHERAPY

Aromatherapy is most simply defined as "the inhalation and bodily application of essential oils." Modern aromatherapy centers on therapeutic treatment based on the chemical components and aromas of essential oils and the experiential knowledge that has been passed down through many traditions. Essential oils are highly aromatic and concentrated substances distilled from specialized cells or glands within certain plants. Examples of essential oils include lavender, eucalyptus, grapefruit, and sandalwood. Essential oils have been found to have both psychological and physical effects on the body. The use of essential oils can support relaxation, reduce inflammation from an injury, and reduce pain.

A common misconception is that aromatherapy refers strictly to treatments involving inhaling the scent of any given essential oil. The truth is, many aromatherapy treatments involve various forms of topical application. Therefore, a professional aromatherapist must have an understanding of human anatomy and physiology as well as the therapeutic properties of essential oils.

The term aromatherapy was first used in 1928 by French chemist René Maurice Gattefossé. Gattefossé devoted his life to researching the healing properties of carefully distilled essential oils. His passion originated from an accidental mishap in his perfume laboratory. After inadvertently lighting his arm on fire, Gattefossé thrust this arm into the nearest cool liquid, which happened to be a vat of lavender oil. He immediately noticed relief from his severe pain, and later noted that his burn healed significantly more quickly than other burns that had not been dipped in lavender. He also noticed that the lavender-drenched burn healed with no scarring and with minimal discomfort. Though many cultures and systems of medicine had use inhalants and aromas for healing centuries before Gattefossé's experiments, Gattefossé conducted the first scientific research regarding the chemical healing properties of essential oils.

In 1964, Jean Valnet, a follower of Gattefossé's research, published his own work, *The Practice of Aromatherapy*. In 1977, Robert Tisserand captured the nation's interest in the healing power of aromas with his book *The Art of Aromatherapy*. It is through scientists like Tisserand and Valnet that aromatherapy has gained mainstream attention and respect as a Western approach to integrative medicine.

Aromatherapy is becoming increasingly popular in the United States. According to the National Association for Holistic Aromatherapy, the American aromatherapy market is over a billion-dollar industry. Clinical aromatherapy within allopathic medicine is already prevalent in many parts of Europe and is becoming more common in the U.S.

Career Information

There are two national organizations in the United States for aromatherapy: the National Association for Holistic Aromatherapy (NAHA) and the Alliance of International Aromatherapists (AIA). In 1999, NAHA's Council for Aromatherapy Schools and Educators formally agreed on Guidelines for Professional Aromatherapy Training. These guidelines have been adopted by schools and independent educators throughout the world. When a student completes a NAHA-approved school's 200-hour certification program, the school provides a certification through NAHA. At this time there is no state or national licensure or laws for aromatherapy in the United States. Many qualified aromatherapists incorporate their aromatherapy training with another profession that they are already licensed in, such as massage therapy, nursing, acupuncture, allopathic medicine, naturopathy, etc. Other aromatherapy students have had no previous training or health care background and begin their holistic health career with aromatherapy. It should be noted that at the time of this publication, the Alliance of International Aromatherapists was in the process of developing educational standards to exceed the 200 hours currently defined by NAHA.

A few examples of potential aromatherapy careers include: aromatherapy consulting, essential oil retail or online sales, custom skin care/body care production, working in a holistic health clinic, writing, and teaching. Aromatherapy can easily complement any form of healing—allopathic or otherwise. Some advocates in the field are discouraged by its lack of licensing, while others appreciate the blessing of not having their practice confined by the limitations of modern medicine.

RESOURCES

PERIODICALS

NAHA Aromatherapy Journal—USA
www.naha.org

International Journal of Essential Oil Therapeutics—France
www.ijeot.com

International Journal of Clinical Aromatherapy—France
www.ijca.net

Aromatherapy Today—Australia
www.aromatherapytoday.com

Aromascents Journal—Canada
www.aromascentsjournal.com

Aromatherapy Thymes—USA
www.aromatherapythymes.com

ORGANIZATIONS

National Association for Holistic Aromatherapy
www.naha.org

Alliance of International Aromatherapists
www.alliance-aromatherapists.org

TRAINING

The National Association for Holistic Aromatherapy approves about seventeen nondegree programs. They include the following areas of study:

- Basic anatomy and physiology
- Essential oil chemistry
- Therapeutic uses of essential oils
- Safety issues
- Blending techniques
- Botany and taxonomy

These programs represent a recommended handful. For a complete listing, see http://www.naha.org/education.htm.

Aromahead Institute, School of Essential Oil Studies
Sarasota, Florida
www.aromahead.com

RJ Buckle and Associates
Mentor, Ohio
www.rjbuckle.com

Institute of Integrative Aromatherapy
The Woodlands, Texas
www.floramedica.com

Aroma Apothecary Healing Arts Academy
Austin, Texas
www.aahaa.info

Atlantic Institute of Aromatherapy
Tampa, Florida
www.AtlanticInstitute.com

Flower Road Natural Therapies
Dallas, Texas
www.flowerroad.net

Institute of Spiritual Healing and Aromatherapy
Arvada, Colorado
www.ISHAhealing.com

The College of Botanical Healing Arts
Santa Cruz, California
www.cobha.org

ART THERAPY

Art therapy is a form of expressive therapy that uses art materials, such as paints, drawing chalk and markers, photography, and sculpture. It combines traditional psychotherapeutic theories and techniques with an understanding of the psychological aspects of the creative process, especially the emotion-inducing properties of the differing art materials and their respective results. Art therapists are able to both diagnose psychopathology via analyzing artwork and offer treatment after diagnosis via other artwork.

Art therapy uses aesthetics and self-expression to foster wholeness. The practice is rooted in the belief that the creative process develops self-awareness and creativity, which are two of the first steps toward integrated psychological well-being. Desired outcomes include: resolving inner psychological conflict, bringing about emotional catharsis, reducing stress, building self-esteem, and fostering the courage to grow and explore.

It can be a technique for licensed health care providers or a larger discipline incorporating other expressive arts, such as dance and vocal therapies. Art therapy works well with children and adolescents because, unlike many adults, they are closely tied to metaphor, symbolism, and their rawest emotions. Impaired, nonverbal populations benefit also, as do "well-adjusted" adults—who may display initial resistance to the childlike nature of the work. Art therapy settings include clinics and psychiatric centers as well as art studios.

Practitioners are most often trained and licensed in some form of clinical psychology or social work. There are also some graduate programs in the wider discipline of expressive art therapy. An art therapist can expect to learn psychodynamic theory in a manner similar to what a more traditional therapist will also learn.

The American Art Therapy Association grants the registered art therapist certificate to those with a master's degree and two years experience with a mentor—at a clinic or in private practice. This association also accredits schools in the few states where art therapy is recognized as a licensed profession.

RESOURCES

PERIODICALS

American Journal of Art Therapy
www.periodicals.com/html/ihp_e.html?ea01689

Art Therapy: Journal of the American Art Therapy Association
www.arttherapyjournal.org

Arts in Psychotherapy
www.elsevier.com/wps/find/journaldescription.cws_home/833/description#description

ONLINE

AATA Student Networking Group
http://groups.yahoo.om/group/AATAStudentNetworking

ORGANIZATIONS

American Art Therapy Association
www.arttherapy.org

The AATA was founded in 1969 and represents some 4,000 professionals and students. It offers a listing of accredited art therapy programs.

Art Therapy Credentials Board
www.atcb.org

The ATCB is an independent organization, which grants postgraduate registration (ATR) after reviewing documentation of completion of graduate education and postgraduate supervised experience.

The National Coalition of Creative Arts Therapies Associations
www.nccata.org

Represents more than 8,000 individual members of six creative arts therapies associations

International Networking Group of Art Therapists
www.adler.edu/ing

Represents professional art therapists, students, and others interested in art therapy in nearly eighty countries

Arts in Therapy Network
www.artsintherapy.com

Provides an online community for therapists and those interested in the healing arts

Expressive Therapy Concepts
www.expressivetherapy.org

Association for Creativity in Counseling
www.aca-acc.org

This integrative organization was established in 2004 as a forum for counselors, counselor educators, and counseling students interested in creative, diverse, and relational approaches to counseling.

National Board for Certified Counselors
www.nbcc.org

United States Association for Body Psychotherapy
www.usabp.org

TRAINING

Albertus Magnus College
New Haven, Vermont
www.albertus.edu

Antioch University
Seattle, Washington
www.antiochsea.edu

Caldwell College
Caldwell, New Jersey
www.caldwell.edu

College of New Rochelle
New Rochelle, New York
www.cnr.edu

Drexel University—Hahnemann Creative Arts in Therapy Program
Philadelphia, Pennsylvania
http://drexel.edu/cnhp/creativearts/default.asp

Eastern Virginia Medical School
Norfolk, Virginia
www.evms.edu/hlthprof/art-therapy.html

Emporia State University
Emporia, Kansas
www.emporia.edu/psyspe/arttherapy/athp.html

Florida State University
Tallahassee, Florida
www.fsu.edu/~are

George Washington University
Washington, DC
www.gwu.edu/~artx

Long Island University
Brookville, New York
www.liu.edu/svpa/art

Lesley University
Cambridge, Massachusetts
www.lesley.edu

Loyola Marymount University
Los Angeles, California
www.lmu.edu/mft

Marylhurst University
Marylhurst, Oregon
www.marylhurst.edu

Marywood University
Scranton, Pennsylvania
www.marywood.edu

Mount Mary College
Milwaukee, Wisconsin
www.mtmary.edu

Naropa University
Boulder, Colorado
www.naropa.edu

Nazareth College of Rochester
Rochester, New York
www.naz.edu/dept/creativearts_therapy

New York University
New York, New York
http://steinhardt.nyu.edu/art/therapy

Notre Dame de Namur University
Belmont, California
www.ndnu.edu

Phillips Graduate Institute
Encino, California
www.pgi.edu

Los Angeles Institute for Art Therapy
Los Angeles, California
www.laiat.com

Pratt Institute
New York, New York
www.pratt.edu

School of the Art Institute of Chicago
Chicago, Illinois
www.artic.edu

School of Visual Arts
New York, New York
www.schoolofvisualarts.edu

Seton Hill University
Greensburg, Pennsylvania
www.setonhill.edu

Southern Illinois University at Edwardsville
Edwardsville, Illinois
www.siue.edu/ART/areas/art_therapy

Southwestern College
Santa Fe, New Mexico
www.swc.edu

Springfield College
Springfield, Massachusetts
www.spfldcol.edu

University of Louisville
Louisville, Kentucky
www.louisville.edu/edu/ecpy/et/et.html

Ursuline College
Pepper Pike, Ohio
www.ursuline.edu

Wayne State University
Detroit, Michigan
www.wayne.edu

AYURVEDIC MEDICINE

Ayurveda's closest translation might be: "the science and knowledge of life." It is probably humankind's most ancient systematized medical tradition, as well as the medical system with the longest continuity of use. Dating back over 5,000 years to India and southeastern Asia, ayurveda was only popularly introduced into the United States in the 1970s. It has yet to attain the public acceptance experienced by traditional Chinese medicine, which was first brought to Westerners' attention during the same decade.

Ayurveda is considered by many medical historians as one of the original models for holistic healing. Although it existed well before the term "holistic" was coined in the twentieth century, ayurvedic medicine embraces all aspects of a patient's life similar to the way in which the Yoga and Hindu religion that forms the basis for ayurveda embraces all other religions as part of its own. It is a highly customized form of medicine. There is no personal detail, physical symptom or structure, emotional tendency, or spiritual thought in a patient that is considered irrelevant to a diagnosing ayurvedic practitioner. This is because every item, action, thought, and feeling has been categorized as being composed of the same five elements (earth, water, fire, air, and ether) as is the human organism itself. By altering the elemental makeup of a patient's lifestyle, the elements that compose the patient can be brought into balance, or inadvertently pushed even farther out of balance.

In ayurvedic medicine, balance equals health—with balance in this case meaning that the elements that currently compose a patient's body-mind are in similar proportion to the way they were when that patient was a healthy newborn. In addition, patients are encouraged to learn to practice preventive medicine and treatment upon themselves as much as possible, with the ayurvedic practitioner serving more as a mentor who guides his or her clients toward simultaneous spiritual, psychological, and physical balance. The major focus of ayurveda is to help patients manifest a continuously changing but balanced elemental flow in harmony with the equally changing elements of their external environments.

Nothing in the universe is static. Everything is in constant motion, although sometimes one has to look all the way to the atomic level in order to detect it. Humans can only manifest well-being when they are able to interact with the changing elements around them yet still keep within themselves the appropriate ratios of earth, water, fire, air, and ether. Thus ayurveda is not only a healing system but also a means toward radical self-knowledge and the deepest levels of self-awareness. At its most refined level, the goals of medical ayurveda and spiritual Yoga unite, with a patient's ultimate health equaling his or her enlightenment.

As would be expected from a medical system that spans multiple millennia of human existence, the methods, techniques, and philosophy of ayurveda have evolved to meet the needs of a dynamic Indian, and global, culture over time. Ayurvedic medicine shares striking similarities with other traditional methods of healing. Scholars explain that the knowledge of ayurvedic medicine spread from India by 100 B.C. and greatly influenced classical and traditional Chinese medicine, the element (or humor)-based medicine practiced by the Greeks, and the Unani medicine of the Persians. Ayurvedic and Chinese medicine then went on to mold the medical systems of the entire Asian continent, including Japan, Korea, Vietnam, and Nepal. Because of the maternal relationship with which ayurveda has nurtured other ancient medical modalities, it is sometimes referred to as the "Mother of All Healing." This concept of maternal healing may also come from ayurvedic medical philosophy, due to its adapting, balancing, forgiving, mediating, and nourishing approach to health care.

It is important to note that India has been the cultural inspirer for not just medicine but also for the religions and martial arts of Asia. In fact, although health care, religion, and fighting are viewed as three separate disciplines today, in ancient India every part of life was included within the spiritual system known then as Vedanta but known at the present time as Yoga/Hinduism.

Legend has it that some 5,000 to 10,000 years ago, holy men and women known as "rishis" amalgamated together various ancient spiritual "texts" from a longstanding oral tradition. These texts became the first recorded scriptures of humankind, known today as the Vedas—"Knowledge" or "the Truths." They became the cornerstone of Vedanta philosophy and gave birth to a remarkably elaborate and complex system of knowledge, combining the science of healthful life with the art of practical divine inspiration. The Vedic sciences, ritual methods for attaining mundane worldly attainment as well as the self-realized enlightenment of deepest universal understanding, are extrapolated from the repetitive hymns of the Vedas.

They are comprised of four main branches or principles that are instrumental in Hindu philosophy: Self-knowledge, Yoga (union with God), Vedic astrology, and ayurveda. Ayurveda encompasses the pragmatic elements of health care, including the medical modalities that address psychophysiological healing via diet, herbs, mantras, meditations, and bodywork. Because ayurveda is part of a larger system of philosophy, it cannot be isolated from the other Vedic principles. In this respect, ayurveda is not merely a system of healing, but also a philosophy, a lifestyle, and a paradigm through which to view the world. Just as a fundamental tenet of ayurvedic medicine insists that body, mind, and spirit cannot be separated, ayurveda cannot be confined in a box by itself. It is simply one part of a much larger spiritual tradition, just as traditional Chinese medicine cannot be accurately severed from its Taoist and Buddhist roots. For the purposes of this book, however, we will not discuss all elements of Vedic philosophy and Hinduism. Rather the terms and techniques that are presented in this section are those deemed relevant to the general understanding of ayurvedic medicine.

Terms

Five Elements: Although ayurveda originally spoke of just three elements (air, fire, and water), centuries ago ayurveda added the elements of earth and ether. Now all forms of existence are boiled down into the five basic elements of earth, fire, water, air, and ether. The knowledge that comes from understanding the interactions between these elements is much greater than what can be derived from their literal meanings. The five-element concept is perhaps better translated as "five guiding principles" with which to understand

and categorize the overlapping physical, psychological, and spiritual worlds of Hinduism and ayurveda. Dr. Karta Purkh Singh Khalsa, a practitioner of ayurveda for many years in Seattle, Washington, explains that the five elements are mostly symbolic. "They are metaphors for classifying the interchangeable matter and energy of the universe. They are also the means toward understanding how subtle forces can and do manifest as relative health or ill health within the human body-mind."

The transformation of water into different states is a frequently used allusion to help demonstrate the interaction of the five elements. Dr. Vasant Lad, another longtime practitioner of ayurveda as well as the founder of the Ayurvedic Institute in Albuquerque, New Mexico, explains it this way: "As a solid, water is ice—a manifestation of the Earth principle. Ice is melted when it comes into contact with fire; once it is liquefied, the earthy expression of water (ice) has transformed into the water principle. Eventually, through transpiration and evaporation, the water becomes steam, which symbolizes the air principle. The steam disappears into ether or space, and thus the five basic elements can been seen even as manifesting within one substance". Ayurveda relies on this type of explanative logic to describe the process of constant change occurring every second within all matter and energy in the universe. If indeed all process of change can be reduced to the five essential elements, then all energy and matter in the universe may be thought of as part of the same basic cosmic process of change. Therefore, the philosophy of "monism," which states there is really only One substance making up all of creation, is a vital theme within the ayurvedic healing and lifestyle guidance that is paramount to ayurvedic philosophy and treatment.

Tri-dosha: The three doshas can be translated as "those elemental combinations which become imbalanced or contaminated." They are also one of the main concepts with which ayurvedic practitioners label, categorize, and diagnose patients and everything else in the universe. The doshas are derived from the Vedic belief that all matter is comprised of five elements or principles, as we've already discussed. These elements combine to form the three doshas, which account for both the structure and function of the entire human organism as well as the organism that is the universe itself. The three doshas are: vata (ether with air), pitta (fire with water), and kapha (water with earth). Although the doshas are omnipresent, they are easier to spot in some places than others, especially within the physical human form. In this regard, they are similar to the way in which the Western mind defines physiques: thin and angular (vata), moderately muscular (pitta), and husky to voluptuous (kapha). Doshas can also be easily sensed by observing any individual body part or function and determining whether it shares more characteristics from the long list of traits that describes vata versus those that describe pitta and kapha. A patient's relative psychological dosha ratios, which may differ from their physiological ratios, can be diagnosed by observing all the elements of a patient's personality. For example, an airy, spacey personality is more vata; a fiery, competitive one is more pitta; and a sweet, possessive type is more kapha.

But the gold standard for overall dosha categorization is pulse diagnosis. By reading at least nine different pulse locations at each wrist, an ayurvedic practitioner determines not only what dosha ratio a patient manifested as a healthy infant but also how that patient has veered into doshic imbalance at the present time. This is nearly identical to the pulse diagnosis of Chinese medicine that allows a doctor insight into the specific interactions taking place between a patient's (slightly different) five-element ratios of earth, water, fire, wood, and metal. An ayurvedic patient's original dosha ratio is considered his or her ongoing constitutional type, or "prakriti." A patient's current ratio illustrates his or her relative imbalance.

A patient's prakriti, or birth constitution (also often confusingly called one's "dosha," as in, "what's your dosha?"), can be thought of as a blueprint that outlines the innate tendencies that are hard-coded into a person's body-mind. The dosha variations of prakriti and constitution that manifest as each person are the explanations as to why some people enjoy activities that others cannot stand (a pitta fire type dislikes hot showers, for example). They are also the explanations as to why people tend to feel differently about similar interpersonal situations, why people react differently to similar environmental stimuli, and why people have individual preferences at all. People with differing dominant doshas receive different kinds of therapeutic treatment.

Practitioners use keen observation skills, far superior to the ayurvedic questionnaires found in books, to determine which doshas are dominant in their patients and thus which treatments are most helpful. Normally prescribed for any patient are specific foods, herbs, massage oils, Hatha Yoga postures, mantras, and meditations. All of these treatments, as everything else in the universe, will themselves express a certain dosha ratio. At this simplest level of ayurvedic treatment explanation, all that is required is to match a patient's dosha imbalance with those modalities whose doshic makeup is in opposition to the patient's imbalance. Many other factors come into play, such as the need to detoxify or rejuvenate a patient.

In total, there are ten major dosha combinations. But there are only three "pure" doshas:

Vata: Vata is the combination of ether and air. It is that force that animates life and motivates the actions of the other two doshas. It is considered dry, light, cold, rough, subtle, and agitated. It directs nerve transmission and respiration and has its primary location in the often gas-filled colon. Vata also governs mental adaptability and creativity. A vata dominant individual tends to be physically thin, angular, and frail, with protruding veins, joints, and facial features. The skin tends to be cool and dry. Mental characteristics of Vata individuals tend to be enthusiasm, with infectious creative and vivacious energy. They are spirituality imaginative, hyperactive, with a tendency toward moodiness, anxiety, constipation, nervous disorders, and muscular cramping. Vata's energy often fluctuates, with jagged peaks and valleys. Vata types also tend to eat and sleep erratically, which helps to explain their susceptibility to anxiety and nervous tics.

Pitta: Pitta is the combination of fire and water. It primarily exists in acid form as the digestive power called "agni" but is responsible for all chemical transformations in the body. It also directs mental "digestion" in the form of clear, accurate perception. Pitta types are regarded as predictable, competitive, clearheaded, and sharp-tongued. They usually have me-

dium to muscular builds, thin fine hair, and warm perspiring skin that is often ruddy and reddish. Pitta types also are usually regimented, organized, and articulate regarding their strong personal feelings. They tend to have quick minds and are characterized by a biting intelligence that can be either critical or endearing. They tend to be motivated by pleasure (including a voracious appetite), passion, and intensity. They are warm and loving but also prone to short temperaments and stressful (for everyone), explosive outbursts. Pitta types often suffer from heartburn, ulcers, hemorrhoids, acne, and other acidic stomach ailments.

Kapha: Kapha is the combination of water and earth and is that force which provides substance and support, making up the bulk of the body tissues. It also provides our emotional depth, from greed to altruistic love. Kapha types have tendencies toward inertia, relaxation, and measured meticulousness. They are often heavyset with thick wavy hair. Their skin tends to be cool, oily, and pale. They eat slowly and sleep deeply. Kapha personality types are compassionate, forgiving, and tolerant of other's opinions. They are ponderous yet graceful, lethargic yet relaxed. They are affectionate and lovable, yet slow to act on emotional feelings. Kapha types have a predisposition to procrastination, obesity, high cholesterol, and heart disease. Wet respiratory symptoms (such as a chest "cough," from the word kapha) or sluggish digestion are also indicative of Kapha types.

Constitution: Without the advent of prakriti constitution we might all be getting the same medicine for the same condition. This is what occurred when eighteenth century allopaths departed from treatments based on the four humors, derived from the ayurvedic doshas, and instead gave the same basic treatments to every patient regardless of how it debilitated them. Given the motley mix of humanity's body types, colors, shapes, and sizes, that period of allopathic medicine could scarcely have been less scientific or logical. Ayurvedic philosophy is designed to tailor therapy and self-care to an individual based on his specific needs—it is not an arbitrary or uniform system of medical care. While the flexibility of care and medicine is largely regarded as one of ayurveda's many strengths, skeptics can also view this notion as lacking standardization, methodology, and scientific reasoning.

Prana: Prana is a focal concept in ayurvedic medicine that describes the vital energy innate within every living being. In fact, ayurveda is the mother all of vitalistic medical systems. Congruent to the Chinese concept of chi, prana is that physical and metaphysical component of life which enlivens the body-mind, unifying it with spirit. This primal pranic energy is also responsible for healing bodily ailments and restoring internal equilibrium. In ayurveda, prana is likened to a nutrient that can be taken into the body for great good and yet cause a host of (usually vata-related, airy) problems if blocked or overflowed toward imbalance. Many techniques in ayurveda are dedicated to receiving an increased amount of prana into the body and, thereby, restoring those deadened areas created by a lack of life force. In fact, within simpler versions of Yogic medicine, patients simply direct life force to ailing areas via muscle tension, relaxation, and visualization as they practice one of humankind's earliest known attempts at panacea.

According to ayurvedic tradition, prana enters the body through the breath. Learning to control this entry via visualizations, mantras, and breathing exercises are thus essential methods of patient self-care, holding an important role in health promotion for all patients of all dosha types. Control of the life force via the breath is a direct way for individuals to build life energy within themselves. Pranayama is the name given to those exercises used for directing prana and enlivening the body-mind. In Chinese medicine, these exercises are known as chi kung. One of the most common pranayama practices is "alternate nostril breathing," during which one closes off one nostril and then the other (with special finger configurations) in order to inhale and exhale out of the one nostril that remains open. Once prana has entered the body, it flows through a network of subtle energy channels. In Sanskrit, these channels are called nadis, the direct precursors to the acupuncture chi meridians of Chinese medicine.

The three major nadis are: the ida (on the left side of the spine and paralleling it), the pingala (right side of the spine), and the sushumna (the central spinal channel, connecting the six or seven major energy wheels or chakras from the coccyx to the cranium). The interaction between prana's often intangible energy flow and its psychophysiological pathways throughout the body-mind is symbolic of the ever-present, but often difficult to perceive, connection between body, mind, and spirit within Vedanta dogma. The same prana that the spiritual practitioner manipulates to achieve enlightenment is manipulated by the ayurvedic practitioner so that it at least flows in the proper channels at the proper rate and helps patients manifest optimal health.

The Rasas: The rasas are the six tastes within food, drink, herbs, etc. that are so important to the ayurvedic doctor because diet and herbal medicine form the core of ayurvedic treatment modalities. These tastes are: sweet, salty, sour, pungent, bitter, and astringent. Each rasa is made up of two elements, just as each dosha is made up of two elements. For example, the strong to mild sweet tastes of pure sugar and whole grains is composed of earth and water. Since the kapha dosha is also composed of earth and water, kapha excess may be created via eating a few too many refined sweets or way too many complex carbohydrates. The salty tastes of pure salt and seaweed are composed of the elements water and fire. So these kinds of foods are ideally kept to a minimum in the diets of pitta types, since pitta is also composed of water and fire. Vata types, already dominated by the elements air and ether, are usually recommended to reduce their intake of bitter herbs, such as aloe and golden seal, that are also composed of mostly air and ether. The other three tastes: sour (earth and fire), pungent (fire and air), and astringent (earth and air) have less impact on pure dosha types.

The Gunas: Within the Taoist traditions that form the backbone of Chinese medicine, the entire universe is divided into relative dark, feminine, passive "yin" and relative light, masculine, assertive "yang." The five elements are then born from this dualistic realm. Similarly, in the Yoga/Hindu traditions that inspire ayurveda, there is a pre-elemental dividing up of the universe that is important to understand in terms of practical patient health care. Instead of yin and yang, Indian Yogis divided the world into three forces, or "gunas": sattva, rajas, and tamas.

Sattva is the spiritual force most attuned with God. It is calm, harmonious, loving, serviceful, wholesome, and positively charged. Rajas is the universal activating force, from the Big Bang to the needs and desires of humankind and beyond. It is exciting, electric, engrossing, insistent, and neutrally charged. Tamas is the inhibitory force, the yin to rajas' yang. It is banal, sluggish, evil, toxic, and negatively charged.

Each dosha type can manifest the full spectrum from sattvic to rajasic and tamasic. For example, a kapha type may at first manifest mostly tamasic lethargy, then evolve a bit to express passionate possessiveness, and finally become a sattvic individual emitting peace, devotion, and loyalty. Similarly, vata types can evolve from fearfulness through hyperactivity and on to energetic creativity. Pitta types can move from hateful anger through aggressive ambition and on to warm and friendly leadership.

Ayurvedic Diagnosis

When a patient visits an ayurvedic doctor, there is the usual oral and written medical history given by the patient, followed by a macro- and microanalysis of the patient's body-mind and any existing symptoms. Instead of prioritizing symptom and disease labeling, ayurvedic doctors are looking to determine a patient's dosha ratio when it is functioning well. This is the same ratio that manifested in the patient when he or she was a healthy child. From that point, the practitioner determines in which direction the doshas have become imbalanced and in what specific body tissues. The practitioner then proceeds to use a variety of techniques to restore that patient's unique elemental balance.

Ayurvedic doctors use all of their senses to determine nearly every aspect of a patient's body-mind (for example, visually assessing overall skin color and freckling, listening to style of conversation, being aware of any specific body aromas, and observing whether the joints are very prominent). Especially important are diagnoses of the eyes, nails, lips, and tongue. Overall, this exam is similar to the "Four Examinations" of Chinese medicine. The doctor mentally computes the likely relative guna and dosha ratios of the patient's current presentation and proceeds to perform the gold standard of prakriti and constitutional determination: pulse diagnosis.

There are three pulse positions to read on each wrist, corresponding to vata, pitta, and kapha. There are also at least two levels of depth to read at each pulse position, corresponding to the superficiality or relative depth of the dosha imbalance. Combining this authoritative final opinion of pulse diagnosis with all of the earlier observations performed by the doctor as soon as the patient was introduced, the doctor now understands what kind of dosha deviation has occurred from what specific prakriti constitution manifested by the patient at conception (hypothetically) and birth.

Treatment

The ayurvedic doctor prescribes specific foods, herbs, and meditations that help to rebalance a patient's doshas and also reduce the amount of ama (toxins) in a patient's body-mind. Because everything—thought, feeling, activity, and item—in the universe is classified as being composed of certain ratios of the five elements as well as certain ratios of the three gunas, an ayurvedic doctor can give guidance to patients regarding the ideal composition of the types of thoughts and feelings they should cultivate as well as the activities they should practice and the items they should surround themselves with. To complement, or even take priority over, their dietary and herbal recommendations for patients, ayurvedic doctors give individualized guidance regarding: what type of oil to use for the daily, full-body self-massage that is recommended for all types; what colors to wear and to place within one's environment; what gems to wear next to the skin, via necklace, bracelet, etc.; and which Yoga postures (asanas), prayers and affirmations (mantras), breathwork (pranayama), and meditations are best suited for each person. Prescribing certain gem and Yoga activities are more specific to the ayurvedic subspecialties of Vedic astrology and Yoga therapy. Thus, most ayurvedic patients may have these items left out of their treatment plans. But a patient should not be surprised to receive gem and Yoga prescriptions from any ayurvedic doctor, since in the practitioner's mind, there is no real separation between medicine, astrology, religion, Yoga, or anything else. In Yoga and Hinduism all is one since all is God. It is only the less-than perfectly accurate perceptions of God's creations that sense separation where there is none. This belief stretches to ayurvedic medicine, in which any part of the whole can be used to balance (or ignorantly imbalance) patients' constantly changing doshas.

Beyond the abovementioned treatment methods, ayurvedic doctors will also often ask their patients to consider an intensive form of treatment called "panchakarma (or the "five actions"). This is especially true if the patient is from a culture that greatly ignores preventive medicine. Panchakarma traditionally lasts for approximately forty-five days, although in the United States it is usually truncated to five to ten days due to convenience and cost factors. Whereas a forty-five day treatment in India will cost around $850, a week-long panchakarma treatment in the U.S. can run several thousand dollars and be heavily altered in order to please Americans squeamish about internal body fluids. The intention behind panchakarma is to remove physical and energetic toxins (called ama) from the body and also to influence the flow of excessive doshas throughout a patient's body-mind so that his or her prakriti balance can be deeply, and more easily, retained for the long term. When this is accomplished, the patient's physical tissues are revitalized. This is why, within ayurvedic medicine, panchakarma is believed to be a premier anti-aging rejuvenative.

Using the formula from the longer lasting, forty-five-day panchakarma still provided in India today, each panchakarma patient first switches to a diet of whole grain rice and cooked mung beans (not mung sprouts). This is one of the classic complementary protein diets (similar to Mexican corn tortillas and pinto beans) that most native cultures have concocted for times when complete protein containing animal products were scarce. It is also an easy and quick-to-prepare dish that is considered "tri-doshic." This means that every prakriti type may eat it and know that it is either improving, or at least not worsening, whatever imbalanced dosha ratio the patient is currently experiencing.

Following these ten days of dietary preparation, a second preparatory treatment begins. Each day, for four to five days, patients receive an invigorating but soothing oil massage called "abhyanga." Abhyanga strokes are more similar to the long, medium-depth,

Swedish-style of massage techniques versus the frequently forceful and painful deep-tissue massage methods popular in the United States. The thirty- to sixty-minute abhyanga massage is designed to mobilize a patient's excess ama and doshas so that they will be easier to expel during the subsequent panchakarma actions that focus mainly on the digestive system. During abhyanga, certain points on the patients are pressed in order to stimulate the balanced flow of life force within the patient. It is these "marma" points that are believed to have later evolved into the acupuncture chi points of Chinese medicine. The main difference that external observers would note if comparing abhyanga to massage as seen in the West is that ayurvedic patients are asked to shift their positions from seated to supine to prone to lying on their sides, etc., as the massage progresses. This allows the practitioner to access the patient's body and manipulate the flow of life force, ama, and doshas from several different angles.

A third pretreatment may be used by an ayurvedic practitioner to open up the marma dotted "nadis," or channels, that allow the life force, doshas, and ama to move in the first place. These nadis are believed to be the precursors of the chi meridians in Chinese medicine, and in panchakarma, they serve as vehicles that lead directly to the stomach and intestines. In ayurveda, a variety of sweat-inducing treatments (swedana) are used to widen the nadis, such as a twenty-minute stint in an enclosed herbal steam bath. The combination of abhyanga massage and swedana sweating has prepared the patient to efficiently expel toxic material starting with the first step of panchakarma proper.

"Vamana," or therapeutic vomiting, is this first step. The ama and excess doshas that have been concentrated in the digestive system from the pretreatments can now be expelled from either direction. Vomiting is usually induced first by having the patient drink a nauseating herbal concoction or salt water. Although Western patients have much distaste for vomiting, either from memories of the flu or food poisoning or bulimia, patients from the East do not typically have such cultural inhibitions. To these patients, occasional vamana is usually experienced as a refreshing release. Western panchakarma clinics, on the other hand, often leave out this important step altogether to avoid the undeniable misgivings of American patients.

When vamana has been judged successful by the practitioner, usually after one to three days, "virichana" purgation begins. This is a procedure in which oral herbal laxatives are given to patients so that the ama and doshas that entered their intestinal tracts can be effectively removed. Once this has been deemed successful after a day or two, "vasthi" enemas are prescribed on subsequent days. The last step is to remove any ama or doshas from the respiratory system via the nose. This is called "nasya" and is performed via the inhaling of hot herbal infusions as well as oiling and massaging the inside and outside of the nose. A sixth treatment, "rakta moksha" or bloodletting, was commonly used in panchakarma until the modern era. Both the East and the West have largely eliminated therapeutic bloodletting from their protocols due to patient distaste and blood borne pathologies, although using blood-sucking leeches to assist in reconstructive surgery is now widely accepted within modern allopathy.

The follow-up, or panchakarma posttreatment, is for patients to follow that specific lifestyle which will keep their dosha imbalancing and toxin formation at bay. This means they are to eat, exercise, herbally medicate, think, and pray in such ways that will be specific to their prakriti. One person's medicine is another person's poison.

One last treatment to mention, among many, many others, is the practice of "shirodhara," or "head flow." This technique is commonly photographed to represent ayurveda, although it is practiced in a minority of cases. Shirodhara involves the pouring of unadulterated or medicated oils or milks upon the forehead of a patient as they lie supine upon a comfortable table. The flow of oil or milk is constant and continues for up to an hour. It is believed to be one of the best treatments for nervous system pathologies, such as anxiety and depression, and it is also used for pain management, chronic headaches, and upper respiratory ailments. It is thought to stimulate the flow of serotonin and melatonin from the pineal gland, located a few inches below the skin surface of the forehead area being stimulated by the flowing oil. Normally, shirodhara is combined with other ayurvedic therapies in true holistic fashion, since any therapy performed in a practitioner's office is less important than a patient's day-to-day habitual activities.

These ancient panchakarma treatments are remarkably similar to the vomiting, purging, and bloodletting days of allopathy that went on for centuries from the Renaissance through colonial times. The main difference between the two systems is that ayurvedic practitioners use panchakarma as an occasional, specialized, and individualized toxin-dispelling treatment. Day-to-day ayurvedic treatments are highly individualized diet, herb, and meditation practices. Conversely, allopaths used these harsh treatments as their main medical modalities without the pretreatment diagnostics of a patient's constitutional type and specific dosha imbalance.

There has been a fair amount of Western science applied to ayurvedic medicine in general as well as to panchakarma in specific. However, much of this research has been sponsored by highly biased organizations such as the Maharishi University of Management in Fairfield, Iowa. This university is part of the transnational empire of the recently deceased Maharishi Mahesh Yogi (the Beatles' short-term guru), whose organization made millions on the sales of ayurvedic remedies over the last two decades. One panchakarma research study resulted from the alliance of Maharishi University and the Colorado State University Department of Environmental Health in 2002. Eighty-eight subjects, aged forty-five and older, had the fat-soluable toxins in their blood measured. Those who had received panchakarma, versus those who had not, carried significantly fewer toxins in their blood compared to the untreated subjects. More impressively, fifteen subjects who received two months of panchakarma treatment were found to have an approximately 50 percent reduction in the two measured fat soluable blood toxins. Although no control group was used for this study, the normal rate for reduction of fat soluable toxins was stated to be only a fraction of 1 percent.

More unbiased and comprehensive research on panchakarma and other ayurvedic modalities is needed. For those desiring scientific backup for their ayurvedic leanings, however, at least the biased studies seem to support ayurveda's effectiveness based upon the Western model of detoxification. Validating alterations of patients' ama and dosha balance will be next to impossible.

Career Information

Holistic education is undoubtedly one of the fastest growing medical economies in the United States. Integrative medicine is now viewed by many as the answer to America's health care crisis as well as the solution to chronic and previously untreatable diseases.

Ayurveda is a large factor in this solution because it emphasizes a true mind-body-spirit model centered on self-responsibility and preventative care. Ayurvedic practitioners may choose to enter or start a private practice, join other practitioners at a wellness center, teach about ayurveda in the public sector, supervise and oversee retreat centers, teach at private holistic institutions, and/or conduct workshops or seminars. Current holistic and nonholistic practitioners can enhance their healing credentials by offering ayurvedic services to their clients. Because it is an extremely flexible discipline—a philosophy as well as a holistic model for health—the future is bright for ayurveda and practitioners who are dedicated to making this ancient wisdom accessible and available.

With that said, ayurveda is just beginning to become known in North America, and its acceptance next to other modalities such as acupuncture has a long way to go. Among 31,000 Americans surveyed, only four-tenths of 1 percent had ever used ayurveda, and one-tenth of 1 percent had used it in the past twelve months. About 750,000 people in the United States have ever used ayurveda and 150,000 in the last twelve months.

Prospective students should take this into account, since there are many other CAM choices that will provide an easier, more lucrative path to career success. A more likely option is to be certified as an ayurvedic practitioner after receiving a base license featured in this book.

Regulation, Licensure, and Certification

There is no ayurvedic license in the United States. The practice is not regulated by state or federal agencies. As a result, standards of competency are defined by institutions and organizations that have received state approval but not accreditation.

Because of these conditions, ayurvedic practitio-

ners are taught how to practice legally within a limited scope so that they *are not* viewed as practicing medicine without a license. Ayurvedic professionals are not legally responsible for their treatment recommendations, and their diagnostic methods and techniques are not regarded as legitimate medical practices in the eyes of the federal government. Ayurveda's status is analogous to the popular conception of Chinese medicine in the early 1970s. Practitioners and enthusiasts alike are convinced that federal recognition and regulation will come within the next ten years, although there is currently no political or legislative evidence to support this belief.

Tuition and Graduation Statistics

Tuition for ayurvedic programs in the United States typically ranges from $1,000 to $2,000 per semester, although less expensive and less rigorous programs certainly exist. Because ayurveda is not nationally recognized as a formal medicine, there is no standardized system of financial aid. Tuition discounts and private aid are available on a school-to-school basis. American schools are typically part-time "certification" courses that take from one to two years to complete.

RESOURCES

BOOKS

Textbook of Ayurveda by Dr. Vasant Lad

Aghora: At the Left Hand of God by Robert Svoboda

Ayurveda and the Mind: The Healing of Consciousness by Dr. David Frawley

PERIODICALS

Ayurvedic Holistic Community
http://ayurvedahc.com/articlelive
A journal on several types of holistic healing

ONLINE

Ayurvedic Health Center
www.ayurvedic.org

This comprehensive site is maintained by the Jiva Ayurvedic Research Institute. Click on "Ayurveda Education" and then "Science of Ayurveda" to read about the origin, definition, basic principles of ayurveda, and causes and treatment for common diseases. Determine your ayurvedic constitution.

HealthWorld Online: Ayurvedic Medicine

www.ayurvedic.com

A detailed site maintained by Dr. Vasant Lad of the Ayurvedic Institute

Dhanvantri Aushadhalaya

www.dhanvantri.com

This site has categorized and detailed information on ayurveda, including a list of ayurvedic practitioners.

Saffron Soul

www.saffronsoul.com

This excellent site offers comprehensive information on ayurveda, Yoga, massage, and panchakarma. It also includes links to related online journals and a directory of professionals.

SpiritWeb

www.spiritweb.org/Spirit/ayurveda.html

This site briefly describes the basic principles of ayurveda and provides a list of related Web sites.

ORGANIZATIONS

National Ayurvedic Medical Association

www.ayurvedic-association.org

NAMA is a nonprofit professional trade association representing the ayurvedic profession in the United States. Its purpose is to preserve, improve, and promote ayurvedic medicine through the provision of leadership within the ayurvedic profession.

American Council of Vedic Astrology

www.vedicastrology.org

This nonprofit educational organization is dedicated to teaching the art and science of Vedic astrology or Jyotish.

California Association of Ayurvedic Medicine

www.ayurveda-caam.org

CAAM provides a unified voice for the advancement of the ayurvedic profession, as well as membership benefits for practitioners in the area.

National Institute of Ayurvedic Medicine

http://niam.com

Established by Scott Gerson, MD, this site provides a definition of ayurveda and a detailed description of the basic principles of ayurveda. NIAM also offers correspondence courses.

Chavarcode Ayurvedic Research Center

www.chavarcode.com

The center provides basic information about ayurvedic medicine as well as consultants and a list of medications for specific illness.

TRAINING

American Institute of Vedic Studies

Santa Fe, New Mexico
www.vedanet.com

Ayurveda Institute of America

Foster City, California
www.ayurvedainstitute.com

Ayurvedic Institute

Albuquerque, New Mexico
www.ayurveda.com

California College of Ayurveda

Grass Valley, California
www.ayurvedacollege.com

College of Maharishi Vedic Medicine

Fairfield, Iowa
www.mum.edu/cmvs/ba

Heritage College

Denver, Colorado
Kansas City, Missouri
Manassas, Virginia
Oklahoma City, Oklahoma
Wichita, Kansas
www.heritage-education.com

Heritage Institute

Fort Myers and Jacksonville, Florida

Kerala Ayurveda Academy and Clinic

Seattle, Washington
www.ayurvedaacademy.com

The National Institute of Ayurvedic Medicine (NIAM)
Brewster, New York
www.niam.com

New England Institute of Ayurvedic Medicine/ International Institute of Ayurveda
Worcester, Massachusetts
ayurveda@hotmail.com

Offers a one-year certification program of classroom instruction in ayurveda and additional programs for internship and advanced training programs. Also runs an ayurvedic clinic for panchakarma and other procedures

Southwest Institute of Healing Arts
Tempe, Arizona
www.swiha.org

BIOENERGETIC ANALYSIS

Bioenergetic analysis is a body-centered psychotherapy. It is based on the balance of energy flow through the body and provides a way of understanding personality. Dr. Alexander Lowen, founder of Bioenergetic Analysis, writes in his book *Bioenergetics*: "Every physical expression of the body has meaning; the quality of a handshake, the posture, the look in the eyes, the tone of the voice, the way of moving, etc. If these expressions are fixed and habitual, they tell a story of past experiences. The interpretation of fixed, physical attitudes and the work upon chronic muscular tensions which underlie them, add a dimension of reality to the therapeutic experience." Successful treatment results in greater patient fulfillment via increased spontancity, creative self-expression, and the inherent feelings of well-being that occur via the smooth, unblocked flow of life force. Requiring greater patient effort and participation than most psychotherapies, body-centered approaches tend to offer quicker results due to treating closer to the root causes of mental illness.

Founded by Alexander Lowen, MD, and John Pierrakos, MD, bioenergetics comes directly from the groundbreaking work of their teacher, psychiatrist and modern-day allopathic vitalist, Wilhelm Reich, MD. Reich was a protégé of Sigmund Freud and a colleague of Carl Jung, and all three devoted their lives to perfecting psychoanalysis in their own way. Reich named his contribution, "orgonomy," from the esoteric sounding word "orgone." This was Reich's name for the same vital force called "prana" in ayurveda, "chi" in Chinese medicine, and a thousand other names before and since. Reich had discovered that chronic patterns of emotional and sexual repression result in chronic patterns of predictable muscular tension occurring in horizontal bands across the body. These bands interrupt the flow of orgone energy from head to toe and result in all known psychopathologies. Because these bands begin developing before children have even begun to talk, Reich believed that this was one reason Freud-style talk-only therapy was so ineffective. Instead, he believed the psychiatrist must aim directly at the site of the original psychopathology: the emotions stored in the patient's muscles.

Reich placed an initial emphasis on understanding and labeling his patients' emotional character traits, writing the classic *Character Analysis* still used by psychologists today. The heart of Reich's work consisted of helping patients re-establish the healthy emotional flexibility of a child while attaining fully grounded success in the world of adults. In general, orgonomy achieves this by helping patients relive and intensely act out previously unreleased emotions while lying on a comfortable padded treatment table. The orgonomist is able to assist patients, via targeted finger pressure on specific "frozen" body parts, to more fully express their unresolved emotions built up since babyhood. Once this occurs repeatedly in therapy, and once this also becomes a regular option for the patient outside of therapy, this is a sign that the patient's chronic muscular bands are dissolving. The patient's orgone is now said to be moving more freely with each session of emotional and physical release, and psychological health improves likewise. Not a mere theorizer, Reich also invented machines to measure his patients' relative physiological relaxation so that he could quantify the effects of his therapy.

In a typical initial bioenergetic session, practitioners try to identify commonly circumscribed human character traits that manifest in their patients' personalities—just as in orgonomy. The six main categories of Reich's original character analysis include: schizoid, oral, masochistic, psychopathic, rigid, and narcissistic. Each occurs due to a different pattern of sexual and emotional repression experienced by the child in response to parents, teachers, friends, and the overall culture.

Once an unyielding character "armor" is detected, bioenergetic treatment helps patients "discharge" their repressed emotions by having them assume various "stress positions" that elicit strong emotions from them. Although these emotions are probably as partially repressed as they were when the patient held them back as a child, the bioenergeticist can then guide these patients to fuller, more healthful expression of these and all other emotions. First, these new skills are learned and embodied in therapy sessions, and soon they are transferred into the patient's entire life. According to Lowen, his stress positions accomplish the identical result as the traditional hands-on approach of an orgonomist, working with a patient on a treatment table. Common stress positions may be as peaceful as taking deep breaths, as challenging as remaining in a deep squatting position, or as violent as beating a pile of mattresses. Therapy is individualized. Although because there are a limited number of character types, the practitioner sees the same body armoring patterns repeatedly. Bioenergetic analysis can be practiced both as an individual and group psychotherapy.

The International Institute for Bioenergetic Analysis (IIBA) certifies and regulates this healing modality. Training programs are available through the institute and exist in two phases: preclinical and clinical. In the preclinical phase, students spend time understanding the philosophy behind bioenergetic analysis and read a lot of Reich and Lowen. In the clinical phases, students learn the pragmatic, manipulative methods. The IIBA will only certify a student as a bioenergetic therapist if he or she has previously attained a valid license to practice psychotherapy.

RESOURCES

ONLINE

BodyPsych
www.bodypsych.com
A great general resource for expressive body psychotherapies

ORGANIZATIONS

The International Institute for Bioenergetic Analysis
www.bioenergetic-therapy.com
The only place in the United States to become certified in bioenergetic analysis

San Diego Institute for Bioenergetic Analysis
www.sdiba.org

Dallas Society for Bioenergetic Analysis
www.bioenergetics-dallas.com

New York Society for Bioenergetic Analysis
www.bioenergetics-nyc.org

United States Association for Body Psychotherapy
www.usabp.org

Chicago Society for Bioenergetic Analysis
www.bioenergetics-chicago.org

Florida Society for Bioenergetic Analysis
www.bioenergetics-society.com

BIOFEEDBACK

Biofeedback was formulated in the West by multiple American scientists and psychologists during the 1960s. It is the process of recording a patient's physiological signals, such as muscle tension, skin temperature, and brain waves, and signaling them back to the patient via sounds or visuals. This is done so that the patient can recognize what it takes to voluntarily alter normally involuntary physiological states, usually related to relaxation and well-being, while training in a treatment room. This is similar to other therapies that help patients become aware of their normally involuntary psychological processes so that they can learn to voluntarily control those as well. Newly learned skills are then transferred into everyday life, giving patients greater control over their general health as well as over the moment-to-moment psychological states. These states always have some correlation to measurable physiological changes. Biofeedback can be an effective nondrug therapy for adjusting deep-seated psychophysiological patterns. Biofeedback is excellent for reducing stress, panic attacks, insomnia, chronic headaches, asthmatic attacks, ADHD, incontinence, and chronic pain. Unlike medication, it fosters a patient's ability to concentrate. Unlike many other manipulative therapies, biofeedback relies on the patient's ability to heal himself or herself. The biofeedback practitioner acts more as a technical guide than a probing therapist. By observing vital signs in real time (such as heartbeat and respiratory rate), clients can learn to consciously change their internal physiological processes. Patricia Norris, former clinical director of the Biofeedback and Psychophysiology Clinic in Topeka, Kansas, equates biofeedback practice to a sport: "With practice, biofeedback skills continue to improve. If you stop taking lessons but continue playing, your game will improve. With biofeedback, it works the same way. The more you practice, the better you get."

In a typical session, electrodes are placed on the skin, and the client is guided through mental techniques (such as counting and visualization). The biofeedback device monitors the patient's skin temperature and tracks brain activity. Patient skill progress can be easily measured as the computer tracks the current session and compares data with past results.

Eastern traditions have known for centuries that normally involuntary physiological processes could be voluntarily controlled via diligent training. Yogis regularly demonstrated their control over pain, respiration, circulation, and mental anguish millennia before Westerners proved that such things were possible via scientific research. Because biofeedback is a form of concentration similar to meditation, practitioners of Eastern faiths believe it can be used for much more than improved health and relaxation. They maintain it can be used to attain full enlightenment if used with spiritual attention. Similar to the Western approach to Hatha Yoga, however, biofeedback has been desacralized and removed from its original spiritual traditions. Has the baby been thrown out with the bathwater?

Certification in biofeedback is provided by the Biofeedback Certification Institute of America. The entry-level prerequisite to become certified is that you are first a licensed health worker of some sort. There are several different educational programs and formats detailed on the institute's Web site.

RESOURCES

ONLINE

HolisticMed Online
www.holisticonline.com/Biofeedback.htm
General resource for information on biofeedback

Biofeedback Network
www.biofeedback.net

ORGANIZATIONS

Association for Applied Psychophysiology and Biofeedback
www.aapb.org
General membership and advocacy organization

Biofeedback Certification Institute of America
www.bcia.org
Various certificate programs

Menninger Clinic
www.menninger.edu
A holistic clinic that pioneered biofeedback, the Menninger Clinic conducts research, treatment, and workshops in many types of psychotherapies.

BODY-MIND CENTERING

Body-mind centering is the work of Bonnie Bainbridge Cohen. Cohen began her research in human development and experiential anatomy in 1959. She holds a degree in occupational therapy; she is certified as a neurodevelopmental therapist by Dr. and Mrs. Bobath in England, as a Laban movement analyst by the Laban/ Bartenieff Institute of Movement Studies in New York, and as a Kestenberg movement profiler by Dr. Judith Kestenberg. Her research and discoveries have been fed by her studies in dance, dance therapy, neuromuscular re-education, Katsugen Undo (a method of engaging in automatic movement), Yoga, craniosacral therapy, and zero balancing.

There is no mention of the influence of Wilhelm Reich, MD, on her life's work. However, the basic principles of body-mind centering are similar to Reich's theories of orgonomy developed from the

1920s through the 1950s in Austria, Sweden, and the United States. This quote of Ms. Cohen unites their work poetically:

> "The mind is like the wind,
> and the body is like the sand;
> if you want to know
> how the wind is blowing,
> look at the sand. "

Individual sessions with a practitioner are customized for each patient. In response to patients' needs, a practitioner chooses from a combination of hands-on work, movement therapy, guided imagery, playful props, and dialogue, based upon the physiological patterns and developmental preferences of each individual. Infant/family/group sessions are also available. Patients discover their postural strengths and weaknesses and learn new ways to think, feel, and move in response to their own, and others', ever-changing psychophysiological states.

In 1973, Cohen founded the School for Body-Mind Centering, now licensed and located in Amherst, Massachusetts. The school offers an intensive four-year practitioner certification program, a rigorous training requiring experiential and academic studies in anatomy, physiology, kinesiology, touch and "repatterning," movement, psychology and counseling, the arts (performance, visual, or literary), nutrition, and mind/spiritual practice. There is also a graduate certification program for teachers and shorter programs leading to certification as a somatic movement educator, body-mind centering and Yoga and infant developmental movement education. Certification programs are offered in Massachusetts and Germany.

The practice is commonly used in conjunction with other movement-based expressive therapies such as dance therapy, voice therapy, music therapy, and art therapy as well as other introspection-based movement therapies such as Hatha Yoga, various bodywork modalities, occupational therapy, and sports massage.

RESOURCES

BOOKS

Sensing, Feeling, and Action: The Experiential Anatomy of Body-Mind Centering by Bonnie Bainbridge Cohen

A Shooting Smile by Piera Teatini

The Practical Application of Body-Mind Centering in Dance Pedagogy by Martha Eddy

Boundaries, Defense and War by Linda Hartley

ONLINE

Bellevue Massage Therapy
www.bellevuemassagetherapy.com/body-mind-centering.html

Robert Schulman
www.schulmanmd.com/html/dr__schulman__body_mind_center.html

Body-Mind Centering by Kate O'Boyle
homepage.eircom.net/~kateoboyle1/bodymind.htm

ORGANIZATIONS

Body-Mind Centering Association
www.bmcassoc.org

The School for Body-Mind Centering
www.bodymindcentering.com

This three-decade-old-school offers a certificate program in practitioner of body-mind centering and teacher of body-mind centering.

Institute for Integrative Bodywork and Movement Therapy
www.ibmt.co.uk/body-mind-centering

Offers workshops in body-mind centering and a plethora of other movement-based modalities

Body-Mind Centering in North Carolina
www.bmc-nc.com

United States Association for Body Psychotherapy
www.usabp.org

This nonprofit membership group advances the art, science, and practice of body psychotherapy.

COLOR THERAPY

Color therapy, also known as chromotherapy, is based on the premise that colors have a variety of effects upon our physical bodies, mental health, and spiritual harmony.

It was invented at least as long ago as the millennia-old founders of ayurvedic medicine in India, classical Chinese medicine, and ancient Egyptian medicine. The latter constructed solariums with interchangeable colored panes of glass so that prescribed light of different colors could shine upon patients in whatever shade deemed therapeutic. Avicenna (980–1037), one of the fathers of scientific Western medicine from the Middle East, used color not only as a treatment but also as a method of diagnosis. He constructed diagnostic charts based on the changing colors of patients' disease symptoms. As late as the nineteenth century, European smallpox victims and their sickrooms were draped with red cloth to draw the disease away from their bodies. Bernard Jensen, DC, American father of iridology, used a color therapy "chapel" for decades at his Hidden Valley Health Ranch through the 1970s.

Color is a form of energy, a property of light—one of the most fundamental aspects of the existential universe. Just as the multigalactic universe has different energy fields, which absorb and reflect light, so color therapists believe that our "body universes" have different energy fields, called chakras within ayurvedic medicine, that respond differently to external light stimuli. Each of the seven major chakras, which line the spine from coccyx to crown, has an associated color that corresponds with the "rainbow" color spectrum.

- **Red:** First Chakra—located at the coccyx.

- **Orange:** Second Chakra—sacrum/pelvis area

- **Yellow:** Third Chakra—solar plexus

- **Green:** Fourth Chakra—heart

- **Blue:** Fifth Chakra—throat

- **Indigo:** Sixth Chakra—medulla; reflects to lower forehead

- **Violet:** Seventh Chakra—top of the head

Each chakra is related to specific states of body-mind-spirit health. If a color therapist assesses that a patient is imbalanced, regarding one or more chakra functions, then the appropriate color can be introduced to the client via light, clothing, and imagery.

Color therapists say that each color has properties that target a specific zone of the body-mind. Color therapy attempts to "tune" the ailing organism so that it may more effortlessly express optimal wellness. The color red, for example, stimulates brain wave activity, increases the heart rate, and excites sexual glands. It is said to be a good color to wear or look at if one has a cold or poor circulation. But color therapy is about keeping a delicate balance; too much red can overstimulate the body and cause stress, making illness worse. High blood pressure, for instance, is an indicator of too much red energy in the body. Blue, on the other hand, is a cooler color, which correlates to the throat chakra. Blue color therapy is thus believed to be a good way to counteract hypertension and treat respiratory illness.

Color therapy is not only practiced by certified practitioners. It is one of many self-therapies that can be used by anyone. Sessions with color therapists might involve focusing meditation on a specific color or writing on the skin with colored markers, as well as the more ancient methods detailed above. This therapy is a controversial modality, as no studies have been done on the correlation between health and color or the efficacy of wearing different colors to enhance mood. Certification programs and training in advanced chromotherapy are available through the institutions listed below.

RESOURCES

BOOKS

Color Medicine: The Secrets of Color/Vibrational Healing by Charles Klotsche

How to Heal with Color by Ted Andrews

Healing with Color Zone Therapy by Joseph Corvo

Colors of the Soul: Transform Your Life Through Color Therapy by June Mcleod

ONLINE

About.com
healing.about.com/cs/colortherapy/a/aa_colortherapy.htm

Self-Help: Color Therapy
www.users.totalise.co.uk/~tmd/color.htm

Features an online color demonstration which relegates colors to specific moods

ORGANIZATIONS

Color Medicine
colormedicine.com/index.htm

Offers courses in color medicine and bio-chakra medicine

The Color Medicine Group
colormedicine.net

BioChakra Research Institute
biochakra.com

Offers training, classes, seminars, and general information about color therapy

Color Therapy Healing
www.colourtherapyhealing.com

An information and networking resource for professional color therapists

Colour Energy Home Page
www.colourenergy.com

A group that sells color-therapy tools for practitioners and patients

Color Therapy: The Power of Color
www.suza.com

Musings on color therapy and the meaning of color. Featuring photography by esteemed color researcher Suza Scalora

Color Therapy and Meditation
http://myth.com/color/opening.html

An interactive online demonstration of color meditation

CORE ENERGETICS

Core energetics is a body-centered psychotherapy that focuses on the totality of a client's health as manifested by his or her physical and emotional expressiveness. It was founded over twenty years ago by John C. Pierrakos, MD, also the cofounder of Bio-Energetic Analysis. Core energetics is inspired by the classical and radical psychoanalytic theories of Wilhelm Reich, protégé of Sigmund Freud and colleague of Carl Jung. The therapy enables patients to discharge repressed sexuality and emotions held within the body musculature in the form of "body armoring." These horizontal bands of armoring are chronic patterns of muscular and emotional rigidity that begin to form in infancy at the latest. This is a premise consistent with many body-centered psychotherapies: the mental and emotional are inextricably linked to the physical. Core energetics promotes deep, transformative, full-body experiences of emotional catharsis. Over time, this leads to increased spontaneity, freedom of movement, creative self-expression, and greater moment-to-moment well-being. Within Reich's "orgonomy" therapy, and Pierrakos's bioenergetics and core energetics, the more extensive the body armoring from earlier sexual and emotional repression, the greater a person's general psychological misery. Rather than tending to individual symptoms, body-centered therapists seek to alter psychopathology nearer its roots within the physical structure.

The Core Energetic Model has concentric circles, which form our layers of energy and defense systems. The center is a pulsing moving energy of life and is called the core. This is our life force, which seeks constantly to expand, grow, and evolve. When in touch with this part of ourselves, we feel love for our fellow creatures and ourselves. It is our connection to our spiritual nature. It is this focus on the spiritual essence of each patient—on each patient as a perfect soul—that separates core energetics from Reich's atheistic work and Pierrakos's previous offering of bioenergetic analysis.

Surrounding the always loving "core" is every person's "primal wound." When, as children, we are not allowed to protest or to express our pain or sexuality, the energy of the primal wound becomes stagnant and produces the next layer of defense. This is the "physical armoring" that can be viewed by the practitioner as muscular rigidity and lack of full emotional spontaneity. The final layer of the "social mask" is what we wear to protect ourselves from rejection from others. It is what we believe we should be like, act like, and think like—but it is not us. It is a false self far removed and out of touch with our divine core.

The process of core energetics is to transform the negativity and distortions of the social mask into the creative and positive energy of the core. This can be likened to turning on the light in a once-scary closet and seeing that the feared monsters are in reality just items of clothing. We don't show our dark, wounded sides to others, because it is very tender. But they are there and quite obvious to a trained observer. The therapist guides patients to discover in their bodies both repressed feelings and the physical blocks associated with those feelings. Core energetics includes a lot of bodywork and energy work, because whatever happens to the child that becomes the patient is registered in the patient's physical body. This repressed energy helps to create the physical body, although in deviant ways. By working to dissolve the physical body's armoring, and by transforming the chronic negative emotions of the dark side via allowing the primal wounds to be fully expressed, patients can free themselves of long-held patterns of psychopathology. The core self can then be experienced as loving, joyful, and connected to all of life. At all times throughout the process, attention to the person's positive qualities of his or her core is paramount. Universal spiritual principles are taught and applied, making this a true transpersonal, yet body-centered psychotherapy.

In sessions, practitioners lead patients through a journey of self-discovery. Core energetics therapists use several diagnostic tools unique to this psychotherapy. Infrared thermography and thermo-vision analysis measure body temperatures. This allows patients and therapist to view energy activity emanating from the body. Therapists might also use a darkfield microcopy of the patient's blood, a diagnostic tool that is said to establish a quantitative analysis of the resistance of the patient's blood cells to the vital force as well as their degree of aging. Otherwise, sessions are similar to those in bioenergetics and orgonomy. Emotional states are induced while the patient is static or moving, followed by the practitioner assisting the patient to express previously repressed emotions in a fuller way (physiologically) than ever before.

Certificate training programs in core energetics are available through a handful of institutes. The standard program is through the Institute of Core Energetics, started by founder Dr. John Pierrakos, which conducts trainings in New York and California. Certification programs last about four years and are intensive compared to other body-psychotherapies. Most practitioners become certified in core energetics after they have a degree in a related field, such as a therapist, psychoanalyst, or medical doctor.

RESOURCES

BOOKS

Core Energetics: Developing the Capacity to Love and Heal by John C. Pierrakos, MD

Eros, Love and Sexuality: The Forces That Unify Man and Woman by John C. Pierrakos, MD

ONLINE

Energetic Balancing—Quantum Resonance Technology
www.energeticbalancing.us/health/core_energetics.html
A good overview on diagnostic tools used by therapists

Core Energetics—A Body-Centered Process to Heal Your Life
www.kateholt.info

ORGANIZATIONS

Core Energetics Alumni Association
www.corealumni.org

The Institute of Core Energetics
coreenergetics.org
Founded by Dr. John Pierrakos two decades ago

The International Institute of Core Energetics
www.coreevolution.com
Connects local core energetics communities worldwide

Core Energetics South
www.core-energetics-south.com

CRANIOSACRAL THERAPY

Just as the connective tissue called "fascia" surrounds all muscles, so does another form of connective tissue surround the brain and the rest of the central nervous system (CNS) from the skull to the sacrum. Within this connective tissue flows the cushioning cerebrospinal fluid (CSF). In the early 1930s, William Sutherland, DO, invented a technique he called cranial osteopathy. Upon examining the separate bones of a cadaver skull, Sutherland noticed that the structures of some of the bones were not congruent with the understood anatomy of his day. He claimed that these bones were "beveled, like the gills of a fish, indicating articular mobility for a respiratory mechanism." By this he meant that the skull bones are not immoveable, as had previously been thought. Instead the bones flex at the joints that connect one skull bone to another. These bones are also somehow involved with human respiration. Upon further investigation, Sutherland deduced that any hindrance in movement of the temporal bones of the skull may be associated with many physiological, especially neurological, dysfunction. By 1935, after Sutherland was convinced of his work's legitimacy, he established the Sutherland Cranial Teaching Foundation as a way to establish his method and further his research. This ultimately led to the genesis of craniosacral therapy.

Using the cranial osteopathy technique, DOs or other practitioners gently hold a patient's head in order to sense the subtle, wavelike fluctuation of CSF around the spine and brain. They also try to detect the slow, synchronized movements of the skull bones and the sacrum. This dual flow of CSF and bones is termed the cranial rhythmic impulse (CRI). Rebalancing CRI is believed to improve the overall health of patients because the CNS controls the functioning of every organ, muscle, and nerve in the human body. CRI becomes dysfunctional due to injury to almost any part of the body, as well as the general stress of daily living. The merits of cranial osteopathy are highly debated within the field of modern osteopathy due to its lack of supportive science. A more popularized version of cranial osteopathy is craniosacral therapy. This is basically cranial osteopathy for nonosteopaths and was named by John Upledger, DO, when he began teaching this technique to nonmedical students.

CST is employed by massage therapists, naturopaths, chiropractors, and osteopaths. It has been used to effectively treat stress, neck and back pain, migraines, TMJ syndrome (a chronic inflammation of the lower jaw bone), and difficult-to-treat nervous conditions such as fibromyalgia.

In a single session, CST practitioners work with subtle flow cycles of various rates, considered pseudo-scientific by most allopaths. These cycles are aptly dubbed "tides," alluding to the ebb and flow of fluids that fluctuate during a treatment session. The tide incorporates a change in cerebrospinal fluid flow as well as a slow oscillation in all body tissues, most notably in the skull.

In 1985, John Upledger, MD, established the Upledger Institute, a health center based in Florida dedicated to the education and certification of practitioners in craniosacral therapy. Since then, many programs have developed in the United States; however, the Upledger Institute is regarded as one of the best. Certification is awarded by the institution where training is received. There are no legal requirements prior to being trained in CST, although most practicing therapists are chiropractors, naturopaths, osteopaths, and medical doctors.

If a practitioner graduates from an approved program, he or she is eligible to apply for registered craniosacral therapists status through the Biodynamic CranioSacral Therapy Association of North America.

RESOURCES

BOOKS

Life in Motion by Dr. Rollin Becker

Wisdom in the Body by Dr. Michael Kern

Craniosacral Biodynamics, Volumes 1 and 2 by Franklyn Sills

Teachings in the Science of Osteopathy by Dr. William Sutherland

ORGANIZATIONS

Biodynamic CranioSacral Therapy Association of North America
www.craniosacraltherapy.org

Oversees certification eligibility and membership

The International Alliance of Healthcare Educators
www.iahe.com

Upledger Institute
www.upledger.com

Leading institution in research and education

The American CranioSacral Therapy Association
www.acsta.com

Radiant Health Center
www.radianthealthcenter.info

Focuses on the integration of psychotherapy, acupuncture, bodywork, and craniosacral therapy

The Polarity Center
thepolaritycenter.com

The International Institute for CranioSacral Balancing
www.icsb.ch/en

BodyEnergy
www.bodyenergy.net

Seminar, workshop, and treatment opportunities

TRAINING

American Institute
Pompano Beach, Florida
www.aimt.com

ATI Career Training Center
Various locations in Texas including Dallas/Fort Worth, North Richland Hills, and Richardson. Campuses also in Florida, New Mexico, and Oklahoma.
www.aticareertraining.edu

Body Therapy Institute
Siler City, North Carolina
www.massage.net

Boulder College of Massage Therapy
Boulder, Colorado
www.bcmt.org

Connecticut Center for Massage Therapy
Campuses in Groton, Newington, and Westport, Connecticut
www.ccmt.com

Diamond Light School of Massage and Healing Arts
San Anselmo, California
www.diamondlight.net

Florida School of Massage
Gainesville, Florida
www.floridaschoolofmassage.com

Institute of Natural Therapies
Campuses in Hancock and St. Ignace, Michigan
www.intherapies.com

International Professional School of Bodywork
San Diego, California
www.ipsb.edu

Irene's Myomassology Institute
Southfield, Michigan
www.imieducation.com

Kaplan College
Campuses in Hammond and Merrillville, Indiana
http://getinfo.kaplancollege.com

Mt. Nittany Institute of Natural Health
State College, Pennsylvania
www.mtnittanyinstitute.com

NAMTI—School of Massage and Bodywork
Prescott and Sedona, Arizona
www.namti.com

New Mexico Academy of Healing Arts
Santa Fe, New Mexico
www.nmhealingarts.org

Upledger Institute
Palm Beach Gardens, Florida
www.upledger.com

Utah College of Massage Therapy
Various locations with schools in Utah, Nevada,
Arizona, and Colorado
www.ucmt.com

World School of Massage and Holistic Healing Arts
Pleasanton and San Francisco, California
www.worldschoolmassage.com

DANCE THERAPY

Dancer Marion Chace is considered the principal founder of what is now dance therapy in the United States.[1] In the 1960s, she founded a training program for dance therapists in New York after being influenced by the work of Carl Jung. In 1966, she founded the American Dance Therapy Association and became its first president. In the United Kingdom, this profession has been renamed dance movement psychotherapy in order to reflect the psychotherapeutic nature of the work.

Laban movement analysis (LMA) is also part of dance movement therapy as it is used to categorize movements, which can be used as an insight into the patient's psychological state. Wilhelm Reich's second wife was an LMA practitioner, and it is believed that Reich combined psychoanalytic character analysis with movement therapy ideas (from LMA and other sources) as he formulated his influential orgonomy system of body-centered psychotherapy.

Dance therapy, or dance movement psychotherapy, is the therapeutic use of movement (and dance) for emotional, cognitive, social, behavioral, and physical conditions. It is a form of expressive therapy, along with music therapy, art therapy, etc. Certified dance therapists normally hold a master's level of training. Dance therapists work in rehabilitation, hospital, psychiatric, and pediatric programs that focus on topics such as chronic pain, substance abuse recovery, and post-traumatic experiences. Some also work with the physically challenged. Regardless of the setting, clients tend to have body-image problems that are not easily ameliorated with traditional talk-therapy modalities.

Dance therapy is founded on the premise that the body and mind are an interrelated continuum and that the state of the body affects mental and emotional well-being in manifold ways. In contrast to artistic dance, which is usually concerned with the aesthetic appearance of movement, dance therapy explores the nature of all movement as related to personal habits and personal growth. Through observing and altering the kinesthetic movements of clients, dance movement therapists diagnose and help to solve various psychological problems. As any conscious person can move on some level, this therapy can work with any population.

Graduates of programs approved by the American Dance Therapy Association are eligible to become a registered dance therapist. The more advanced registered American dance therapist is granted after acquiring more professional experience. Students with extensive movement backgrounds may combine their experience with study in a related field such as social work or clinical psychology as an alternative path leading to certification.

RESOURCES

BOOKS

Stern's Books
www.sternsbooks.com

PERIODICALS

American Journal of Dance Therapy
www.springerlink.com/content/0146-3721

The Arts in Psychotherapy

www.elsevier.com/wps/find/journaleditorialboard.
cws_home/833/editorialboard?navopenmenu=1

General expressive arts professional publication

At Health Newsletter

www.athealth.com

Mental health journal for practitioners and consumers

ORGANIZATIONS

American Dance Therapy Association

www.adta.org

The ADTA is a membership and advocacy group that sets dance therapy eligibility standards. It provides a list of seven graduate training programs, including specific education requirements, and publishes the American Journal of Dance Therapy.

Authentic Movement Community

www.authenticmovementcommunity.org

Community for expressive therapists with a focus on dance and movement therapy

Arts in Therapy Network

www.artsintherapy.com

A community for creative arts therapists

Expressive Therapy Concepts

www.expressivetherapy.org

A group dedicated to the art and culture of expressive therapies

Association for Creativity in Counseling

www.aca-acc.org

ACC was established in 2004 as a forum for counselors, counselor educators, and counseling students interested in creative, diverse, and relational approaches to counseling.

National Board for Certified Counselors, Inc.

www.nbcc.org

National Coalition of Creative Arts Therapies Associations

www.nccata.org

United States Association for Body Psychotherapy

www.usabp.org

The USABP is a nonprofit membership association dedicated to developing and advancing the art, science, and practice of body psychotherapy.

National Dance Association

www.aahperd.org/nda

Promotes and supports creative, artistic, and healthy lifestyles through quality services and programs in dance and dance education

National Dance Education Organization

www.ndeo.org/index.asp

Defines standards of excellence within the field of dance education. Also a resource to locate dance seminars and conferences in your area

TRAINING

Graduate Degree Programs in Dance and Movement Therapy

The American Dance Therapy Association approves the following programs. Graduates are eligible for registry in dance therapy.

Antioch University
Keene, New Hampshire
http://antiochne.edu/ap/dmt

Columbia College
Chicago, Illinois
www.colum.edu/graduate/graddance.html

Drexel University
Philadelphia, Pennsylvania
www.drexel.edu/cnhp/creativearts

Lesley University
Cambridge, Massachusetts
www.lesley.edu/gsass/56etp.html
www.lesley.edu/faculty/estrella/dance.html

Naropa University
Boulder, Colorado
www.naropa.edu

Pratt Institute
Brooklyn, New York
www.pratt.edu/ad/ather

Nondegree Graduate Programs

These programs exist in states where dance therapy is not a regulated medical profession. The ADTA recognizes these programs as an alternate route to registry provided that individuals with extensive dance and movement backgrounds might employ a master's level education in a related field such as social work, psychology, counseling, and special education.

California Institute of Integral Studies
San Francisco, California
www.ciis.edu

John F. Kennedy University
Orinda, California
www.jfku.edu

Marylhurst University
Marylhurst, Oregon
www.marylhurst.edu

Dance Therapy Institute of Princeton
Princeton, New Jersey
(609)-924-3520
(818)-783-3630

Kinections
Rochester, New York
www.kinections.com

The Moving Center
Mill Valley, California
www.movingcenterschool.com

The Center for Creative Counseling and Dance/ Movement Therapy Studies
Greensboro, North Carolina
larmeniox@triad.rr.com

Undergraduate Dance/Movement Therapy Coursework

These courses help students evaluate their interest and may serve as prerequisites for graduate study.

Brookdale Community College
Lincroft, New Jersey
www.brookdale.cc.nj.us

Goucher College
Townson, Maryland
www.goucher.edu

Manhattanville College
Purchase, New York
www.manhattanville.edu

Marymount College
Tarrytown, New York
http://web.archive.org/web/20011128090531/http://www.marymt.edu

Naropa University
Boulder, Colorado
www.naropa.edu

Queens College, City University of New York
Flushing, New York
www.qc.cuny.edu

Red Rocks Community College
Lakewood, Colorado
www.rrcc.edu

Russell Sage College
Troy, New York
www.sage.edu

University of the Arts
Philadelphia, Pennsylvania
www.uarts.edu

University of Wisconsin-Madison
Madison, Wisconsin
www.wisc.edu

ENERGY MEDICINE

Energy medicine is a broad category within holistic medicine that encompasses many nonmanipulative, noninvasive forms of therapy, including chromotherapy, healing touch, magnetic therapy, chi kung, reiki, and therapeutic touch.

According to the National Institutes of Health, there are two types of energy medicine: veritable and putative.

Veritable energy therapies usually employ mechanical vibrations (i.e., sound), electromagnetic forces, and/or other types of specific measurable wavelengths to treat patients. These methods of healing, such as magnetic therapy, employ the use of machines, where the practitioner becomes interpreter of data much like a biofeedback therapist.

Putative energy medicine is based on the premise that illness is a result of disturbed energy within the body. This energy, referred to by many names, such as "prana," "chi," "orgone," and the "vital force," is unquantifiable in a scientific paradigm, yet paramount in therapies such as healing touch or reiki. Putative energy practitioners can allegedly detect subtle energies that are not measurable by scientific equipment and then manipulate these energies to promote health, fight disease, and restore balance in their patients' body-minds. Putative energy medicine dates back several thousand years: mummified bodies from around 3000 B.C. were found to have tattoos in the exact pressure points indicated by Chinese medicine for treating lumbar spine arthritis. Veritable energy medicine, due to the nature of the technological tools involved, is not nearly as old. Yet the essential philosophy behind these therapies is virtually the same.

Because energy medicine is such a broad category that includes several different healing modalities, there are few educational programs that cover more than one modality. There is, however, considerable skepticism among scientists as to the efficacy of both veritable and putative energy therapies—due to a lack of scientific evidence. Skepticism is faced with anecdotal accounts of how specific healing modalities have saved the lives of individuals.

For more information on specific types of energy medicine and training in a particular modality of energy therapy, consult sections on chi kung, healing touch, therapeutic touch, or reiki.

RESOURCES

BOOKS

Energy Medicine by Donna Eden

The Field by Lynne McTaggart

Energy Medicine in Therapeutics and Human Performance by James L. Oschman

The Promise of Energy Psychology by David Feinstein

ONLINE

Energy Medicine and Bioenergetic Fields
www.colorado.edu/philosophy/vstenger/Medicine/EnergyMed.html

A well-informed and academic article by Victor Stenger, PhD, explaining the more complicated theory behind energy medicine, bioenergetic fields, quantum healing, and its relationship to auras, spirit, and other energetic discharges

Energy Connections
www.energy-connections.com

Articles and news about energy medicine and energy psychology

Energy Medicine Directory
www.energymedicinedirectory.com

A worldwide directory of practitioners and events

Energy Medicine: Hands-On Healing
www.transitiontoparenthood.com/janelle/energy

ORGANIZATIONS

The Energy Medicine Institute
www.energymed.org

Offering training, certification programs, and practitioner membership in the general category of energy medicine

Akamai University Energy Medicine Program
www.akamaiuniversity.us/EnergyMedicine.html

Offers a master's and doctorial degree in energy medicine, as well as certificate programs and general classes

Innersource
www.innersource.net

Offers training, informal certification, and products—all for energy medicine. This site also has home study programs, articles about different philosophical approaches to medicine, and a free online newsletter.

Energy Medicine University
www.EnergyMedicineUniversity.org

Energy Medicine University is a distance learning institution offering graduate degree programs in integrative holistic health and other programs and classes.

The International Society for the Study of Subtle Energies and Energy Medicine

www.issseem.org

An interdisciplinary organization for the study of the therapeutic applications of subtle energies. It hosts a conference.

Academy of Intuition Medicine

www.IntuitionMedicine.org

The academy offers career training in medical intuition and intuition medicine counseling. Institution and faculty approved by State of California Bureau of Postsecondary Education.

Association for Comprehensive Energy Psychology

www.energypsych.org

ACEP is a nonprofit, professional organization dedicated to the research, education, and promotion of energy psychology among health professionals

ESSENTIAL MOTION

Essential motion is a movement-based body-oriented psychotherapy developed by Karen Roeper, a Rosen Method bodywork practitioner and teacher. It is a derivative of the Rosen Method in that it fuses dance therapy with a deep understanding of the mind-body connection. The result is a synthesis of mental and physical exercises that promote general health as well as ameliorate stress-related ailments.

Essential motion relies upon the body's intelligence as the practitioner attempts to have his patients inhabit their bodies more fully, moving through the day with ease, power, and grace. By remaining conscious of how one moves in day-to-day life, one can detect physical imbalances that often correspond to psychological ones. Essential motion utilizes noninvasive self-therapy to restore balance within the body.

Similar to almost all body-centered psychotherapists, Roeper believes that in childhood we express the natural ease and spontaneous playfulness of our authentic, unique selves. Our minds may forget, but our bodies remember this relative freedom and well-being. Essential motion reconnects patients with their bodies as their source of aliveness, creativity, and wisdom. Watching patients move, practitioners observe where their patients' bodies are stuck and where they are free to move uninhibitedly. The more unhibited the physical movements, the more flexibly healthy the patient's psyche is believed to be.

Through gentle probing, suggestions, directions, and coaching, practitioners allow patients to explore their psychological resistance and emotional limitations. By guiding patients' bodies to a place of internal listening, essential motion helps them to discover and remember how they long to move—both physically and psychologically. Within the deep dialogue between the body and its expressive movements, patients can dissolve their bodies' unconscious, rigid movement patterns and move beyond the constraining beliefs that controlled their lives.

There are several different types of training available for students. Certificate programs are available at a few institutions across the United States ranging from coaching and supervision certificates to leadership and senior teaching programs. As essential motion is a relatively new methodology, there is but a small community of associations and organizations.

RESOURCES

ORGANIZATIONS

Essential Motion, Inc.
Manitoba, Canada
www.essentialmotion.ca

Classes, training, and certificate programs

Essential Motion
www.essential-motion.com

This organization was started by Karen Roeper, the founder of essential motion, and is the largest training and resource center for essential motion in the United States. It holds conferences and seminars around the country.

Fortuna Life
www.fortunalife.com/movement.php

In addition to certifying essential motion instructors, Fortuna Life offers classes and workshops for the public.

Invisible Elephant
www.ielephant.com/program-essentialmotion.html

Certifies essential motion instructors and offers classes in essential motion

EYE MOVEMENT DESENSITIZATION REPROCESSING

Developed by psychologist Francine Shapiro in 1987, eye movement desensitization reprocessing (EMDR) is an "information processing" modality used primarily by mental health professionals for the treatment of stress, anxiety, and trauma. Using an alternative approach to psychosomatic medicine, the EMDR model hypothesizes that difficult memories and periods of life are unconsciously suppressed and held by the bodies of those undergoing these stressors. Holding in feeling and emotions usually becomes detrimental to psychological health, as Western psychotherapists began understanding in the early twentieth century. In Wilhelm Reich's "orgonomy," practitioners lead supine patients through eye movements in order to elicit repressed emotions and to give the doctor information on the muscular "armoring" around the eye region. This is the first of seven body segments treated within Reich's seminal body-centered psychotherapy. Without giving any nod to Reich's work with eye movements and their relation to both repressed emotions and overall psychological health, EMDR proponents say that their modality is solely based on Shapiro's observation that eye movements can reduce the intensity of disturbing thoughts. Shapiro subsequently formulated a method of eye-based psychotherapy that involves recalling a stressful past event and reprogramming—or desensitizing—the memory in light of a more positive self-aware attitude. This psychological exercise is coupled with rapid close- or open-eyed movements to both relax the patient and elicit suppressed memories. EMDR therapists may accompany eye movement therapy by waving one or two fingers in front of their clients' eyes, while talking to them in a calm voice.

EMDR's most unique aspect is an unusual component of bilateral (both-sided) stimulation of the brain, such as eye movements, bilateral sound, or bilateral tactile stimulation coupled with cognitions, visualized images, and body sensation. EMDR also utilizes dual attention awareness to allow the individual to vacillate between the traumatic material and the safety of the present moment. This prevents retraumatization from patient exposure to their disturbing memories.

EMDR is a multiphase therapy process; typical treatment plans are about four to seven sessions long. EMDR requires a fairly complicated vocabulary and understanding of memory, trauma, and psyche.

Though it has been scientifically researched, there is no definitive explanation as to how EMDR works. Empirical support and anecdotal evidence is overwhelming, especially in treating personality disorders, anxiety disorders, dissociative disorders, post-traumatic stress disorders, and general emotional dysregulation in both children and adults. There are several theories about the relationship to deliberate rapid eye movements and REM sleep, yet EMDR researchers and holistic psychologists still seek to understand why EMDR works. According to Dr. Gary Peterson, EMDR has had "more double-blind, placebo-controlled studies published in peer-reviewed journals than any other psychotherapy method" for the treatment of post-traumatic stress disorder.

It rose in popularity around 1999 as an effective treatment for trauma victims when the American Psychological Association and the International Society for Traumatic Stress Studies approved the treatment as a valid therapy for post-traumatic stress disorder. Since then, education, literature, research, and professionalism in the field has grown significantly.

EMDR training is available through several different programs in the United States. Since it is a relatively new field, certification programs are limited. There are two structurally different programs that can lead to certification in EMDR: students who are enrolled in an approved mental health field such as social work, clinical psychology, and psychiatry may concurrently enroll in an EMDR program. Medical doctors and registered nurses must first demonstrate training in psychology. Certification in EMDR is completed by the EMDR International Association.

RESOURCES

BOOKS

EMDR: The Breakthrough "Eye Movement" Therapy for Overcoming Anxiety, Stress, and Trauma by Francine Shapiro and Margot Silk Forrest

Eye Movement Desensitization and Reprocessing (EMDR), Second Edition: Basic Principles, Protocols, and Procedures by Francine Shapiro

A Therapist's Guide to EMDR: Tools and Techniques for Successful Treatment by Laurel Parnell

EMDR Solutions: Pathways to Healing by Robin Shapiro

Transforming Trauma: EMDR: The Revolutionary New Therapy for Freeing the Mind, Clearing the Body, and Opening the Heart by Laurel Parnell

ONLINE

Help Guide
www.helpguide.org/mental/emdr_therapy.htm

A useful resource for general information on EMDR

EMDR Web-links
www.emdr-therapy.com/emdr-info-links.htm

A portal that contains links to many Web sites with information on EMDR, as well as a query that will locate practitioners in your area

ORGANIZATIONS

EMDR Institute, Inc.
www.emdr.com

This general resource organization for practitioners of EMDR worldwide provides information on training programs, certification requirements, and EMDR-related state laws.

EMDR International Association
www.emdria.org

The EMDR International Association is a professional association where practitioners and researchers seek to create the highest standard for clinical use of EMDR through recognized certification requirements, research projects, and practitioner networking.

EMDR Network
www.emdrnetwork.org

The EMDR Network provides access to information to clients and clinicians. The organizations listed on this Web site are well-established and supposedly professionally scrutinized.

American Psychological Association
www.apa.org

Based in Washington, DC, the APA is a scientific and professional organization that represents psychology in the United States. With 148,000 members, it's the largest association of psychologists worldwide.

EMDR Humanitarian Assistance Programs
www.emdrhap.org

Trains mental health professionals serving traumatized communities

International Society for Traumatic Stress Studies
www.istss.org

Promotes the advancement and exchange of knowledge about severe stress and trauma

EMDR-CERTIFIED TRAINING PROGRAMS

EMDR Institute, Inc.
Watsonville, California
www.emdr.com/train.htm

John F. Kennedy University
Pleasant Hill, California
www.jfku.edu/ce/psychology_health/emdr

Alliant International University
San Francisco, California
www.alliant.edu

Philip Manfield, PhD
Berkeley, California
emdr_dr@practicemagic.com

DaLene Forester, PhD
Redding, California
www.emdrtrainingyou.com

Laurel Parnell, PhD
San Rafael, California
www.emdrinfo.com/index.php/training

The Traumatic Stress Network
Corona, California
www.webpages2000.com

Molly Gierasch, PhD
Boulder, Colorado
www.mollygierasch.com

Julie K. Greene, MA, LPC
Boulder, Colorado
www.juliegreene.com

Sandra A. Tinker-Wilson, PhD
Colorado Springs, Colorado
drswilson@msn.com

EMDR Humanitarian Assistance Programs
Hamden, Connecticut
www.emdrhap.org

Diane Clayton, LCSW
Fort Myers, Florida
http://emdrtrainer.com

Adler School of Professional Psychology
Chicago, Illinois
www.adler.edu

EMDR of Greater Washington
Bethesda, Maryland
www.emdrgreaterwashington.com

Child Trauma Institute
Greenfield, Massachusetts
www.childtrauma.com/tremdr.html

Mel Rabin, EdD
Needham, Massachusetts
mrabin101@aol.com

Natalie S. Robinson, MSW, LICSW
Boston, Massachusetts
www.natalie-robinson-licsw.com

Boston University, Professional Education Programs
Boston, Massachusetts
www.bu.edu/ssw/training/pep/programs/certificate/emdr/index.shtml

Bender-Britt Seminars
Montclair, New Jersey
BenderBritt@optonline.net

University of Buffalo (SUNY)—School of Social Work
Buffalo, New York
www.socialwork.buffalo.edu/fas/smyth/Personal_Web/Courses/Courses_taught_EMDR.htm

Mark Dworkin, MSW
East Meadow, New York
mdworkin@optonline.net

Sandra E. Kaplan, LCSW
Syracuse, New York
skaplan3@twcny.rr.com

Upstate Medical University
Syracuse, New York
www.upstate.edu

William M. Zangwill, PhD
New York, New York
www.emdrandtraining.com

Rick Levinson, LCSW
Austin, Texas
rick@radiancetx.org

Carol York, MSSW, LMSW-ACP
Austin, Texas
cyorkmssw@aol.com

Barbara A. Parrett, RN, MS
Lynnwood, Washington
bparrett@jps.net

FELDENKRAIS METHOD

Moshe Feldenkrais was a Ukrainian physicist who, similar to one of his inspirations, F.M. Alexander (of Alexander Technique fame), had a personal physical trauma in his life that led to his subsequent development and promotion of a new movement therapy. As a middle-aged man serving on a slippery submarine in World War II, Feldenkrais reaggravated an old soccer knee injury. Instead of receiving the recommended surgery, Feldenkrais employed his knowledge of judo, physiology, anatomy, psychology, neurology, and especially self-observation, toward seeking an alternative therapy that would reverse his impairment and allow him to simply walk without pain.

Feldenkrais studied himself closely and watched how the healthy parts of his muscle system compensated for the injured ones. The idea of "self-image" is a central component within both the Feldenkrais Method and the Alexander Technique. According to Feldenkrais himself, "Each one of us speaks, moves, thinks, and feels in a different way, each according to the image of himself that he has built up over the years. In order to change our mode of action, we must change the image of ourselves that we carry within us."

Feldenkrais's discoveries led him to begin sharing with others through lectures, experimental classes, and one-on-one teaching. His self-rehabilitation also enabled him to continue his judo practice. From his position on an international judo committee, he began to scientifically study this newly developed martial art, incorporating the knowledge he had gained through his self-rehabilitation. In 1949, he published the first book on the Feldenkrais Method, *Body and Mature Behavior: A Study of Anxiety, Sex, Gravitation and Learning*. During this period he studied the work of mystic and movement expert G.I. Gurdjieff, F. Matthias Alexander, gymnast Elsa Gindler, and William Bates, MD (of the Bates Method of natural vision improvement via conscious eye muscle relaxation). He also traveled to Switzerland to study with Heinrich Jacoby. Jacoby was Gindler's colleague who helped her develop the body psychotherapy she named "Arbeit am Menschen," roughly translated as "People Work." This system joined Wilhelm Reich's orgonomy and Jungian Arnold Mindell's dream body work to form the three main sources of body therapy used today.

Feldenkrais developed two approaches for working with students and clients: one implements group therapeutic techniques and the other is focused individually, utilizing hands-on touch and movement. He dubbed the group therapy, "Awareness Through Movement," as he guided participants through infinitesimal movement sequences designed to replace old patterns of movement with new ones. The individual therapy, named "Functional Integration," is more intense than the group "floorwork" process. The practitioner actively directs the patient's body through specialized movements that cater to the individual's needs, essentially simulating new ways in which the client can move for optimal well-being. As with many other forms of CAM therapy, the patient's relationship with the practitioner can make or break the patient's "faith" in the therapy. This can create the "nocebo," or negative placebo effect, when a client's belief that a therapy will be ineffective results in a self-fulfilling prophecy. Placebo and nocebo can be the most important factors for determining the effectiveness of holistic medicine.

One central tenet of the Feldenkrais Method holds that improving one's ability to move freely, unbound by subtly damaging movement habits, can improve one's overall well-being. Because they are not usually licensed doctors of any kind, practitioners of the Feldenkrais Method generally refrain from diagnosis and do not refer to the Feldenkrais as conventional therapy.

In 1951, Feldenkrais returned to the recently formed Israel, as he had lived from age seven until fourteen in Palestine. After directing the Israeli Army Department of Electronics for several years, in 1954 he settled in Tel Aviv where he began to teach his healing method full time. In 1957, he gave lessons in the Feldenkrais Method to David Ben-Gurion, the prime minister of Israel, enabling him to stand on his head in a Yoga pose! Throughout the 1960s, 1970s, and into the 1980s, he presented the Feldenkrais Method throughout Europe and in North America. This included an "Awareness Through Movement" program for human potential trainers at Esalen Institute in 1972. Late in life, he rehabilitated himself from consecutive strokes over three years until he finally succumbed and died in his home in Tel Aviv. There are well over 2,000 practitioners of his method teaching throughout the world today.

Over the years, there have been various extensions to Feldenkrais's original method. Voice movement integration, a new modality of healing under the guise of Feldenkrais treatment, incorporates spoken words into therapy sessions. Patients are encouraged to actively talk about how the therapy is making them feel during the sessions themselves. The Feldenkrais Method, as a result, is not a single fixed methodology but an evolving approach to health that incorporates new forms of body-mind communication as it grows in practice.

RESOURCES

BOOKS

Awareness Through Movement: Easy-to-Do Health Exercises to Improve Your Posture, Vision, Imagination, and Personal Awareness by Moshe Feldenkrais

Feldenkrais: The Busy Person's Guide to Easier Movement by Frank Wildman

The Potent Self: A Study of Spontaneity and Compulsion by Moshe Feldenkrais and Mark Reese

Relaxercise: The Easy New Way to Health and Fitness by David Zemach-bersi

Awareness Heals: The Feldenkrais Method for Dynamic Health by Stephen Shafarman

Body and Mature Behavior: A Study of Anxiety, Sex, Gravitation, and Learning by Moshe Feldenkrais and Carl Ginsburg

The Feldenkrais Method: Teaching by Handling by Yochanan Rywerant and Moshe Feldenkrais

Master Moves by Moshe Feldenkrais

ONLINE

The Feldenkrais Method: Flowing Body, Flexible Mind

www.flowingbody.com/felden.htm

A useful introductory resource on the philosophy and practice of the Feldenkrais Method. Includes a lesson of the month as well as course plans for practitioners

Achieving Excellence

www.achievingexcellence.com

Articles, books, and audio tapes for purchase on the Feldenkrais Method

Mirko Michael Kadelc's Home Page

www.feldenkraismethod.ca

General consumer-targeted information about the Feldenkrais Method from the perspective of an experienced practitioner

Posture Page

www.posturepage.com/feldenkrais/index.html

An article about postures used in the Feldenkrais Method

InteliHealth: Feldenkrais

www.intelihealth.com/IH/ihtIH/WS/8513/34968/358818.html?d=dmtContent

Aetna's Web site is dedicated to the Feldenkrais Method's relationship with health insurance companies.

Readings about Feldenkrais Method

www.feldnet.com/ArticlesabouttheMethod/tabid/58/Default.aspx

A collection of various journal articles and research done on the efficacy of Feldenkrais treatment

ORGANIZATIONS

The Feldenkrais Method of Somatic Education

www.feldenkrais.com

The largest online organization dedicated to the Feldenkrais Method. Includes publications, conference listing, practitioner classes, and general resources

The International Feldenkrais Federation

http://feldenkrais-method.org

The International Feldenkrais Federation is the coordinating organization of most Feldenkrais guilds and associations and other key Feldenkrais professional organizations worldwide. The aim of the federation is the development of the international Feldenkrais community, through promoting effective cooperation and communication in the spirit of the Feldenkrais Method.

Feldenkrais Resources

www.feldenkrais-resources.com

An organization dedicated to networking and helping therapists find training options

Feldenkrais Movement Institute

www.feldenkraisinstitute.org

Includes a rigorous training program and semiannual workshops and conferences

FLOWER ESSENCES AND BACH FLOWER REMEDIES

Flower essences are a submodality of homeopathy and aromatherapy. They are used to address emotional and spiritual dysfunctions such as depression, anxiety, low self-esteem, and insomnia. Homeopathic-like dilutions of flower "essences" are placed under the patient's tongue or inhaled. This method is used independently, in combination with other naturopathic modalities, or as an adjunct to psychotherapy or massage therapy.

Flower essences were developed by Englishman Edward Bach, MD, in the 1930s. Bach had been a house surgeon and casualty medical officer, in charge of 400 hospital beds in World War I. Turning toward alternative medical modalities, such as homeopathy, at midlife Bach formulated thirty-eight flower essences based solely on his intuitions. He could supposedly judge the healing effect of a flower just by walking past it or by placing it on his tongue. According to Bach ("batch," not "bock"), the core foundation of flower remedies revolves around the premise that "true healing involves treating the very base of the cause of suffering. No effort directed to the body alone can do more than superficially repair damage. Treat people for their emotional unhappiness, allow them to be happy, and they will become well." Bach believed that all diseases resulted from conflict between the soul's duty and the ego's desire to do differently. After extensive trials and personal research, Bach decided that his flower essences were the key to treating all psycho-spiritual conditions that also commonly resulted in physical disease.

The flower essence method of diagnosis is a unique process in which the practitioner asks the patient a series of questions and selects one remedy or a mixture of several that will treat the patient's general psychological state. These remedies are usually in liquid form and preserved in alcohol. Practitioners dilute two drops of each remedy into a 30ml dropper bottle filled with mineral water and instruct patients to take four drops four times a day, either on the skin or tongue. Remedies are sometimes mixed to match daily changes in mood or mental atmosphere. Rescue remedies (as they are often called) are designed to be effective almost immediately and have both long- and short-term stress-reducing benefits. Flower essences, a term which may be used interchangeably with Bach flower remedies, has been used for treatment of chronic emotional problems, clinical depression, and anxiety disorders, though the evidence to support its efficacy is largely anecdotal.

Education in Bach flower remedies in not limited to homeopaths and aromatherapists because there aren't many prerequisites for students before enrolling in one of the few programs available. Most training programs consist of three training levels. The first teaches the basics of the system, including a definition of each flower essence. Level two courses build on the philosophies behind the flower essence paradigm. The third and final level of education is for aspiring practitioners who want to work professionally with remedies. Some students of flower essences prefer to take only the first two levels of study. Certification for those who have completed the third level is available through the Bach International Education Program (associated with Nelson Bach USA). A list of certified training programs and organizations can be found grouped in the organizations section.

A Sampling of Bach Flower Remedies and Their Uses

1. Beech—intolerance

2. Cerato—lack of trust in one's own decisions

3. Chicory—selfish, possessive love

4. Elm—overwhelmed by responsibility

5. Mustard—deep gloom for no reason

6. Olive—exhaustion following mental or physical effort

7. Pine—guilt

8. Rock Water—self-denial, rigidity, and self-repression

9. Star of Bethlehem—shock

10. Wild Rose –resignation, apathy

RESOURCES

BOOKS

Encyclopedia of Bach Flower Therapy by Mechthild Scheffer

Bloom by Stefan Ball

Heal Thyself by Dr. Edward Bach

Bach Flower Remedies to the Rescue by Gregory Vlamis

Advanced Bach Flower Therapy by Gotz Blome, MD

ONLINE

Aetna InteliHealth
www.intelihealth.com

Contains studies regarding efficacy

Rainbow Crystal Resource Guide to Flower Essences
www.rainbowcrystal.com/bach/bach.html

Pet Synergy
www.petsynergy.com/flower.html

Hpathy: Flower Remedies
www.hpathy.com/bachflower

ORGANIZATIONS

My Bach Remedies
www.mybachremedies.com

Sells videos, tutorials, and tinctures, and offers general information

Dr. Edward Bach Centre
www.bachcentre.com

Based out of the United Kingdom, this organization is the largest worldwide association dedicated to training practitioners and raising international awareness about Bach flower remedies.

BachFlower.com
www.bachflower.com

Sells tincture for animals, children, and adults, and offers useful information

Bach Flower Education
www.bachflowereducation.com

This program is designed to teach the healing system as taught by Dr. Edward Bach.

The Bach Flower Research Programme
www.edwardbach.org

Dedicated to scientific research about flower essences

The Flower Essence Society
www.flowersociety.org

The society is an international membership organization of health practitioners, researchers, students, and others interested in deepening knowledge of flower essence therapy. Its objectives include promoting research, conducting training and certification seminars, disseminating educational material, and networking.

Bach Wiki Project
www.bachwiki.com

An ongoing effort to compile all relevant information and research on flower remedies

Bach Remedies
www.bachremedies.co.uk

A U.K.-based educational organization with connections to training centers in the United States

FOCUSING

"Focusing" is a naturally occurring human coping mechanism that was first observed and described by psychotherapist-philosopher Eugene Gendlin. In 1953, at the University of Chicago, Gendlin observed that differences in psychotherapy techniques usually *did not* determine their success or failure regarding successful patient treatment. Gendlin hypothesized that most of the healing came from something the patients did themselves during therapy sessions. Gendlin called this an inner act a "felt sense": an intuitive body-mind self-awareness that senses both how emotional upsets are felt and also how they can be visualized as occurring at specific points within the body. These points change in feeling and imagined appearance when the emotions resolve, and are usually located between the head and the pelvis rather than the limbs.

Gendlin developed the focusing method in order

to induce inward body awareness for his many patients who did not already have the ability to sense changing physical sensations due to their changing emotions. He first had patients "clear a space" by listing for the practitioner, in a ritualized manner, their perceived imperfections in life. When the patient can no longer think of any more complaints, he or she usually senses a clearer peace of mind. Patients are then asked to choose one issue to work on for the therapeutic session. The therapist proceeds to assist their closed-eyed patients to tune into their physical sensations for the remainder of the session, reporting any feelings or visuals that come up in relation to the problems being discussed. If a session is successful, the physical sensations and/or visuals reverse from painful to pleasant, and the corresponding emotional issue feels resolved—for the moment; and with enough psychotherapy, for good.

Focusing is usually classified as a form of body-mind psychotherapy. It is not a set of ideas but an experimental process. Acknowledging that everyone's emotional constitution is different, practitioners cater focusing sessions to the individual patient and the subject at hand. Focusing may be done as a self-therapy, but more often it is practiced as an adjunct technique during psychotherapy.

Certification is given out on an individual basis through the Focusing Institute, which offers a comprehensive directory of certified trainers.

RESOURCES

BOOKS

Focusing by Eugene Gendlin, PhD

Focusing-Oriented Psychotherapy by Eugene Gendlin, PhD

Focusing-Oriented Therapy by Neil Friedman, PhD

Person-Centered Therapy: The Focusing-Oriented Approach by Campbell Purton, PhD

Let Your Body Interpret Your Dreams by Eugene Gendlin, PhD

The Power of Focusing: A Practical Guide to Emotional Self-Healing by Ann Weiser Cornell, PhD

The Radical Acceptance of Everything: Living a Focusing Life by Ann Weiser Cornell, PhD (featuring Barbara McGavin)

Felt Sense: Writing with the Body by Sondra Perl, PhD

ONLINE

Inner Relationship Focusing
www.innerrelationship.com

Includes a directory of practitioners and workshops

Inner Wisdoms Recovery Focusing
www.innerwisdoms.com

Anecdotal accounts of focusing sessions, with poetry, art, and information about focusing for emotional recovery

Body-Links Home Page
www.biospiritual.org

Do Focusing
www.dofocusing.com

Easily accessible information on the benefits of focusing. Includes essays and archived projects

ORGANIZATIONS

The Focusing Institute
www.focusing.org

For a detailed list of training programs available in the United States, consult this Web site. It is the largest international organization of its kind.

The International Association for Focusing Oriented Therapies
www.focusingtherapy.org

This organization provides links to training programs in the United States and information on combining focusing with other therapies such as EMDR.

New England Focusing
www.newenglandfocusing.com

Association for Humanistic Psychology
ahpweb.org

Founded in 1962, the AHP hosts events, workshops, and publishes a journal on humanistic psychology.

United States Association for Body Psychotherapy

www.usabp.org

The USABP is a nonprofit membership association dedicated to developing and advancing the art, science, and practice of various body psychotherapies.

Focalizing

focalizing.com

A permutation of focusing pioneered by Michael Picucci, MD, focalizing is defined as a "dynamic and effective process that allows us to respectfully set aside familiar thoughts and feelings to access our innate intelligence."

Foundation for Human Enrichment

www.traumahealing.com

This education organization helps victims of post-traumatic stress disorder as well as other trauma-related mental injuries.

The Institute for Authentic Process Healing

www.theinstitute.org

The Omega Institute

http://omega-inst.org

Offers training, retreats, and conferences in many body-mind psychotherapies including focusing

GUIDED IMAGERY

Imagery is the natural way the nervous system stores and categorizes information. Though we still are not able to scientifically express exactly how the brain functions in every instance, we know that the mind has the ability to evoke powerful images that have physical ramifications. Just as fear, happiness, and passion manifest physically in the body, focusing the mind's eye internally upon particular images can often help reduce stress, elevate mood, slow heart rate, stimulate the immune system, reduce pain, and potentially assist in the treatment of all psychosomatic ailments. Guided imagery is founded on the premise that the imagination is commonly a person's least utilized health resource. Through the expertise and methodology of a trained psychotherapist, guided imagery seeks to develop patients' imagination for the express purpose of healing.

Guided imagery has been effective in many chronic cases ranging from tension and headaches to life-threatening diseases. While this process makes no scientific claims to heal in the allopathic sense, a series of imagery sessions can relax patients, change their attitudes toward their conditions, and ultimately teach them to relax in moments of pain and discomfort, much as biofeedback does. Proponents of guided imagery believe that many illnesses are physical expressions of emotional problems. The theory goes that by lessening tension in the mind, patients often experience relief from their superficial symptoms.

Training in guided imagery is primarily available through the Academy for Guided Imagery. Students must enroll in the first level thirteen-hour program before moving on to advanced programs. The Interactive Guided Imagery course is designed for individual study. To practice guided imagery professionally, you must complete the certification program, which includes a total of about 150 hours of study and training.

RESOURCES

BOOKS

Guided Imagery for Self-Healing by Martin L. Rossman

Anxiety Relief: Guided Imagery Exercises to Soothe, Relax and Restore Balance (Guided Self-Healing Practices) by Martin Rossman, MD

Guided Imagery for Groups: Fifty Visualizations That Promote Relaxation, Problem-Solving, Creativity, and Well-Being by Andrew E. Schwartz

Relaxation Body Scan and Guided Imagery for Well-Being by Carolyn McManus, PT MS MA

Deep Relaxation by Sandy McDermott

Staying Well with Guided Imagery by Belleruth Naparstek

ONLINE

Holistic Online

www.holisticonline.com/guided-imagery.htm

Includes definitions of visualizations and tips on personal imagery

The Healing Mind: The Art and Science of Mind-Body Healing

www.thehealingmind.org

Information on treatment for chronic life-threatening conditions

ORGANIZATIONS

Academy for Guided Imagery

www.academyforguidedimagery.com

This is the largest national organization dedicated to education, research, training, and networking in the area of guided imagery.

Imagery International

www.imageryinternational.org

A professional organization of practitioners, it hosts conferences, speakers, and workshops.

The Institute of Transpersonal Psychology

www.itp.edu

Founded in 1975, the institute is a private nonsectarian graduate school that is dedicated to teaching holistic approaches to psychotherapy. It offers master's and doctoral degrees in a range of related disciplines.

Guided Imagery Incorporated

www.guidedimageryinc.com

A good general resource for integrated psychotherapy, including information on the efficacy of guided imagery in treating physiological conditions

Association for Music and Imagery

www.ami-bonnymethod.org

The AMI is made up of members who have been trained in the Bonny Method of Guided Imagery and Music. Consult the Web site for information on training programs in this method of psychotherapy, which combines music therapy and guided imagery.

The Bonny Institute

www.bonnyfoundation.org

Founded by Helen Lindquist Bonny, this method is a hybrid psychotherapy, which includes guided imagery and music therapy.

HAKOMI

Hakomi is a relatively new method of body-mind-spirit healing developed by Ron Kurtz in 1970. The word comes from the Hopi language, meaning: "How do you stand in relation to these many realms?" or "Who are you? What is your source?" Hakomi incorporates various body-centered psychotherapeutic methods along with Eastern concepts of mindfulness for the purpose of continuous inner peace. Hakomi is a noninvasive touch-therapy, which borrows techniques from massage, structural alignment from chiropractic, movement exercises from dance therapy, and subtle energy work from energy medicine. The hakomi method is an efficient and powerful process for discovering and then studying body-mind patterns and core beliefs as the patient experiences them. As in any psychotherapy, the main reason to study one's own body-mind patterns is to change those which are subjectively impeding one's progress toward interpersonal happiness, fulfillment, and self-actualization. According to the Hakomi Institute Web site, this journey proceeds from "Who are you?" to "Who you are!" given the therapist's skill and the patient's willingness to change. As for the results of hakomi, "At the end, you have consistency and vision. You know your needs and direction. You can say, 'This I will do, and this I won't!' You have resolved many conflicts in which one part of you wants something and another part is against it. It's not a final place you reach. The journey itself becomes a way of life. If it ends at all, it ends in enlightenment." This spiritual intention sets hakomi in the same category as core mastery, regarding the inherent transpersonal focus of these two body-centered but spirit-aimed, psychotherapies.

At its most basic level, hakomi is the therapeutic expression of a specific set of universal principles: mindfulness, unity, mind/body/spirit holism, nonviolence, and organicity. Because all of these principles hail from Yogic/Buddhist/Taoist philosophy, one can say that hakomi blooms from the fertile soil of the "perennial philosophy" of our earliest human civilizations. It also draws from modern body-centered psychotherapies such as psychomotor, Reichian, bioenergetics, Gestalt, Feldenkrais, structural bodywork, focusing, Ericksonian hypnosis, and neurolinguistic programming. Hakomi is a synthesis of philosophies, techniques, and approaches that has its own unique artistry, form, and organic process. It can be used within most therapeutic situations, including work with individuals, couples, families, groups, movement, and bodywork. Like the inclusive philosophy from which it springs, hakomi serves everyone at all times of their lives.

As a holistic fusion discipline, it is difficult to define exactly how a hakomi practitioner will treat any given patient. Founder Ron Kurtz distinguishes hakomi from other disciplines this way: "The unique contribution of the hakomi method is this: the method contains as a necessary element precise experiments done with a person in a mindful state, the purpose being to evoke emotions, memories, and reactions that will reveal or help access those implicit beliefs influencing the client's nonconscious habitual behavior."

Throughout each session, patients are taught to maintain mindful self-awareness and to inform the practitioner about what is happening in their bodies during their manipulative therapy. When the patient reaches this internally reflective—almost meditative—state, the practitioner uses positive statements, called "probes," to conjure up personal insights and emotions. The simultaneous mindful and manipulative work has a certain synergy, Kurtz claims, with recipients' emotional attentiveness and sensitivity. Patients of hakomi learn to release unhealthful coping mechanisms (such as nervous habits and self-destructive tendencies), as they gain deeper understanding of how their bodies interact with their minds and souls. Hakomi is mostly characterized and separated from other similar forms of body-centered psychotherapy by its compassionate, gentle, and soothing approach to health. Although hakomi is not regulated or licensed, certification programs are available through a limited number of professional institutions.

RESOURCES

BOOKS

Body-Centered Psychotherapy: The Hakomi Method: The Integrated Use of Mindfulness, Nonviolence and the Body by Ron Kurtz

Grace Unfolding: Psychotherapy in the Spirit of Tao-te ching by Greg Johanson and Ron Kurtz
Body-Centered Psychotherapy by Ron Kurtz

Body-Mind Psychotherapy: Principles, Techniques, and Practical Applications by Susan Aposhyan

ONLINE

Wikipedia: Hakomi
http://en.wikipedia.org/wiki/Hakomi

Contains a useful step-by-step analysis of hakomi's procedural method

Flowing Body, Flexible Mind
www.flowingbody.com/hakomi.htm

General information about hakomi

ORGANIZATIONS

The Hakomi Institute
www.hakomiinstitute.com

The Hakomi Institute was founded in Boulder, Colorado, in 1981 by Ron Kurtz and a core group of trainers. Now it is a membership organization as well as a training center. It offers courses of varying length ranging from master's degree programs through PhD programs. It also publishes a professional journal.

Ron Kurtz Hakomi Training
www.ronkurtz.com

The Web site from the founder of Hakomi

United States Association for Body Psychotherapy
www.usabp.org/

The USABP is a nonprofit membership association dedicated to developing and advancing the art, science, and practice of body psychotherapy.

Hakomi Institute of San Francisco
www.sfhakomi.org

This institute offers weekend workshops, hakomi method training, consultations, and seminars in the San Francisco Bay Area.

Hakomi Institute of Atlanta
www.hakomiatlanta.org

This institution offers weekend workshops, hakomi method training, consultations, couples therapy, and seminars in the Atlanta area.

HERBAL MEDICINE

Herbalism has been around since before the dawn of medicine, which is also the dawn of humankind. Even chimpanzees, and other animals, use specific plants to treat ailments and elevate mood. So too, the earliest human tribal communities around the globe used plant preparations that were found in the wild to aid their own natural healing processes. This tradition continues today, from still "undiscovered" Amazonian tribes to counterculture (and now increasingly mainstream), modern, allopathy-based, first world nations. Herbology as it is known is an ancient art that is also on the cusp of cutting-age medicine, as governments and naturopathic institutions continue to put more and more research focus on the science behind our archaic planetary folk medicines.

Even though herbalism has accompanied every human generation on Earth, it comes as a big surprise to many Americans that most prescription drugs in the United States have been derived from plants. The relatively sterile, chemical-based world of modern medicine has done a masterful job of convincing Americans that what is invented by modern men is safer and more effective than the herbal medicines that got us so far in the first place. Yet the healing power of herbs is well established worldwide, and herbalism works well as a relatively noninvasive complement to other methods of healing.

Modern herbalism (also known as herbal medicine) is a system of healing that utilizes whole plants, plant extracts, and natural products containing plant ingredients for the treatment of almost every conceivable health concern. It is simultaneously a healing art and a science. Herbalists are responsible for diagnosing and treating patients, understanding and producing existing herbal remedies, and inventing new herbal formulas by combining and mixing new herbs with old ones. Herbalism rests on a basic premise that all the ingredients necessary to heal a person already exist in nature; cures do not need to be created in a lab, synthesized by a scientist, or performed by a surgeon. Instead, our natural world has both the intrinsic power to create life and heal life, as well as to destroy it. With the accumulated knowledge and wisdom of various plants and their medicinal functions, ingestion of carefully selected herbs and remedies can help to cure illness and restore bodily homeostasis. If we accept that diseases are a manifestation of the natural world, isn't it logical to expect that their cure will also be found in the natural world?

Herbalism has a particularly patchwork history because it has been used to varying degrees within the many forms of traditional medicine. In the American colonies, herbalism developed out of family home remedies derived from the combination of European and Native American folklore. Most forms of herbalism were based on a system of elements, such as within ancient ayurvedic, Chinese, and Greek medical systems. Only within the last hundred years or so has this elemental system been almost entirely dropped from herbal medicine, even by those who claim to be preserving traditional herbal medicine. Except for the manipulative, nonmedicinal therapies, most forms of healing that use any type of medication are in some way based upon the herbalist tradition. With plants making up such a high percentage of the human diet for millennia, it was nearly automatic that the trial-and-error approach to plant ingestion would also result in highly plant-based medical systems around the globe. Today, allopathic scientists around the world are still researching the healing properties of plants in order to synthesize cures for diseases such as cancer, HIV/AIDS, and psychological disorders. As the world forests continue to be decimated by encroaching technologies, these scientists understand that we are also losing our richest treasure of biochemical medicines within this disappearing sector of the plant kingdom.

The herbalist's philosophy is rooted in a deep-seated respect for the earth. Plants and herbs are valuable entities and are to be honored for their medical value as well as their inherent right to exist. While specific plants are used for specific ailments, many herbs are also believed to support the human immune system and ideal cellular function in a variety of ways. In this sense, herbal treatment can be curative, preventive, and perhaps even rejuvenative. Herbalism can also work in complement with other treatments for patients at risk of side effects. For instance, patients receiving chemotherapy or taking heavy doses of antibiotics will often seek herbal treatment not as an alternative to allopathy but to work in complement with their primary allopathic treatments. Not only can such complementary practices speed the healing process; they can also help to prevent side effects from allopathic protocols (or, in rare cases, promote them).

Herbalism in Practice

There are five basic routes of administering herbal remedies within the field of herbal medicine. Each method has its distinct advantages and disadvantages, and the method chosen is usually a collaborative effort between the practitioner and the patient:

Tinctures are alcohol/glycerin and water extracts of one or more herbs. The herbs to be extracted are first pulverized and then soaked for at least several hours in whatever liquid ratios are most appropriate for ideal extraction of the plant's constituents. The filtered solutions are then dissolved into water, around a teaspoon at a time, and drunk by the patient several times a day. Echinacea extract is one such example. Tinctures can also come in concentrated powders within pills or gel-caps.

Infusions and decoctions are hot-water extracts of herb. These are medicinal herbal teas but normally far more concentrated than those drunk for everyday thirst-quenching. Dried bits of herbs are placed into hot water and either simmered for a longer time to make decoctions from roots, barks, and stems, or for a shorter time to make infusions from leaves and flowers. Because there is no alcohol in teas, plants with mostly water-soluble constituents are most appropriate in this form. Those with fat-soluble constituents are best taken whole or in alcohol extract form. Teas are drunk after the water has absorbed as much as possible of the active ingredients in the plants being simmered.

Topical application of herbal concoctions is another method of administering herbal medicine. Oils are mixed with herb constituents and hardened into salves and ointments for absorption of plant medicines through the skin. Sometimes the herbs are designed to treat surface skin lesions, and sometimes they are designed to penetrate all the way to the bloodstream for systemic healing. Placing plant essential oils upon the skin is primarily practiced in aromatherapy.

Suppositories are a subset of topical medications that are better absorbed through the anus and rectum or vagina than through another body orifice. Usually herbs are mixed into a waxy base that slowly melts upon the skin. Herbs for the treatment of hemorrhoids or vaginal yeast infections are two such examples. Another important usage is for those individuals with poorly functioning digestive systems. Since these patients aren't able to comfortably ingest any herb orally, suppository dosing is an effective alternative for herbal medicine absorption.

Raw herb consumption is "chewing the plant directly" and is the oldest, easiest method of administration— if you can stand the taste. Medicinal roots and shoots have long been chewed and swallowed by patients of indigenous healers to promote healing. And this method is still used today, although most patients take their raw herbs within relatively tasteless tablets and capsules. This provides most of the medicinal benefits while removing any patient dislike regarding eating the unaltered plant. Many herbalists argue that consuming an entire plant part is the most beneficial way to ingest an herb. They believe that the multiple ingredients in plants work synergistically. This is opposed to the normal allopathic model, which isolates the perceived active chemical or chemicals within an herb and uses that part alone for medical treatment.

Insufflation is the last major method of administering herbal medicines. This is primarily used in aromatherapy, such as during the inhalation of essential oils. Herbal medicines for treating upper respiratory symptoms are sometimes most effective when taken into the nose. The current discovery in the U.S. of the ayurvedic "neti pot" for nasal lavage is one way in which insufflation is being used today. In India, herbs are often added to the neti pot salt water mixture so that extra healing can occur where the solution washes over any inflamed mucous membranes.

Career Opportunities

Currently, most herbalists in the United States are self-employed. Some offer educational herb walks for local laypersons or general health advice as they carefully avoid practicing medicine without a license. Some choose to run small manufacturing companies and create their own herbal products to sell to larger distribution plants or retail stores. There are various teaching positions in herbology available at nontraditional medicine colleges. Some herbalists will go to work for the more entrepreneurial herbalists (mentioned above), and jobs can range from growing herbs to extracting plant constituents. The best way to find jobs within the field of herbology is to attend herbal conferences, oriental medicine seminars, and ayurvedic workshops. Since few of these positions are advertised conventionally (classifieds; online job sites), networking is key. The resources herein can help you begin a career as a herbologist.

In addition, there is a branch of anthropology entitled "ethno-botany." Ethno-botanists study the use of plants in native cultures for food, medicine, religious practice, home crafts, etc. Research opportunities and other various academic jobs are sometimes available in this field. Most of this type of work, though it is not necessarily involved with the practice of medicine, is found through university or private institutions. Typically, academic positions are reserved for undergraduate and graduate students within the field of ethno-botany.

Economics and Herbalism

One common answer to the question, "How much money can I make as an herbalist?" is: "As much as you want." As usual, this normally means, "Not much, but if you have excellent business skills anything can happen!" Many working herbalists choose to live away from civilization and "off the grid," closer to their plant allies. Others make comfortable capital working as counselors, teachers, writers, or holistic practitioners within urban confines still rife with hardy medicinal plants. Most herbalists have more than one job or are also certified practitioners in other healing modalities. Herbalism is often a wonderful complement of knowledge for an already established healer.

A Note on Regulation and Licensure

Herbalists tend to fall under state regulations governing a small business owner rather than under laws concerned with medicinal practice. Herbalists who grow herbs for the use of others, or who manufacture products from raw herbs, are under the jurisdiction of laws governing the safe production of foods and food supplements. Some states restrict the sale of certain herbs, which are considered harmful—ephedra, comfrey root, and chaparral being three recently restricted herbs. The American Herbal Products Association (www.ahpa.org) is one organization that helps herbalists conform with state regulations. In general, the scope of herbal medicine practice is dictated by how the herbal treatment is used. For instance, a licensed massage therapist may be able to use herbs in her practice, but only as it is relevant to muscle tension and/or chronic pain.

Eligibility Requirements for School

Most herbalists begin training by taking correspondence courses or reading any number of instructive books on herbalism. After gaining a general understand of the methods and techniques used, students can move on to "one-on-one" herbal apprenticeship training with other professionals. Most correspondence courses have few eligibility requirements, and there is a plethora of nonprofessional classes that are available to just about anyone.

Independent teachers offer a more pragmatic approach to herbal medicine via field trips, hands-on activities, and weekend classes. Some courses will speak of herbal medicine in the same context as allopathic drug therapy (how much herb to prescribe for which symptom); some will focus on plant energetics and Shamanism. Others will focus on botany or fieldwork, and some will teach students how to prepare various plant medicines from raw herbs. "Wildcrafting"—the art of identifying and picking herbs in the wild—is one type of activity that makes education in herbalism far different from modern, lecture-oriented classroom education.

There are also other workshops and retreats that are structured as continuing education for current practitioners. Often CAM professions that require a continuing education component (such as massage or chiropractic) will offer credit for classes or seminars in herbal medicine.

Tuition, Aid, and Graduation

There is a wide array of herbalist programs, which run from weekend seminars (a few hundred dollars) to yearlong certification programs. The latter, more intensive programs can be as expensive as $4,000 per year. As a rule, financial aid is usually not available to these nonaccredited and nonrecognized institutions. Currently, there is no formal or standardized system of accreditation for herbalism schools. If the herbology course is being offered at a larger institution that *does* offer financial aid (such as a community college or university), then financial aid is a more realistic possibility. Most courses are structured to take less than a year. Schools in the United Kingdom offer four-year degree programs in herbalism, but this is true for the minority of herbology programs.

Professionalism in the Field

The American Herbalists Guild (AHG) offers a type of professional membership. The AHG welcomes members after a peer-reviewed processing of each applicant via an admission committee. Applicants submit personal and professional biographies outlining their experience, training, and knowledge of herbalism. Typically, professional members of the AHG have several years of experience in herbal medicine, complete the AHG essay requirements, provide letters of recommendation or reference from other professional herbalists, and pay an application fee. Once accepted into the AHG, applicants are granted permanent membership after they submit their curriculum vitae. The advantage to membership is not to gain larger clientele directly; rather, the AHG is a wonderful network for communication with dedicated professional herbalists. It is also a good place to access information about herbology seminars, scientific studies, and new methods and breakthroughs.

RESOURCES

BOOKS

The Master Book of Herbalism by Paul Beyer

Encyclopedia of Herbal Medicine by Andrew Chevallier

Natureae Medicina and Naturopathic Dispensatory by A.W. Kuts-Cheraux

Comprehensive Monographs on Ayurvedic and Chinese Herbs by Kerry Bone

ONLINE

International Bibliographic Information on Dietary Supplements
ods.od.nih.gov/Health_Information/IBIDS.aspx

This resource boasts more than 400,000 scientific citations and abstracts on dietary supplements.

ORGANIZATIONS

American Botanical Council
www.herbalgram.org

An independent, nonprofit research and education organization dedicated to providing accurate and reliable information for consumers, health care practitioners, researchers, educators, industry, and the media

American Herbal Pharamacopoeia
www.herbal-ahp.org

The declared mission of the AHP is to promote the responsible use of herbal medicines and ensure they are used with the highest degree of safety and efficacy as is achievable.

American Herbalists Guild
www.americanherbalistsguild.com

The AHG was founded in 1989 as a nonprofit, educational organization to represent the goals and voices of herbalists specializing in the medicinal use of plants. Its primary objective is to promote a high level of professionalism and education in the study and practice of therapeutic herbalism.

Herb Research Foundation
www.herbs.org

The Herb Research Foundation is the authority on health benefits and safety.

NONDEGREE TRAINING IN HERBALISM

Alchemy Botanicals
Ashland, Oregon
www.alchemybotanicals.com

Australasian College of Health Sciences
Portland, Oregon
www.achs.edu

Northwest College for Herbal and Aromatic Studies
Willow Spring, North Carolina
www.theida.com

Avena Institute
West Rockport, Maine
www.avenainstitute.org

Bastyr University
Kenmore, Washington
www.bastyr.edu

Blazing Star Herbal School
Shelburne Falls, Massachusetts
www.blazingstarherbalschool.org

Blue Heron Academy
Six schools in Michigan and one in Indiana
www.blueheronacademy.com

Blue Ridge School of Herbal Medicine
Asheville, North Carolina
www.BlueRidgeSchool.org

Boston School of Herbal Energetics
Arlington, Massachusetts
www.bostonherbalstudies.com

California School of Herbal Studies
Forestville, California
www.cshs.com

Centre for Natural Healing
Ashland, Oregon
www.centrehealing.com

Chicago College of Healing Arts
Chicago, Illinois
www.chicagocollegeofhealingarts.com

Clayton College of Natural Health
Birmingham, Alabama
www.ccnh.edu

David Winston's Center for Herbal Studies
Broadway, New Jersey
www.herbalstudies.org

EarthSong Herbals
Marblehead, Massachusetts
www.earthsongherbals.com

East West School of Herbology
Ben Lomond, California
www.planetherbs.com

Florida School of Herbal Studies
Orlando, Florida
www.floridaherbalschool.com

Foundations in Herbal Medicine
Albuquerque, New Mexico
www.fihm.com

Foundations of Herbalism
Williams, Oregon
www.foundationsofherbalism.com

Greenfingers Foundation for Studies in Herbal Medicine
Phoenix, Arizona
greenfingersherbs@copper.net

Heart of Herbs
Springfield, Vermont
demetria@demetria.com

Herb Pharm HerbaCulture Work/Study Program
Williams, Oregon
www.herb-pharm.com/Education/workstudy_fs.html

Herbal Medicine for Women
Cheshire, Connecticut
E-mail: avivajill@aol.com

Institute of Aromatic and Herbal Studies
San Francisco, California
www.jeannerose.net

Midwest School of Herbal Studies
New Brighton, Minnesota
www.midwestherbalstudies.com

NAMTI School of Botanical Studies
Sedona, Arizona
www.namti.com

Northeast School of Botanical Medicine
Ithaca, New York
www.7song.com

Philo School of Herbal Energetics
Philo, California
www.herbalenergetics.com

Pipsissewa Herbs
Bloomington Springs, Tennessee
www.pipsissherbs.com

PrairieWise Herbal School
Kansas City, Missouri
www.prairiewise.com

Professional Herbalists Training Program
St. Petersburg, Florida
www.acuherbals.com

Red Moon Herbs Educational Center
Black Mountain, North Carolina
www.redmoonherbs.com

Sierra Institute of Herbal Studies
Big Oak Flat, California
www.sierra-institute.com

Southwest Institute of Healing Arts
Tempe, Arizona
www.swiha.org

Southwest School of Botanical Medicine
Bisbee, Arizona
www.swsbm.com

Tai Sophia Institute
Laurel, Maryland
www.tai.edu

The North American Institute of Medical Herbalism
Boulder, Colorado
www.naimh.com

The North Carolina School of Holistic Herbalism
Asheville, North Carolina
www.HerbsHeal.com

The School of Natural Healing
Springville, Utah
www.snh.cc

Tree of Light
St. George, Utah
www.treelite.com

HOLOTROPIC BREATHWORK

This is perhaps the only healing modality to directly result from governmental repression of scientific research into the use of psychedelic ("mind-manifesting") medicine for the study and treatment of psychopathology. Used for millennia for initiation rites, group bonding, mystical insights, and practical guidance by many native cultures around the world, psychedelics were introduced to the West when chemist Albert Hofmann of Switzerland accidentally absorbed some lysergic acid diethylamide (LSD) through his skin at work one day in 1943. Although Hofmann had been seeking for ways in which LSD could be of general pharmaceutical use, soon practitioners and researchers within the field of psychology realized that a new, extremely powerful class of chemicals was at their disposal. These chemicals seemed to create a temporary psychosis in nearly every recipient; yet depending on the mind-set and the external environment ("set and setting") of the patient, this altered state was subjectively experienced on a spectrum from exhilarating, liberating, and enlightening to devastating and terrifying.

Most psychologists and psychiatrists, from the late 1940s to mid-1960s, placed a great deal of attention on the potential therapeutic use of these now-called "entheogens." Stanislav Grof, MD, was no exception. Grof became one of the leading LSD doctors in the world, treating hundreds of psychiatric patients from 1957 until LSD became illegal around 1966 due to "off-label" recreational use. Grof noted that LSD's extreme effects were useful not just for treating the ill; they could also assist those who were thought to be psychologically "normal." Rapturous reports from LSD-inspired individuals were found to be indistinguishable from reports of mystical ecstasy from religious figures throughout the ages. And LSD "trips" also began to reproduce what seemed to Grof and his patients to be prenatal and perinatal memories in some patients, helping to relieve them of chronic psychopathologies. From these experiences, Grof synthesized an overarching belief that mental illness is based more on spiritual disconnect and birth trauma than anything else.

When LSD was made illegal, not only was the catalyst for his life's work no longer available for research, it was demonized by governments, and those practitioners who had used it tended to pretend that it had never existed in the first place out of fear for their career reputations. Over the last two decades, there has been an increasing tide of research on LSD and other psychedelics, especially due to the impressive work of Rick Doblin, a Harvard PhD from the Kennedy School, and his Multidisciplinary Association for Psychedelic Studies. This did not occur fast enough for Grof, however, who needed to find a new modality that would legally elicit psychedelically similar altered states of consciousness in his patients. And though Grof has stated that his answer never really approached the power of LSD, he simply did the best he could: enter holotropic breathwork.

Holotropic breathwork is itself a powerful, holistic, experiential method that integrates aspects of anthropology, transpersonal psychology, depth psychology, Eastern spiritual practices, and consciousness research. It is a psychotherapeutic approach that allows clients to access nonordinary states of consciousness without the use of synthetic drugs or plant medicines. The word, "holotropic," is derived from the Greek *holos*, "wholeness," and *trepein*, "moving in a particular direction."

The method is relatively simple and quite comparable to some forms of meditation. Practitioners instruct patients to accelerate their breathing, while concentrating on evocative music in a peaceful external setting and lying on one's back with eyes closed. Holotropic breathwork is more common in group settings. Participants usually work in pairs and have a distinct role as the "breather" and the "sitter." The latter's responsibility is to focus compassionate attention toward the breather and to assist, but not interfere, with the breather's experience.

Bodywork upon breathers and expressive drawing by breathers may also occur depending on felt needs. Participants in holotropic breathwork sessions report a wide variety of experiences. From observations of

people in these nonordinary states of mind, Grof developed what he considers to be a "cartography" of the psyche, which describes four main categories of experience:

Sensory and somatic: This realm of experience includes various hallucinatory phenomena, such as visualizing images or geometrical patterns. More commonly, participants report a greater awareness of and ability to act out somatic processes and bodily impulses, such as assuming postures, dancing or moving in specific ways, and making sounds. They may also claim to feel where energy is blocked or streaming, consistent with the belief in vitalism.

Biographical and individual unconscious: As in more traditional therapies, participants may revisit unresolved conflicts, repressed memories, and nonintegrated traumas. Compared to talk therapies, the unconscious material is more likely to be reexperienced than merely remembered. Participants report that this deeper processing can be more effective at clearing trauma, especially as it relates to subtle ways that trauma is held in the body.

Perinatal: In disagreement with Freud's claim that the infant after birth is basically a blank slate, Grof believes that the birth process is a traumatic event that leaves powerful residue in the psyche (see further description below). Participants in holotropic breathwork sessions report having images, emotions, physical sensations, and cognitions that convince them that they are remembering aspects of their own birth. Sometimes details can be verified with medical records. Some claim that these experiences help them release the birth trauma, including deeply held negative beliefs about themselves and the world.

Transpersonal: Referring to the possibility of accessing information outside the normal boundaries of the ego and body, transpersonal experiences reported in holotropic breathwork sessions include past-life memories, experiential identification with other life forms, out-of-body experiences, oneness with Nature or another aspect of God, encounters with spiritual archetypes, and connection with the human collective unconscious.

At the end of each breathwork session, it is important that each breather feel well grounded and that the session has come to a successful resolution. Bodywork upon the breather is one way to help an unresolved session come to a relaxed completion. At this stage it is common for the breather to experience spontaneous "violent shaking, grimacing, coughing, gagging, vomiting, a variety of movements, and a wide range of sounds that include screaming, baby talk, animal voices, talking in tongues or a language foreign to the client, Shamanic chanting, and many others." These are all considered to be external manifestations of emotional pain that will subside if they are allowed to express without inhibition.

Contraindications to this practice are similar to those for psychedelic therapy in general: avoid holotropic breathwork if a potential breather has serious cardiovascular problems, severe psychiatric illness, and/or pregnancy; special precautions are recommended in the case of epileptics. Grof points out that caution is required in the case of individuals with a history of psychiatric hospitalization, "If the process gets to be too active and extends beyond the framework of the sessions, it can require special measures." Elsewhere, Grof writes that "experiential work with severely disturbed individuals requires a special residential facility with trained staff where continuous support is available for twenty-four hours a day, it should not be conducted on an outpatient basis."

Holotropic breathwork can be a complementary addition to a psychospiritually oriented therapy practice. It also may have application within massage therapy, or any kind of manipulative bodywork, especially if the practitioner is experienced with the spectrum of altered states of consciousness.

There is an extensive training and certification program for facilitators through Grof Transpersonal Training. For those who wish to become certified, there are two tracks: educational and practitioner. Both cover training in transpersonal psychology (including psychopathology, spiritual emergency, and addictions), as well as the theory and practice of holotropic breathwork. The training also includes ten hours of consultation with a certified practitioner and 150 total hours of participation in holotropic breathwork workshops led by Stanislav Grof or a certified practitioner. In addition, those wishing to become independent workshop leaders (practitioners) must apprentice at least four times at workshops with previously certified practitioners before leading groups of their own. There are currently more than 1,000 trained facilitators located throughout the world, including clinicians, businessmen, psychotherapists, etc.

There is also an Association for Holotropic Breathwork International, which promotes professional and ethical practices governing holotropic breathwork. Other institutions may offer Grof-accredited training programs; consult their Web sites for more specific information.

RESOURCES

BOOKS

Exploring Holotropic Breathwork by Kylea Taylor

The Breathwork Experience: Exploration and Healing in Nonordinary States of Consciousness by Kylea Taylor

The Adventure of Self-Discovery by Stanislav Grof

ONLINE

Holotropic Breathwork Links
primal-page.com/holo.htm

Provocative information on its historical use in conjunction with LSD psychotherapy. Includes academic article by Dr. Stanislav Grof

Holistic Med Online
www.holisticmed.com/inner/breath/holotropic.html

Good summary of general information on holotropic breathwork

ORGANIZATIONS

The Association for Holotropic Breathwork International
www.breathwork.com

Supports the practice and integrity of holotropic breathwork

Grof Transpersonal Training

www.holotropic.com

Provides training programs in holotropic bodywork and other spiritually based transpersonal disciplines

Holotropic Breathwork in Seattle

holotropicbreathwork.net

Seminars, education, training, practitioner networking, and general conferences regarding transpersonal psychology in the Seattle area

The Association for Transpersonal Psychology

www.atpweb.org

The Institute of Transpersonal Psychology

www.itp.edu

Holotropic Breathwork in California

www.holotropicbreath.com

Seminars, education, training, practitioner networking, and general conferences concerning holotropic breathwork throughout California

Stanislav Grof's Home Page

www.stanislavgrof.com

The personal Web page by the founder of holotropic breathwork

Dia Lynn's Home Page

www.dialynn.com/breathwork.htm

Dia Lynn is a certified practitioner and trainer of holotropic breathwork

HOMEOPATHY

The history and philosophy of homeopathy is one of medicine's strangest and deserves special attention for its audacious claims and global worldwide usage, as well as for its practitioners' frequent claims regarding their patients' near instantaneous relief from a myriad of symptoms.

Homeopathy sprouted from the mind of one allopath in 1796: Samuel Hahnemann, MD, a German physician and chemist. He was one of many MDs at the time who were disillusioned with the side effects of the staple treatments of the time, such as debilitating blood letting via leeches, toxic oral mercury and opiate concoctions, and powerful irritating laxatives. These allopathic standards often worsened symptoms and sometimes even killed people. George Washington is widely believed to be one of these fatalities.

One day Hahnemann was disagreeing with a certain medical claim regarding an herbal tree bark treatment in one of his textbooks. He swallowed some of this Cinchona bark, used effectively and safely for malaria treatment at the time. After a time, he began to feel fever, shivering, and joint pain, the same symptoms that herald the onset of malaria. From this event alone, he began to hypothesize that the best cures would come only from products that were extreme dilutions of those *same substances* that cause symptoms in *healthy* individuals. In other words, "Like cures like." He then quickly coined two terms, "homeopathy," meaning, "like cures disease," and "allopathy," meaning, "difference cures disease." To Hahnemann, the word "allopath" was a slur, and no "regular doctor," as they were called at the time, would have ever agreed to label himself an "allopathic doctor." To Hahnemann, he alone had discovered the secret to correct medical protocol. All others were allopathic fools.

Of course, Hahnemann made many MD enemies very quickly and had to move geographically around during his life to escape persecution. But Hahnemann also was an MD: he had impressive writing and debating skills and was quickly piling up a significant number of converts. One reason for this was because by simply removing the blood letting, etc., from patient care, this significantly improved the survival rate from certain diseases (such as bronchitis, the simple ailment that began Washington's tragic deathbed scenario). Patients and their families were also thrilled to be able to take small, sweet, candy-like homeopathic pills or liquid and recover from their ailments at often even better rates than before.

Within 120 years, homeopathy would become so popular in Europe and the United States that by 1915 approximately 15 percent of medical practitioners were officially homeopaths. Schools abounded on both sides of the Atlantic. Hahnemann's "Organon (System) of Rational Therapeutics" was published in 1810 to promote all of his discoveries, and its 1921 sixth edition is still one of the bibles of modern homeopathy. Yet by 1920, all homeopathy-only medical schools in the U.S. had closed. In between, this sometimes furious medical battle between homeopaths, "regular" allopaths, "eclectic" herbalists, naturopaths, chiropractors, and osteopaths experienced many dramatic twists and turns as each treated their respective patients' scourges of influenza, small pox, malaria, and other regularly lethal illnesses. Practitioners of each medical modality were trying to prove that their system was the best, providing preventative medicine and cures with the fewest side effects possible.

Not until the allopathic medical industry was able to combine with the U.S. Federal Government and begin to close the majority of their competitors' schools (via the Flexner Report of 1910) did the contest come to a quick conclusion. Homeopathy became a fringe medical modality from this point on in the United States, becoming part of the complementary and alternative medicine community up until the present time. Homeopathy in Europe continued to flourish, however, despite virulent criticism from Queen Victoria's royal physician at the time.

Ironically, the British Royal Family has become one of the strongest proponents for homeopathy in postmodern times, and one of England's ex-colonies—India—has become the main purveyor of cutting-edge homeopathic philosophy. When the medical practitioners and spiritual searchers of India came in contact with the vitalistic, energetic, invisible, panacea-like, instantaneous, life force manipulating, and inexpensive medicine emanating from Europe, they quickly merged it with their own ayurvedic and Yogic beliefs. Today millions of Indians use homeopathy as their primary form of first-line treatment and homeopaths as their general practitioners; equal millions of Americans use homeopathic remedies via their health food stores or their CAM practitioners. Someday we may even understand if homeopathy works, and, much more difficult, how it works. For now, homeopathy remains arguably the most popular, yet mysterious, medical modality in use today.

The first principle behind homeopathy is the law of similars: for the perfect medicine, use the same substance that will produce the exact same symptoms as you are experiencing now and want to get rid of. The second principle was the law of infinitesimals: use but an infinitesimally small dilution of whatever medicine you choose.

The third principle is prescribe these diluted medicines, as much as possible, not only based on detailed symptom descriptions but also on the intricate details of each patient's lifestyle and temperament. Because each patient is unique, his or her vitalistic life force flow is presumed to be unique. Therefore, the ideal remedy might be unique and difficult to determine. Because many different substances produce similar symptoms in a healthy person, one way to distinguish remedy sources was to also determine what kind of activities and mind-set a person generally experiences if he or she takes those same substances, like Cinchona bark, at full strength. If greater fastidiousness appeared after ingestion of some full-strength herb, then that diluted herb was better for treating a normally fastidious person versus an herb that at full strength produced greater sloppiness in a healthy person.

Why would a healthy person take these full-strength substances in the first place? To help the cause of homeopathy, or simply to be a paid research subject. These testings are called "proving," and they still occur to this day via homeopaths who choose to further their craft by testing a substance that has not yet been "proved." Once it has been proved, it can enter the official textbooks that have been formulated since Hahnemann's time.

Confused or astounded yet? It gets much stranger, sometimes bordering on a "beyond the looking-glass" adventure. Not to say that homeopathy doesn't work, but here are some rational questions that homeopathy will have to answer as long as scientific research to date ranges from ambivalent to negative regarding homeopathic treatment effectiveness:

Why does each remedy, often diluted to the point that no measurable amount of the original substance can be detected anymore, have to be "succussed," or shaken or beaten in such a way before the remedy is effective? Hahnemann believed that succussing loosened the vital force from the substance being diluted and allowed the substance to become an invisible, immeasurable, quick-acting medicine. Hahnemann is reported to have joked that a suitable procedure for dealing with an epidemic would be to empty a bottle of poison into Lake Geneva if it could be succussed sixty times.

Why do homeopathic remedies become more potent the more diluted they become? The more deeply a symptom picture has invaded the body-mind-spirit complex that Hahnemann believed made up a human organism, the more dilute the remedy should be. This leads to another questions: What is the *spiritual mechanism* in action that systematically increases a remedy's action the more it is diluted in water and succussed?

What is the mechanism behind the homeopathic belief that using allopathic medicine in opposition to symptoms automatically suppresses those symptoms, likely to return in a more severe, transmogrified form? If this belief is true, why do the vast majority of people in the West, raised with allopathic medical treatments, live as long and as healthily as homeopaths do? Most of us should be "basket cases" next to the radiant homeopaths and homeopathic patients around us.

Why does taking a homeopathic dilution of an allopathic drug only decrease the side effects of that drug, as claimed by homeopaths? Why doesn't it also remove the general effects of that drug? How does the substance, diluted into a spiritual form, know which effect to alter?

How can provings, which used to be assessed using full-strength substances, now be done with astronomically dilute substances, yet still be claimed to give the same results? How can these "30C" dilutions, or 1:10 to the sixtieth power, be considered so strong that patients are warned to be careful using such a remedy unless they bring on negative "proving" symptoms instead of the healing they thought was on the way?

How could the allopathic suppression of scabies symptoms lead to such diverse future ailments as epilepsy, cancer, deafness, and cataracts? Hahnemann believed that there were three main categories of suppression early in life that later led to predictable diseases, and that these diseases could be avoided if folks would just wake up and use only homeopathy. Suppressing itching symptoms in general, and especially scabies, was the biggest category of all. Yet there is no known link between allopathic treatment of scabies, eczema, or any other itchy disease, with ailments such as cancer and cataracts.

The list of questionable elements of homeopathy dogma is longer than this. There are many other vitalistic, yet *allopathic*, medical modalities you can learn, such as ayurvedic and Chinese medicine. These systems also oppose symptoms with their full-strength medications, similar to American MDs.

Even chiropractors and osteopaths oppose their patients' symptoms by, for example, pushing bones in the opposite direction and back from where they deviated. One does not have to be a homeopath to be a vitalist; in fact, almost every other vitalistic system is at least partially allopathic in nature. Homeopathy is unique and requires a greater leap of faith from practitioners and patients than many CAM therapies. If you are not of an overly scientific mind-set, and if you are content with your medical modality having an utterly unknown mode of action given our current modern understanding of physics and chemistry, then homeopathy might be for you. If you are of a strongly rational mind-set, however, homeopathy's principles and rationales will leave you shaking your head time and time again.

With a more ancient medical system such as ayurveda, a modern scientist can at least test one of its treatment herbs for inflammation and prove it helpful according to modern science. This is the case for the common kitchen herb, turmeric. Scientists can then say to themselves that, even though the ancient vitalistic dogma behind ayurveda isn't believable to them, many ayurvedic remedies work when tested with scientific rigor. Homeopathic medicines usually don't even exist, however, other than the water and sugar that "carries" the infinitesimal dose of the original substance. And when research doesn't show that homeopathic remedies successfully treat specific ailments better than placebo, homeopaths complain that this is because you have to choose a specific remedy for the whole person not just the ailment symptoms. Immediately, homeopathy becomes nonduplicatable, because the choice of the right remedy is all based on the skill of the practitioner choosing the right remedy. Current science cannot measure such subjectivity, and so at the present time, we have a standstill: research scientists claiming that the only way they can test homeopathy results in insignificant effects from homeopathic remedies versus placebo, and homeopaths claiming that homeopathy only works if the homeopath chooses the right remedy at the right dose to be administered for the right amount of time.

Techniques

Even by homeopaths, it is said that a sizeable portion of patient healing can come from the interaction of homeopath and patient alone—long before a remedy is given. This is because a typical homeopathic medical intake is more rigorous and detailed than any other medical exam. In this case, there is no physical examination, just a lengthy oral intake combined with the homeopath taking in as much unspoken information as possible from the patient regarding his or her habits. Everything from the patient's normal sleep position to whether the patient can't stand the sour flavor to whether he or she urinates in a forked stream may be questioned—if it helps the practitioner narrow down which exact diluted remedy is the best for the patient at that specific time (some substances cause a person to urinate in a forked stream if taken at full strength, according to homeopathic provings). At the same time, the patient's general health and energy level is assessed, including how long his or her symptoms have persisted and which major symptoms (such as itching) may have been suppressed in the past. These interviews are so comprehensive that patients often leave feeling listened to, and verbally cared for, more than any other treatment modality.

Sometimes homeopaths will do a quick assessment on the spot and offer what they feel is the appropriate remedy from the hundreds of pills and liquids they have in stock. Sometimes this remedy is just a temporary general remedy to start the healing process before the homeopath spends more time figuring out the perfect medicine to match the patient's overall presentation. And sometimes the temporary "remedy" is a purposeful sugar pill with nothing on it, even according to a homeopath, so that the patient feels he or she is being immediately treated on the spot.

Unless homeopaths get a quick and clear picture of the right remedy to use, they usually turn to specific reference books for help. These list either all of the "proving symptoms" of thousands of substances in a materia medica, or all the substances connected with specific symptoms in a reperatory. Using these two opposing angles, and combining these with texts equating specific substances with specific personality types, homeopaths can generally come up with a likely remedy of even the most difficult cases within a couple of hours of study.

Some homeopaths believe that one remedy, chosen perfectly, should heal the patient of most of what ails him or her for an indefinitely long time. If this is the case, the homeopath is usually practicing constitutional homeopathy. The homeopath is searching for a patient's deepest set constitution rather than the patient's current acute symptom picture, as the homeopath is aiming for the deepest healing possible. Other homeopaths take their patients on a journey, giving one remedy to treat one symptom layer, then another and another as other symptom layers appear. Such homeopaths believe that such a process will eventually heal every layer of the patient: body-mind-soul. Often they produce engrossing case studies detailing their patients' experiences briefly reliving old disease symptoms from the past as they heal layer after layer.

Although Hahnemann bucked the allopathic trends of his time in recommending excellent diet and regular exercise for his patients, modern homeopathy rarely mentions the importance of doing much of anything regarding using any modality other than homeopathy for treatment. And, although modern naturopathy has effortlessly brought homeopathy under its huge CAM umbrella, homeopathy remains an oddball alongside most of the other umbrella residents. Both naturopaths and homeopaths tend to "look the other way" and not discuss the wide philosophical gap between their two forms of vitalism. Instead, they bond over the perceived common enemy of MD allopathy, not considering much that modern naturopathy can be very allopathic in its makeup. Treating a bacterial infection with bacteria-killing goldenseal herb is but one of many examples. Within homeopathic philosophy, this is pure allopathic medicine, even though it is also naturopathic. As such, one would think that homeopaths would condemn both naturopathy and MD allopathy. This is just one of the paradoxical conundrums one encounters through the diluted and succussed looking glass of homeopathy.

If homeopathy works as claimed, we may be on the verge of fully implementing an already intricately designed system of medicine far more advanced than any other in existence. This medical modality will treat us on all levels of our being, using the most inexpensive (because so dilute) medical treatments known to humankind, based on some as yet unknown energetic, spiritual, or "to-be-later-understood" physical mechanism that we simply cannot measure yet. Homeopathy has certainly not been disproved, and proponents can always claim that any individual or society is not yet evolved enough to understand the subtle metaphysics behind its healing power. Proponents of ayurvedic and Chinese medicine can claim the same as well. One difference is that our present science hasn't yet shown us how acupuncture works, but the U.S. Governement does now publish a long list of ailments shown to be helped by acupuncture treatments. The same type of validation may come for homeopathy, too, followed in some future society with answers regarding how it works that current homeopaths can only guess at. However, unlike acupuncture, the majority of studies regarding homeopathy are not in favor of the homeopaths. Unless researchers can come up with a scientifically reasonable way to test its effectiveness, homeopathy may find itself one of the odd men out as the newly forming field of integrative medicine unites folk medicine and evidence-based medicine.

If this is the case, then receiving a certification in homeopathy may only allow you to treat a small subset of the American population. This subset of homeopaths and their patients are often supportive, however, forging a bond over the hypothetical healing mysteries at the borderlines of body, mind, and spirit.

RESOURCES

BOOKS

Homeopathy: A Frontier in Medical Science by Paolo Bellavite, MD, and Andrea Signorini, MD

Science or Myth? by Bill Gray, MD

The Organon of the Medical Art by Samual Hahnemann, MD, and W.B. O'Reilly

Kent's Repertory of Homeopathic Materia Medica by J.T. Kent, MD

The Science of Homeopathy by George Vithoulkas

ONLINE

Archibel
www.archibel.com
Software and books for homeopathy

HomeopathyHome
www.homeopathyhome.com
A large portal Web site providing information, health news, homeopathic remedies, and books

Homoeosite
http://homoeosite.7p.com
Provides all the essentials including a wealth of homeopathic related resources to make you familiar with this good and gentle medicine, as well as information about professional training courses in Pakistan

The Homeopathic Archives
www.julianwinston.com/archives
Historical information about homoeopathy compiled by Julian Winston

Homeopathic Educational Services
www.homeopathic.com/articles/research/scienti.php
Scientific evidence for homeopathic medicine compiled by Dana Ullman

Ask Dr. Shah
http://askdrshah.com
Dr. Rajesh Shah, MD, an internationally acclaimed physician and teacher, practices in Mumbai, India. He has studied homeopathy intensively for twenty years. Over the years he has conducted seminars and workshops for practitioners and students in England, Holland, Belgium, the Czech Republic, Greece, Sweden, U.S.A., Ireland, Croatia, and Norway.

ORGANIZATIONS

The National Center for Homeopathy
www.homeopathic.org
www.nationalcenterforhomeopathy.org

The NCH is an open-membership organization whose mission is to promote health through homeopathy. By providing general education to the public about homeopathy, and specific education to homeopaths, its members hope to make homeopathy available throughout the United States.

The American Institute of Homeopathy
www.homeopathyusa.org

The AIH is a professional trade association of medical and osteopathic physicians, dentists, advanced practice nurses, and physician assistants dedicated to the practice, promotion, and improvement of homeopathic medicine. The organization places great emphasis on the dissemination of homeopathic medical knowledge through publishing, public speaking, and education.

Homeopathic Academy of Naturopathic Physicians
www.hanp.net

The HANP, affiliated with the American Association of Naturopathic Physicians, intends to further the excellence and success of homeopathic practice in the naturopathic community. The organization is a vehicle for outreach into both communities. It has an extensive membership and hosts annual symposia for the advancement of homeopathic philosophy in naturopathic practice.

The American Association of Homeopathic Pharmacists
www.homeopathicpharmacy.org

The AAHP is an alliance of homeopathic product manufacturers, importers, and exporters. All AAHP members manufacture and/or sell homeopathic drugs in the United States.

North American Society of Homeopaths
www.homeopathy.org

NASH was originally founded in 1990. The organization's mission is to "set standards of competency and to certify individuals in the practice of classical homeopathy in order to inform and protect health care consumers in search of homeopathic treatment."

Council for Homeopathic Certification
www.homeopathicdirectory.com

In 1991, the CHC was formed in response to a new vision for the future of homeopathy as a unified profession of highly trained and certified practitioners. To date, it has certified more practitioners than any other professional homeopathic organization. Consult CHC's Web site for the specific aspects and requirements of homeopathic certification.

Homeopathic Nurses Association
www.nursehomeopaths.org

The HNA is a professional organization for nurses who are pioneering the practice of homeopathy in nursing and choosing to help their clients through personal and family health challenges. Using the science and art of homeopathy, nurses act as educators, primary health practitioners, and/or consultants for clients interested in using this holistic modality. The organization's membership group provides a vast network of homeopathic nurses throughout the United States.

The International Association for Veterinary Homeopathy
www.iavh.org

The IAVH was founded in 1986 with the goal of maintaining and promoting understanding in the area of homoeopathic veterinary medicine.

The Homœopathic Pharmacopœia of the United States
www.hpus.com

The HPUS is the official compendium for homeopathic drugs in the U.S. It has been in continuous publication since 1897, when it was first published by the Committee on Pharmacy of the American Institute of Homeopathy.

HOSPICE WORKER

As midwifery is to the birthing process, so hospice is to the dying process. Midwives work to lessen the potential negative side effects of the natural "symptoms" of pregnancy and birth as they compassionately smooth the way for mothers, fathers, babies, and extended families to healthfully begin a life together with as few pharmaceutical interventions as possible. Hospice workers work to lessen the potential negative side effects of the natural symptoms of terminal illness as they compassionately smooth the way for patients and their support systems to "healthfully" complete a patient's life with as few pharmaceutical interventions as possible.

Both of these modalities take stances not accepted by the allopathic mainstream: midwives state that pregnancy and birth is a common physical event that usually results in a healthy mother and child; it is not a medical condition to be feared and overmedicated. Hospice workers state that the dying and death of the terminally ill physical body is an even more common physical event that always results in permanent, complete withdrawal of the life force and subsequent physical decomposition. It is also not a medical condition to be feared and overmedicated. Being birthed by a midwife, treated by holistic practitioners throughout life for nonemergency ailments, nurtured by holistic allopaths for more life-threatening ailments, then tended and inspired by hospice workers if physical death is inevitable would be one worthy model for a lifelong system of integrated medical care.

Hospices used to be places for travelers to rest during long journeys and were conceived of around 300 B.C. In the nineteenth century, the first hints of hospice care for the dying appeared in religious orders in Ireland and England. But modern hospice developed from the work of physician, Dame Cicely Saunders, of London. Her St. Christopher's Hospice, founded in 1967, became the standard for international hospices as she taught her fellow allopaths how to ease the psychophysiological traumas commonly experienced by dying patients and their loved ones. Two major discoveries also emerged from her initial hospice program. One was "Brompton's Cocktail," a mixture of several medicines that was given as an elixir for the relief of pain. The second came as a result of working in collaboration with psychiatrist Stanislav Grof, MD (see Holotropic Breathwork), as he taught Saunders the importance of the holistic, body-mind-spirit approach for the relief of emotional and spiritual suffering of the terminally ill and their caregivers.

Even before founding her own hospice, Saunders introduced the idea of specialized care for the dying to the United States during a 1963 visit to Yale University. Her lecture, given to medical students, nurses, social workers, and chaplains regarding the concept of holistic hospice care, included photos of terminally ill cancer patients and their families. These photos showed the dramatic differences before and after the compassionate, symptom-control care that she believed should be offered to every patient in need.

In 1969, Elizabeth Kübler-Ross, MD, published a book based on 500 interviews with dying patients. *Death and Dying* became an international bestseller that introduced the public for the first time to the five stages of terminal illness (or any intensely stressful and grief-producing process):

1. **Denial:** "This can't be happening."

2. **Anger:** "Why me? It's not fair."

3. **Bargaining:** "Just let me live to see my children graduate."

4. **Depression:** "I'm so sad, why bother with anything?"

5. **Acceptance:** "It's going to be okay."

Kübler-Ross's book also made a plea for home care for the terminally ill, as opposed to treatment in an institutional setting. She argued that patients should have a choice in this decision as well as all others that affect their destiny stating, "We [in the U.S.] live in a very particular death-denying society. We isolate both the dying and the old, and it serves a purpose. They are reminders of our own mortality. We should not institutionalize people. We can give families more help with home care and visiting nurses, giving the families and the patients the spiritual, emotional, and financial help in order to facilitate the final care at home."

From the 1970s through the 1990s, hospice care was transformed in the United States from an all-volunteer movement to being embraced by individual states and then the national medical industry. In Britain, hospice care always began with "palliative" care, or the compassionate reduction of pain, nausea, and other troublesome symptoms for those with slim to no chance of recovery. In the U.S., this didn't occur until the 1990s, as American allopaths were often more concerned that their patients would become addicted to pain medications than suffering without pain medications. Cutting-edge research in this field includes patient use of psychedelic therapy via LSD or psilocybin for the reduction of anxiety associated with terminal illness. The palliative care debate has also been extended to the realm of physician-assisted suicide as a final act of compassionate medical care. So far, only the state of Oregon has legalized assisted suicide in the U.S., whereas Switzerland, Belgium, and the Netherlands are the only countries to offer this particular route out of a painful existence. Although the U.S. has not agreed to this most extreme example of palliative care, there are now more than 1,200 hospitals in the U.S. that offer palliative care for all patients, regardless of whether they have a terminal illness or not. This is a direct result of the efforts of Saunders, Kübler-Ross, and thousands of hospice workers around the world.

Currently, the U.S. offers Medicare and Medicaid hospice benefits that consist of two ninety-day periods of care followed by an unlimited number of renewable sixty-day periods. Patients experiencing a number of end-stage diseases, such as congestive heart failure, chronic obstructive pulmonary disease, renal failure, Parkinson's disease, and late stage Alzheimer's disease qualify for hospice care.

Hospice uses a team approach to care for people with life-limiting illnesses. The hospice team includes professional staff, trained volunteers, and the patient's family and friends. Staff always includes an allopathic medical director, nurse, social services specialist, home health aide, chaplain, volunteer, grief support specialist, and children's specialist, as needed. Increasingly common are CAM providers offering holistic care that meshes well with the holistic ideals of hospice philosophy. The patient's family and/or friends provide most of the daily care to the patient. Hospice staff regularly visit the family to train them on how to better care for the patient, including learning simple medical care, monitoring medications to ensure pain and symptom control, assisting with physical needs, and offering emotional and spiritual support to the patient and their loved ones. Hospice nurses are on call twenty-four hours per day to assist patients and their families.

In 2005, more than 1.2 million individuals and their families received hospice care. Hospice is the only Medicare benefit that includes pharmaceuticals, medical equipment, twenty-four hour/seven day a week access to care, and support for loved ones following a death. Most hospice care is delivered at home. Hospice care is also available to people in home-like hospice residences, nursing homes, assisted living facilities, veterans' facilities, hospitals, and prisons.

Today there are more than 3,200 hospices across the country—some are part of hospitals or health systems, others are independent; some are nonprofit agencies, others are for-profit companies. According to the National Hospice and Palliative Care Organization, in 2000, about one in every four Americans who died received hospice care at the end of their lives.

Unlike the midwifes (and their lesser-trained "doula" assistants), who receive a particular certification for their skills after a specialized course, the hospice worker can be a volunteer or one of many medical professionals. In this way, a hospice worker differs from other entries within this reference book. However, the holistic, integrative, and "CAM-completing" nature of this work necessitates its inclusion here. Before the 1960s, nearly every person in the developed world experienced terminal illness in an allopathic setting. But now allopaths and CAM practitioners work together to offer the terminally ill the smoothest transition from this life to whatever does or does not happen next. Prospective students can thus choose any avenue within the field of health care and transform it into the life-affirming, pain-reducing, anxiety-lowering, unconditionally loving career of hospice care. Minimal specialized training is needed for the maximum career fulfillment that can be attained.

While volunteers are not required to be licensed to work in a hospice care setting, certification is available through the National Association for Home Care and Hospice (NAHC). Nurses, therapists, and physicians are all subject to examination and board certification pursuant to their career path. Physicians are able to receive board certification from the American Board of Hospice and Palliative Medicine upon completion of education and examination requirements.

RESOURCES

BOOKS

Final Gifts: Understanding the Special Awareness, Needs, and Communications of the Dying by Maggie Callanan and Patricia Kelley

The Hospice Handbook: A Complete Guide by Larry Beresford and Elisabeth Kübler-Ross

Hospice, a Labor of Love by Denise Glavan, Cindy Longanacre, and John Spivey

Hospice and Palliative Care Handbook: Quality, Compliance and Reimbursement by Tina M. Marrelli

Study Guide for the Generalist Hospice and Palliative Nurse by Hospice and Palliative Nurses Association

A Healing Touch: True Stories of Life, Death, and Hospice by Richard Russo

Hospice and Palliative Care: Concepts and Practice by Denice C. Sheehan and Walter Forman

A Practical Guide to Palliative Care by Jerry L. Old and Daniel L. Swagerty

Core Curriculum for the Generalist Hospice and Palliative Nurse by Hospice and Palliative Nurses Association

Notes on Symptom Control in Hospice and Palliative Care by Peter Kaye

The Hospice Choice: In Pursuit of a Peaceful Death by Marcia Lattanzi-Licht, Galen W. Miller, and John J. Mahoney

ONLINE

HealthCare Training
www.healthcare-trainingcenter.com/programs-hospice.asp
General information on hospice education, training, certification, and job opportunities

Medline Plus: Hospice Care
www.nlm.nih.gov/medlineplus/hospicecare.html
A general resource and information site on the tenets of hospice care and practice. Intended for the public

ACS: What Is Hospice Care?
www.cancer.org/docroot/ETO/content/ETO_2_5X_What_Is_Hospice_Care.asp?sitearea=ETO
The American Cancer Society's article on hospice care and its history

ORGANIZATIONS

Hospice Foundation of America
www.hospicefoundation.org
The HFA provides leadership in the development and application of hospice and its philosophy of care with the goal of enhancing the U.S. health care system and the role of hospice within it. The organization was founded in 1982 and expanded its scope in 1990 to a national level.

National Association for Home Care and Hospice
www.nahc.org
NAHC is the nation's largest trade association representing the interests and concerns of home care agencies, hospices, home care aide organizations, and medical equipment suppliers. It is dedicated to making home care and hospice providers' lives easier.

American Hospice Foundation
www.americanhospice.org
The AHS is a nonprofit membership association for hospice workers. It seeks to improve the quality of hospice care via public education, professional training, and consumer advocacy. The foundation trains and certifies practitioners and educates managers and employers about the needs of grieving employees. It supports research initiatives in hospice medicine.

The Institute for Palliative and Hospice Training, Inc.
www.ipht.org
The IPHT, based in Alexandria, Virginia, was established in 2000 to promote and implement training in palliative care for paraprofessional, volunteer, and family caregivers of people with cancer and other chronic or terminal illnesses. The institute, which received 501(c)3 status as a not-for-profit education and research organization in 2001, is an advocacy, educational, and research organization.

American Academy of Hospice and Palliative Medicine

www.aahpm.org

The academy is the professional organization for physicians specializing in hospice and palliative medicine. Membership is also open to nurses and other health care providers who are committed to improving the quality of life of patients and families facing life-threatening or serious conditions. Originally organized as the Academy of Hospice Physicians in 1988, the academy began with 250 charter members and has grown to well over 3,300 in 2008.

The National Association of Complementary Therapists In Hospice and Palliative Care

www.helpthehospices.org.uk/NPA/
complementarytherapists/index.asp

The NACTHPC was established to promote a greater understanding of the use of complementary therapies to enhance the quality of life of people living with progressive illness, and to support complementary therapists in their care.

Children's Hospice International

www.chionline.org

CHI provides education, training, and technical assistance to those who care for children with life-threatening conditions and their families.

Hospice Choices

www.hospicechoices.com

HospiceChoices is the first national job board/career center that is offered exclusively to the hospice community. It forms part of a wider strategy by its parent organization, Choices Healthcare Solutions, to bring unique technologies to serve the hospice community.

Americans for Better Care of the Dying

www.abcd-caring.org

A small yet passionate organization for the advancement and implementation of hospice care for those who cannot afford it

International Association for Hospice and Palliative Care

www.hospicecare.com

The IAHP's vision "is to increase the availability and access to high quality hospice and palliative care for patients and families throughout the world. We do this by promoting communication, facilitating and providing education, and becoming an information resource for patients, professionals, health care providers, and policy makers around the world."

Volunteer Hospice Network

www.growthhouse.org/hospice/vhn.html

The VHN is an affinity group composed of more than 150 volunteer organizations in the United States that provide a wide variety of free health care to the terminally ill and their families. Members of this network include volunteer hospices, grief support programs, and other groups that focus on care for the dying.

HYPNOTHERAPY

Hypnotherapy is any form of psychotherapy practiced in conjunction with hypnosis. Hypnotherapy is therapy that is undertaken with a subject in hypnosis. Hypnosis is not a new modality. The Celts and Druids practiced hypnosis. Ancient Egyptians used "sleep temples," in which curative suggestions were given, and many sections of the Bible allude to hypnotic phenomena.

Little attention, however, was given to hypnotic states until the early sixteenth century, when Paracelsus described how he believed that magnetic fields came from the stars and influenced human behavior. In 1646, the German mathematician, Athanasius Kircher, described a cure for what he thought was disease-causing "animal magnetism" using a process called "magneto therapeutics." Franz Mesmer (1734–1815) is considered by some to be the modern inventor of hypnosis as a treatment technique because he was the first to describe animal magnetism, or an invisible magnetic field, as a therapeutic tool. Working in a room containing a tub of iron filings known as a banquet, he walked in circles around his patients. Some of these individuals entered into a stuporous trance state and were then allegedly cured of their afflictions. Mesmer's popularity resulted in an official investigation appointed by King Louis XVI of France and headed by Benjamin Franklin. The commission concluded that any reported effects of "mesmerism" were due to imagination. Mesmer was denounced as a quack and eventually died in relative obscurity.

What Mesmer had fraudulently claimed was an occult force found a new life as "mesmerism" in Europe up until the 1840s, when Scottish neurosurgeon,

James Braid, studied supposed animal magnetism and coined the phrase "neuro-hypnotism." This he took from Greek words meaning "sleep of the nervous system." Later, after concluding that hypnosis was a state of mental activity rather than sleep, he changed the term to "monoideism." By that time, however, the term hypnosis was already popular among its users, and the word remains in use today.

James Esdaile, an English surgeon, later used hypnosis on all of his patients while practicing in India during the middle 1800s. He performed 3,000 operations, 300 of which were major procedures, and discovered that the mortality rate dropped from 50 percent to 5 percent when his patients were in a hypnotic state. In addition, many of these patients recovered more quickly than normal, had increased resistance to infection, and experienced greater comfort during the surgical procedure. Esdaile presented his findings to the Royal Academy of Physicians in London but was denounced as blasphemous because, "God intended people to suffer."

In France, Hippolyte Bernheiam, a famous neurologist, was mortified that a local family physician was using hypnosis on a patient. Feeling only contempt, he visited the physician but was so overwhelmed after observing the therapeutic effects of hypnosis that the two doctors later collaborated. Together they formed a hypnotherapy clinic at the psychoanalytic School of Nancy, where Freud would later study. In 1885, another famous neurologist, Jean Martin Charcot, taught his students hypnosis in Paris. Freud studied under Charcot and later worked with Josef Breuer using hypnotic techniques. In 1895, Freud and Breuer published, *Studies of Hysteria*, in which hypnosis was used to discover the source of "conversion reactions"—physical symptoms for which a physiological cause can be found. Although Freud's opinion of hypnosis vacillated throughout his life, neo-Freudians became so entrenched in their new psychoanalytic philosophies that they mostly disregarded any potential benefits to be derived from hypnosis.

Hypnosis dropped into obscurity until World War II, when dentists began to use hypnosis with soldiers in combat situations. Spurred on by the studies of American behavioral psychologist and researcher, Clark Hull, in the 1930s, interest in hypnotic phenomena continued to grow. While disproving most extravagant claims, Hull's experiments illustrated the reality of some classical phenomena such as hypnotic *anaesthesia* and *post-hypnotic amnesia*. Hypnosis was also shown to induce moderate increases in certain physical capacities as well as change the threshold of sensory stimulation. Attenuation (or the lessening of perceived sound) effects could be especially dramatic. Hull is famous for his signature hypnotic induction in which he would look at someone straight in the eyes until they were induced.

In 1955 the British Medical Association endorsed hypnosis as an acceptable method of treatment. In 1958, the American Medical Association recognized hypnosis as a therapeutic adjunct, and the American Psychiatric Association endorsed it in 1961. Despite its acceptance into the medical model, however, many physicians remain skeptical. This is mainly because of their misconceptions regarding its usefulness within the therapeutic process.

A person who is hypnotized displays certain unusual characteristics and propensities compared with a non-hypnotized subject, most notably hyper-suggestibility. Clark Hull, probably the first major empirical researcher in the field, wrote, in *Hypnosis and Suggestion*: "If a subject after submitting to the hypnotic procedure shows no genuine increase in susceptibility to any suggestions whatever, there seems no point in calling him hypnotised." Hypnotherapy is often performed upon a patient in order to modify his or her behavior, emotional content, attitudes, and a wide range of conditions including dysfunctional habits, anxieties, stress-related illness, pain management, and general personal development. British and American medical research studies have continued to give approval for the use of hypnosis for the treatment of many conditions.

In 1955, the British Medical Association stated: "The subcommittee is satisfied after consideration of the available evidence that hypnotism is of value and may be the treatment of choice in some cases of so-called psychosomatic disorder and psychoneurosis. It may also be of value for revealing unrecognized motives and conflicts in such conditions. As a treatment, in the opinion of the subcommittee it has proved its ability to remove symptoms and to alter morbid habits of thought and behavior . . .

In addition to the treatment of psychiatric disabilities,

there is a place for hypnotism in the production of anesthesia or analgesia for surgical and dental operations, and in suitable subjects it is an effective method of relieving pain in childbirth without altering the normal course of labor."

By 2001, the British Psychological Society affirmed: "Enough studies have now accumulated to suggest that the inclusion of hypnotic procedures may be beneficial in the management and treatment of a wide range of conditions and problems encountered in the practice of medicine, psychiatry, and psychotherapy."

But hypnosis is difficult to define just because of its many different applications as well as the current, vague understanding of what physiological effects constitute the hypnotic trance versus other observed trance states—religious, sexual, TV-oriented. At its lowest common denominator, the hypnotic technique involves a relationship between a hypnotist and at least one other person. At some point during this time together, the patient lapses into a trance and suggestions made by the hypnotist affects the person's cognition, perceptions, and memory.

Direct hypnotherapy has been the most common approach throughout history, as represented by the direct statement, "You are feeling sleepier and sleepier . . ." However, indirect trance induction is also a common human experience. This tendency was developed into a psychotherapeutic system by psychiatrist, Milton Erickson, MD, starting in the 1930s. Not only would Erickson put patients in a trance via indirect methods, such as interrupting the usual human handshake ritual. He would also give indirect hypnotic suggestions: "You can learn to be a nonsmoker," versus its direct suggestion opposite, "You will stop smoking." Many of Erickson's techniques were then included with those of psychiatrist Fritz Perls and psychologist Virginia Satir in the creation of neuro-linguistic programming (NLP).

Once patients are in a hypnotic trance, they are much more susceptible than normal to making changes in their thoughts, perceptions, emotional reactivity, and actions. If these changes can then be suggested to remain in place after the session, a permanent change of habits can be effected.

There appears to be little research on the relationship between hypnotic trance states and psychospiritual techniques such as Yogic meditation techniques, Grof's holotropic breathwork, and Michael Harner's Shamanic counseling practices which, like hypnosis, induce nonordinary states of consciousness and allow access to latent insights, feelings, and memories. Just as in hypnotherapy, these other techniques result in seemingly spontaneous healings from a variety of psychosomatic ailments and, according to the reports of entranced persons, greater overall functioning.

Many questions remain as to how these altered states of consciousness differ from one another. One researcher even claims that this normal waking state is merely a "consensus trance," one neither better nor worse than any other trance we could have unconsciously chosen to be the norm for our human communities. If this is so, can we now agree to choose another "group trance" if a new one will allow our global community to thrive within a more healthful ecology than the one that exists for us now? These are just a few of the thoughts and promises that present themselves upon closer study of trance in general, and hypnosis in specific.

Hypnotherapy training requirements vary greatly worldwide, with the key determining factor being whether the use of hypnotherapy is state-recognized in any given area. In many parts of the world, there are no requirements, and, in theory, anyone can name himself or herself a hypnotherapist and begin practicing. Other districts, however, define and legislate hypnotherapy, and the qualifications in these districts can vary greatly. In the most extreme cases, hypnotherapy is only allowed to be practiced by a qualified medical professional of another area of expertise such as psychology, psychotherapy, or psychiatry. This in effect rules out hypnotherapy as a stand-alone profession in the affected areas. Generally, this strict approach is rare, and in most parts of the world, it's up to the individual to ensure that his or her training meets a suitable standard.

Suitable training will generally require a minimum of 300 hours of education. Some hypnotherapists are trained in a specialty, such as smoking, and receive much less training. Hypnotherapy is about working with people, so in a proper learning environment, trainees have the opportunity to practice on their fellow classmates and teachers with full support from the staff while they learn. This experiential approach to hypnotherapeutic training is essential in order to be able to work effectively with clients in a real therapeutic setting. Some hypnotherapy schools do offer distance learning courses in the form of video DVDs or audio CDs, but the value of learning in person for a skill as subtle as hypnotherapy cannot be overstated.

In the United States, hypnotherapy is being taught by many medical and dental schools, intern and residency programs, and in training programs across the country. Many doctors and psychologists also have incorporated clinical and experimental hypnosis into their practices. A number of research grants have been awarded to such institutions as the University of Pennsylvania and Stanford Medical School to continue investigating the efficacy of hypnotherapy for just about every ill that ails the human organism.

RESOURCES

BOOKS

Hypnotherapy by Dave Elman

The New Hypnotherapy Handbook: Hypnosis and Mind-Body Healing by Kevin Hogan, Kathy Hume Gray *Hypnotherapy Scripts Second Edition* by Ronald A. Havens

Cognitive Hypnotherapy: An Integrated Approach to the Treatment of Emotional Disorders by Assen Alladin

Scripts and Strategies in Hypnotherapy: The Complete Works by Roger P. Allen

Life Between Lives: Hypnotherapy for Spiritual Regression by Michael Newton

Hypnosis and Hypnotherapy: Basic to Advanced Techniques for the Professional by Calvin D. Banyan and Gerald F. Kein

Hypnosis in Clinical Practice: Steps for Mastering Hypnotherapy by Rick Voit and Molly DeLaney

The Secret Language of Hypnotherapy by John Smale

Hypnotherapy: An Exploratory Casebook by Milton H. Erickson and Ernest L. Rossi

ONLINE

Clinical Hypnotherapy Information
www.clevelandclinic.org/health/health-info/docs/3700/3779.asp?index=9930
A consumer FAQ about hypnotherapy

Katherine Fox's Home Page
http://hypnotherapy.net
Accomplished and certified practitioner Katherine Fox's Web site contains useful facts, articles, and history of hypnotherapy practice

ORGANIZATIONS

American Association of Professional Hypnotherapists
http://aaph.org
The AAPH is a worldwide organization that promotes communication between professionals for the promotion and development of ethical methods, techniques, and standards in the field of hypnotherapy.

The International Association of Counseling Hypnotherapists
www.hypnotherapyassociation.org
The IACH is "committed to creating an international organization of professional hypnotherapists and those interested in this healing modality to continue to increase public awareness, acceptance, and support in the therapeutic and ethical use of hypnotherapy through education and promotion."

The National Board for Certified Clinical Hypnotherapists
www.natboard.com
The NBCCH was organized in 1991 as an educational, scientific, and professional organization dedicated to professionalizing the mental health specialty of hypnotherapy. It certifies professionals including addictions and substance abuse counselors, chiropractors, marriage and family therapists, mental health counselors, pastoral counselors, psychiatric nurses, physicians, psychiatrists, psychologists, school counselors, and social workers.

American Council of Hypnotist Examiners

www.hypnotistexaminers.org

Created in 1973, this nonprofit professional organization engages in self-regulation of all who utilize hypnosis/hypnotherapy as an integral part of a professional practice. The primary focus is on formal and appropriate education and training followed by a comprehensive written examination and a practical demonstration of hypnosis skills before a board of examiners. Examination and registration is done by regional examining boards, while certification is by the national parent body, the American Council of Hypnotist Examiners.

Hypnotherapy Training Institute

www.hypnotherapy.com

Established in 1978, this program is one of the original institutes that started teaching hypnotherapy. It has the largest alumni of any licensed hypnotherapy school.

Transpersonal Hypnotherapy Institute

www.transpersonalhypnotherapy.com

Anne Salisbury, PhD, MA, MBA, NLP, CCHt, founded the instituted in 1990 after completing her MA in transpersonal psychology and making an extensive study of hypnotherapy. Over the next few years, Salisbury and Yukio Hasegawa, MA, NLP, CCHt co-developed the system that is known today as transpersonal hypnotherapy. Thousands of certifications were awarded to individuals who came to study from around the globe. Then in 1996 home study programs were introduced, utilizing the professional video recording of live classes. Because of its effectiveness, all programs are home study today.

American Hypnosis Association

www.hypnosis.edu/aha

The AHA is a national association of hypnotherapists, other professionals, and private persons interested in hypnosis and related fields.

American Psychotherapy and Medical Hypnosis Association

www.apmha.com

Formed in 1992, APMHA is a group of licensed therapists who advocate a multidisciplinary forum for the ethical use of hypnosis and hypnotherapy. APMHA provides an online newsletter, the Eye-Witness News, and an e-mail list group, which both serve as forums for the exchange of professional information and hypnosis-related articles. Through the e-mail list group and newsletter, APMHA provides networking and announces events and practice offerings of members of American Psychotherapy and Medical Hypnosis Association. This also gives members an opportunity to publish their writing.

International Medical and Dental Hypnotherapy Association

www.imdha.com

The IMDHA is a referral service dedicated to providing the community with excellently trained certified hypnotherapists. Certified hypnotherapists work harmoniously with allied health care professionals to aid individuals in dealing with specific challenges and procedures. Its Web site includes a membership directory, standards of practice, and a code of ethics for practitioners.

Oregon Hypnotherapy Association

http://hypnosis-oregon.com

The OHA is a not-for-profit educational corporation in the State of Oregon. Founded in Salem, Oregon, in 1995, the OHA is a professional organization comprised of dedicated individuals committed to preserving professionalism in the field of hypnotherapy.

The International Hypnosis Association

www.hypnosiscredentials.com

This association provides credentialing and certification worldwide for hypnotists, hypnotherapists, and NLP practitioners based upon knowledge and skill level.

The Banyan Hypnosis Center for Training and Services

www.hypnosiscenter.com

The BHCTS certifies hypnotherapists nationally. It is based in southern California and has campus locations in several locations.

IRIDOLOGY

Iridology, also known as iridodiagnosis, is a holistic technique that analyzes patterns, colors, and other unique characteristics of the iris as a measure of a patient's systemic health. By way of color charts, sectional iris zones, and differences in appearance, iridologists view the eyes as a window into the body-mind's state of internal health. Iridology can be used, much like reflexology, to identify problematic, inflamed, or otherwise distressed areas of the entire body by examining a much smaller piece—in this case, the eye. Similarly to many other focused healing modalities, iridology is based on the holistic premise that every organ in the human body has a corresponding location (within the iris) by which the health of that relative organ can be determined by analyzing its related section in the eye. Because our eyes usually play an integral and inextricable role in the way we experience the world, they may be thought of as microcosms of our physical and emotional health. Within the field of iridology, this hypothetical thought has been transformed into an empirically well-researched healing art. Perhaps due to its Hungarian origin, most of the attempts to apply the scientific model to iridology have occurred in Europe. In America, iridology is currently a mostly unused modality within both traditional/folk, and modern/clinically based, naturopathic medicine.

Although iridology is at present a mostly unknown practice, "eye diagnosis" (as it was first called) has an interesting and provocative history that dates back to nineteenth century Hungary. Ignatz von Peczely, a prominent Hungarian physician, allegedly was the first to discover a connection between bodily health and eye color after he noticed similar, newly formed streaks in the irises of both a man he was treating for a broken leg and the iris of an owl that had accidentally broken its leg. His initial claims—about a potential correspondence between bodily health and eye patterns of both the colored irises and the "whites" of the eye, or scleras—were largely unscientific and dismissed by the medical community. In the early 1900s, German minister and folk healer Pastor Felke developed a type of homeopathic treatment specific for treating illness diagnosed by analyzing particular marks in the iris.

Iridology gained its popularity in the 1950s in the United States when Bernard Jensen, a well-known chiropractor with a popular California residential health retreat, Hidden Valley Health Ranch, began offering classes in his own method of iridology. Jensen, a charismatic chiropractor and skilled natural healer, stressed the harmful effects of exposure to toxins and the positive effects of daily fresh air, sunshine, pure water, freshly squeezed juices, raw foods, and goat milk. He perceived the iris as an effective health indicator, using magnified photographic analysis to determine deficiencies in the body. Jensen and other iridologists simply photograph the eyes of patients before treatment; apply a treatment protocol for days, weeks, or months; then rephotograph the irises. Patients' iris colors and surfaces are said to change when the corresponding organs, tissues (and even psychological traits within some modern versions of iridology) are successfully treated. Because iris colors can appear at birth or anytime throughout life as a predictor of future ailments, a patient may not have experienced symptoms yet when he is told by an iridologist that he has some likely "sub-clinical" or future inflammation. If the corresponding iris area changes to a more healthful appearance with medical treatment, that patient is said to have had his hypothetical illness treated or prevented. A powerful medical detection and treatment system, if true!

Since Jensen's peak popularity in the 1970s, some medical researchers have published academic studies on some nonvisual functions of the eye, although iridology is still subject to much scientific criticism. Currently, the field of iridology lacks appropriate funding, testing, and science-based factual evidence. This doesn't mean its basic health philosophy is untrue, just that to date no scientific body has spent much time or money to prove or disprove the holographic nature of animal bodies and their many parts.

Iridology is a holistic modality of healing—not a licensed medical profession. It is utilized by naturopaths, homeopaths, and other types of natural healers, and is still taught at the introductory level at accredited naturopathic medical schools. It is rarely used within the clinics of these same schools, however. Iridology training and certification programs are available through private programs. It is not recognized as a legitimate form of medicine within the Western allopathic model. The International Iridology Practitioners Association offers two levels of certifications classes totaling thirty-five hours. Advanced seminars and master classes are possible through iridology workshops.

RESOURCES

BOOKS

Visions of Health: Understanding Iridology by Bernard Jensen

Practical Iridology: Use Your Eyes to Pinpoint Your Health Risks and Your Particular Path to Well-being by Peter Jackson-Main

For Your Eyes Only: A Fascinating Look at the Art and Science of Iris Diagnosis by Frank Navratil

Science and Practice of Iridology by Bernard Jensen

ONLINE

Healing Facts—Iridology
www.healingfeats.com/whatis.htm

History, efficacy, methodology, and practice of iridology. An extended introduction for nonpractitioners.

ORGANIZATIONS

The International Iridology Practitioners Association
http://iridologyassn.org

The IIPA is a nonprofit organization founded in 1982 and run by a board of iridology practitioners. Standard education programs, certification, and membership groups are all available through the IIPA.

Through the Eye International
www.equineiridology.com

An organization dedicated to providing training and information about animal iridology.

Benard Jensen International
www.bernardjensen.org

An excellent resource for information on nutrition, iridology, and holistic health. The creators are dedicated to continuing the work of Bernard Jensen, DC, an instrumental figure in the history of iridology in America.

Iridology Courses with IIPA-Certified Instructors
http://members.shaw.ca/iridologycourses/

A Web portal for more specific information about field training with certified iridologists.

OTHER TRAINING IN IRIDOLOGY

Clayton College of Natural Health
Birmingham, Alabama
www.ccnh.edu/about/programs/iridology_theory_and_practice.aspx

Westbrook University
www.westbrooku.edu/distance_education_degrees.htm

ONLINE PROGRAMS

Southwest Institute of Healing Arts
Tempe, Arizona and Flagstaff, Arizona
www.swiha.edu

School of Natural Healing
Springville, Utah
www.snh.cc

JUNGIAN PSYCHOLOGY

Carl Gustav Jung (1875–1961), a Swiss psychiatrist, broke from mentor Sigmund Freud in 1913 and later founded the discipline of analytic psychology. By the 1980s, Jungian psychology had crossed the threshold from esoteric obscurity to mainstream popularity. This rapid growth has happened despite the fact that there is no centralized Jungian organization in the United States or any standardized requirements among the seven training institutes. Although the Jungian psychology of today has changed little since its inception, James Hillman, a contemporary neo-Jungian scholar, has developed a theory of archetypal psychology that represents the first departure from the traditional Jungian perspective.

According to Jungian analyst and C.G. Jung Institute of Boston faculty member, Pamela Donleavy, JD, "Jungian analysis includes methods of dream interpretation and makes use of the therapeutic relationship between therapist and client for better client self-understanding. Initially, the work involves clients freeing themselves from unconscious patterns that interfere with effective relationships, appreciation of life, and creative development. The goal of the analysis is to allow the unique individuality of the client to unfold so that life becomes more creative, vital, and meaningful."

Jung developed his own model of understanding and healing individual human psyches. Jungian analysis is based on a comprehensive model of the human psyche, one that offers a psychotherapeutic approach to psychological healing that facilitates mature development of the personality. It also provides a theoretical body of knowledge with wide applicability for social and cultural issues.

The process of Jungian analysis usually involves weekly, hour-long, face-to-face meetings with an analyst in his or her office. As a client, you may bring your life experiences, conflicts, and problems to the hour as well as your fantasies and dreams. One of the premises of Jungian work is that our conscious selves are only a part of a larger consciousness, a whole that includes our forgotten experiences as well as our as yet unlived life potentials. The aim of Jungian analysis is to create a space where the unconscious processes involved both in our suffering and in our healing may be explored. In this way not only may past difficulties be addressed but also future pathways may be discovered and activated in the service of realizing more fully the unconscious potential in our lives. In analysis, you may find an opportunity to explore your relationship with your own religious tradition, as well as how to allow your own unique values to unfold in your life. In addition, Jungian analysis may become a journey that leads to a deepened sense of transpersonal, spiritual meaning and fulfillment.

To become a Jungian analyst, an individual must acquire a certificate from one of the many certifying training institutes in either the United States or abroad. Although admission requirements vary considerably, at least 100 to 250 hours of personal Jungian analysis and an advanced degree in social work, psychology, or psychiatry, or some other prior clinical training, are common prerequisites. Curricula at the various institutes also differ. Some institutes offer seminars and supervision on a weekly or monthly basis, with training lasting anywhere from three to six years.

Academic programs have shied away from offering specialized training in Jungian psychology, preferring to focus on the development of theory and research. Texas A&M University and Pacifica Graduate Institute, however, offer unusual clinical psychology programs in that they allow students to specialize in depth psychology, which, by definition, incorporates Jungian concepts.

According to Jerome Bernstein, a Jungian analyst, there is some confusion outside the Jungian community regarding terminology. He notes that Jung referred to the field as "analytical psychology." The term "Jungian analysis," which essentially describes the same thing, only became popular after Jung's death. Bernstein also notes that the term "Jungian therapist" is misleading to the general public, as it incorrectly implies that the person using the label has undergone all of the requisite training. When applicable, the term "Jungian-oriented therapist" is admissible, as it does not imply that the person is a Jungian analyst. Nevertheless, there are no licensing laws regulating the use of the word "Jungian," just as there is no regulation of the term, "psychoanalysis."

The lack of a centralized Jungian organization in the United States is reflected by the fact that there are few national conferences.

RESOURCES

BOOKS

The Beginner's Guide to Jungian Psychology by Robin Robertson

A Primer of Jungian Psychology by Calvin S. Hall and Vernon J. Nordby

The Handbook of Jungian Psychology: Theory, Practice, and Application by Renos K. Papadopoulous

Depth Psychology and a New Ethic by Erich Neymann

Jung, Irigaray, and Individuation by Frances Gray

Introduction to Jungian Psychotherapy by David Sedgwick

PERIODICALS

Journal of Jungian Theory and Practice

www.junginstitute.org/journal/PageId/9/ParentPageId/0/

One of the most widely read journals in the Jungian community. Published twice yearly by the C.G. Jung Institute of New York.

Chiron Clinical Series

www.chironpublications.com/clinical.html

The series consists of journal-type publications that focus on Jungian topics.

In Touch Centerpoint

www.centerpointec.com

This national Jungian newsletter contains interviews and articles as well as a schedule of programs held at Jungian organizations around the United States and Canada. It also provides a list of regional Jungian societies across the United States.

Journal of Analytical Psychology

www.blackwellpublishing.com/journal.asp?ref=0021-8774&site=1

This academic publication is in its fifty-second volume. Commissioned by the Society of Analytical Psychology in London, the editorial board includes leading analysts from the UK and the USA in collaboration with Jungian analysts from around the world.

Jung at Heart

www.innercitybooks.net

In addition to producing this Jungian-oriented newsletter, Inner City Books is the only publishing house devoted exclusively to the work of Jungian analysts.

Psychological Perspectives

www.junginla.org/psychological_perspectives.htm

This Jungian journal seeks to integrate psyche, soul, and nature. It offers essays, articles, short fiction, poems, visual art, and current research. Published by the C.G. Jung Institute of Los Angeles.

Quadrant

www.junglibrary.org/jungcenter.htm

This newsletter includes current and noteworthy contributions to Jungian psychology. Published by the C.G. Jung Foundation for Analytical Psychology based in New York City.

Spring: A Journal of Archetype and Culture

www.springjournalandbooks.com/cgi-bin/ecommerce/ac/agora.cgi

Located in New Orleans, Louisiana, Spring is the oldest Jungian psychology journal in the world. It is published twice a year, and each editorial features a cultural or philosophical theme.

ONLINE

RobertAziz.com

www.robertaziz.com

Dr. Robert Aziz is one of the leading experts on the work of Jung, Freud, and other disciplines within analytical psychology. His homepage archives his publications, consulting work, blogs, and reviews of popular works in analytical psychology.

The Jung Page

www.cgjungpage.org

Contains amateur and professional articles on psychology, culture, and life. Membership is available.

Fonda's Jung Notes: Summary of Jung's Psychology

www.religiousworlds.com/fondarosa/jung03.html

An interesting in-depth synopsis of Jung's work by scholar and psychoanalyst Marc Fonda. First published in 1996.

A Brief Outline of Jungian Psychology

www.csulb.edu/~csnider/jungian.outline.html

Another simple synopsis of Jung's analytical psychology in outline format. Taken in part from Clifton Snider's The Stuff That Dreams Are Made On: A Jungian Interpretation of Literature.

Carl Jung Resources for Home Study and Practice

www.carl-jung.net

A site designed to offer online resources to advance and promote nonprofessional study about Carl Jung.

ORGANIZATIONS

Harvest Analytical Psychology Club

www.jungclub-london.org/frameset.htm

This club, formed in 1922 by associates of Carl Jung, keeps alive the community and original values of Jungian analysis. Though its members meet in London, there are forums and reading groups that psychotherapists participate in from abroad.

Center for Sacred Psychology

www.sacredselfcenter.com

Founded in 1972, Centerpoint offers nondegree courses, publishes the newsletter In Touch, and sponsors an annual harvest conference held in New Hampshire.

Fairfield County Jung Society

http://practiceofpresence.com/schedule.html

The FCJS at the Temenos Institute sponsors lectures and courses about application of Jungian concepts upon a number of mental health topics and fields.

The Imagination Institute

www.imagination-institute.com

The institute is a nonprofit organization founded in 1987 to foster imagination in all areas of life. Its activities are currently centered in Baltimore, Chicago, and western Massachusetts and include conferences, lectures, workshops, seminars, and ongoing programs in imagination studies. It also publishes Primavera and, in association with Lindisfarne Press, a book series featuring seminal works in the history, theory, and practice of imagination.

International Association of Analytical Psychology

http://iaap.org

IAAP headquarters are located in Zurich, Switzerland, where Jung graduated from medical school in 1902. It is a professional organization open to all certified Jungian analysts. This organization charters and certifies the various Jungian training institutes throughout the world and holds a congress every three years.

The International Association for Jungian Studies

www.jungianstudies.org

The International Association for Jungian Studies provides a forum and focus for the exciting and important work being done in Jungian and post-Jungian studies all over the world. The IAJS is equally open to academics, analysts, therapists, practicing artists, students, and candidates in training.

Journey into Wholeness

http://journeyintowholeness.org

JIW combines Christian spirituality and the psychology of Carl Jung. It publishes an annual resource guide, which is now available online. The organization has officially closed, yet its Web site and archives remain online.

Jung Society of Washington

www.jung.org

JSW is a nonprofit educational membership society open to amateur and professional Jung enthusiasts alike. It is dedicated to helping any interested party learn more about the psychology and methodology of Carl Jung.

TRAINING

Pacifica Graduate Institute

Carpinteria, California
www.pacifica.edu

Carl G. Jung Foundation

New York, New York
www.cgjungny.org

The Center for Religion and Advanced Spiritual Studies

New York, New York
http://spiritcentral.org

Dallas Institute of Humanities and Culture

Dallas, Texas
www.dallasinstitute.org

Process Work Center of Portland

Portland, Oregon
www.processwork.org

Texas A&M University Department of Psychology

College Station, Texas
http://psychology.tamu.edu

C.G. Jung Institute of Chicago

Chicago, Illinois
www.jungchicago.org

C.G. Jung Institute of Dallas

Dallas, Texas
www.cgjungpage.org/dallasinst.html

C.G. Jung Institute of Los Angeles
Los Angeles, California
www.junginla.org

C.G. Jung Institute of New York
New York, New York
www.junginstitute.org

C.G. Jung Institute of San Francisco
San Francisco, California
www.sfjung.org

C.G. Jung Institute of Boston
Boston, Massachusetts
http://www.cgjungboston.com

MIDWIFERY

Midwifery and assisted childbirthing is one of the oldest medical practices in recoded history. The word *midwife* is derived from Old English and literally means, "with woman." Centuries ago, before modern hospitals and medical technology, all women (who could afford it) had midwives to help them remain healthy during pregnancy a difficult and physically stressful time for many women. Due to suppression from the allopathic medical industry, midwifery is far less popular in the United States than it is in foreign countries. While midwives are responsible for nearly 80 percent of births worldwide, American midwives are only responsible for a mere 5 percent of births in the United States.

Because childbirth is an extremely powerful, even spiritual experience, for a woman, midwifery has been a holistic art since its inception. Modern midwives encourage women to design their own birth process and tend to act more as advisors than authorities despite their specialized medical skills. Generally speaking, there are two different types of midwives: lay (independent, direct-entry) midwives and certified nurse-midwives. Lay midwives primarily work in domestic settings, while certified nurse-midwives usually work in hospitals. This section will primarily deal with the former type of profession. For more information on nurse practitioners, consult the Holistic Nursing chapter.

Lay midwives' clients are usually mothers who are interested in having a "natural home" birth. Lay practitioners are trained in all aspects of maternity care—pelvic exams, pap smears, health status exams, fetal heart rate monitoring, and blood work—though they are seldom affiliated with a particular hospital. Additionally, there are private midwifery practices where several practitioners will work together in order to expand their patient base.

It is important to note that the term "lay midwife" has been used to designate an uncertified or unlicensed midwife. Because the practice of midwifery is antiquated, there are many practitioners who are educated in informal programs, such as self-study or apprenticeship. There are formal programs to educate midwives who are not nurses, but this does not best describe lay midwifery practice. A lay midwife does not necessarily connote a low level of education or experience, just that the midwife has either chosen not to become certified or that there was no professional certification available in the practitioner's state. This latter reason has recently been made obsolete by the advent of the certified professional midwife credential—a nationally recognized license to practice midwifery that does not necessarily require traditional coursework. Other terms used to describe unlicensed midwives include: traditional midwife, birth attendant, granny midwife, and independent midwife.

Under the umbrella of "direct-entry midwife" there are even more distinctions within the lay midwife community:

A Certified Professional Midwife (CPM) is a knowledgeable, skilled, and professional independent midwifery practitioner who has met the standards for certification set by the North American Registry of Midwives (NARM) and is qualified to provide the midwives model of care. The CPM is the only international credentialing body that requires knowledge about, and experience in, out-of-hospital settings. At present, there are approximately 900 CPMs practicing in the United States.

A Licensed Midwife (LM) is a midwife who is licensed to practice in a particular state. Currently, licensure for direct-entry midwives is available in twenty-four states.

The American College of Nurse-Midwives (ACNM)

also provides accreditation to non-nurse midwife programs, as well as colleges that graduate nurse midwives. This credential, called the **Certified Midwife (CM)**, is currently recognized in only three states (New York, New Jersey, and Rhode Island). All CMs must pass the same certifying exam administered by the American Midwifery Certification Board for CNMs. At present, there are approximately fifty CMs practicing in the US.

RESOURCES

BOOKS

Hearts & Hands: A Midwife's Guide to Pregnancy and Birth by Elizabeth Davis, Linda Harrison, and Suzanne Arms

Spiritual Midwifery by Ina May Gaskin

Baby Catcher: The Chronicles of a Modern Midwife by Peggy Vincent

Varney's Midwifery (4th edition) by Helen Varney Burst

Holistic Midwifery: A Comprehensive Textbook for Midwives in Homebirth Practice by Anne Frye

Anatomy & Physiology for Midwives by Jane Coad and Melvyn Dunstall

The Art of Midwifery by Hilary Marland

PERIODICALS

Journal of Midwifery and Women's Health
www.elsevier.com/wps/find/journaldescription.
cws_home/620773/description#description

A bimonthly peer-reviewed journal dedicated to original research in midwifery.

MIDIRS Informed Choice
www.infochoice.org

Provides the best scientifically available evidence in support of midwifery including twenty-one articles and titles about pregnancy, childbirth, and postpartum experience.

RCM Midwives Journal
www.midwives.co.uk

A British professional, peer-reviewed journal for midwives. Available internationally.

Midwifery Digest
www.midirs.org

A general interest magazine for midwives.

Midwifery Today: The Heart and Science of Birth
www.midwiferytoday.com

A quarterly journal for midwives, nurses, childbirth educators, doctors, parents, and mothers-to-be. Consumer friendly.

ONLINE

Midwives Online
www.midwivesonline.com

A general consumer-oriented midwife network.

Nucleus Medical Art
www.nucleusinc.com/medical-animations.php
Two- and three-dimensional artistic renderings of childbirth and fetuses in utero. Good for medical reports, journal articles, and pictorial representations of research.

The Doe Report
www.doereport.com

Another professional organization that creates custom medical illustration, animation, and anatomical models for reports, exhibits, and arbitrations.

ORGANIZATIONS

North American Registry of Midwives
www.narm.org

NARM is an international certification agency whose mission is to establish and administer certification for the Certified Professional Midwife (CPM) credential. CPM certification validates entry-level knowledge, skills, and experience vital for responsible midwifery practice. This international certification process encompasses multiple educational routes of entry including apprenticeship, self-study, private midwifery schools, college- and university-based midwifery programs, and nurse midwifery. Created in 1987 by the Midwives Alliance of North America, NARM is committed to identifying standards and practices that reflect the excellence and diversity of the independent midwifery community in order to set the standard for North American midwifery as a whole.

Midwifery Education Accreditation Council

http://meacschools.org/index.php

This nonprofit organization is responsible for accrediting all educational midwifery institutions in the United States and is approved by the U.S. Secretary of Education as a nationally recognized accrediting agency. To become a certified lay midwife (in contrast to a nurse practitioner midwife), one must attend and complete one of MEAC's accredited programs—all of which can be found on its Web site.

Midwives Alliance of North America

www.mana.org

MANA's self-proclaimed goal is "to unify and strengthen the profession of midwifery, thereby improving the quality of health care for women, babies, and communities." Led by a board of certified practitioners, MANA was established in 1982 as a professional advocacy organization. As a membership group for both practitioners and mothers, MANA helps midwives connect with their clients, fostering a warm and vast community. It also hosts an annual conference for midwives.

The National Association of Certified Professional Midwives

www.nacpm.org

NACPM is a general advocacy and membership group for both professionally certified midwives and students of the profession. It seeks to educate legislators and policy makers about the practice of midwifery by defining a national standard of practice (available in full on its Web site), which serves to promote excellence within the profession. It also has a large practitioner directory, which is helpful for finding a certified midwife practitioner in your area.

Citizens for Midwifery

http://cfmidwifery.org/index.aspx

The only national consumer-based group, it promotes the Midwives Model of Care and provides general advocacy and midwifery information for the public.

Foundation for the Advancement of Midwifery

www.formidwifery.org

The mission of this fund-raising group is to increase awareness and fund education, research, and policy initiatives within the midwifery community.

The International Confederation of Midwives

www.internationalmidwives.org

ICM hosts conferences and workshops for mothers-to-be and midwives. It is a general advocacy group with a motley group of related Web links.

International Center for Traditional Childbirth

www.blackmidwives.org

A nonprofit advocacy and networking organization, it emphasizes cultural diversity and spirituality within the midwifery profession.

Mothers Naturally

http://mothersnaturally.org

A consumer-based advocacy/information group.

American College of Nurse-Midwives

www.acnm.org

Dedicated to nurse-midwives, this group publishes a journal and supports research within the field of nurse-midwifery.

The Coalition for Improving Maternity Services

www.motherfriendly.org

A general membership organization that offers resources, news, and projects within the midwife community.

DIRECT-ENTRY MIDWIFERY TRAINING PROGRAMS ACCREDITED BY THE MIDWIFERY EDUCATION ACCREDITATION COUNCIL

Bastyr University

Kenmore, Washington
www.bastyr.edu/academic/naturopath/midwifery

Miami Dade College

Miami, Florida
www.mdc.edu/medical/Nursing/Programs/Midwifery_Prog/main.htm

Birthingway College of Midwifery

Portland, Oregon
www.birthingway.edu

Birthwise Midwifery School

Bridgton, Maine
www.birthwisemidwifery.org

Florida School of Traditional Midwifery
Gainesville, Florida
www.midwiferyschool.org

Maternidad La Luz
El Paso, Texas
www.maternidadlaluz.com

Midwives College of Utah
Salt Lake City, Utah
www.midwifery.edu

National College of Midwifery
Taos, New Mexico
www.midwiferycollege.org

National Midwifery Institute
Bristol, Vermont
www.nationalmidwiferyinstitute.com

Seattle Midwifery School
Seattle, Washington
www.seattlemidwifery.org

MINDFULNESS-BASED STRESS REDUCTION

Mind-based stress reduction (MBSR) was developed by Jon Kabat-Zinn, PhD, at the University of Massachusetts Medical Center. The technique brings together Buddhist-style "mindfulness" meditation and Hatha Yoga, accomplishing a synergy of mind-body balance and promoting overall mental and physical health. Practiced in the United States since 1979, it is an excellent practice for cultivating greater awareness of normally unconscious feelings and behaviors by attuning the conscious mind to be cognizant of both psychological and physical subtleties. MBSR has been anecdotally shown to benefit patients suffering from chronic medical conditions, as well as to alleviate daily stress. MBSR sessions may also include mindfulness-based cognitive therapy, which encourages patients to link physically problematic zones with emotional imbalance and unrest with the help of a therapist. By changing the way they mentally perceive and label life events, patients can simultaneously improve well-being in the always fused body and mind. Over the last few years, the National Institute of Health's National Center for Complementary and Alternative Medicine (NCCAM) has provided a number of grants to research the scientific efficacy of MBSR therapy for the treatment of chronic medical conditions. Examples of these studies may be found below.

Certification in MBSR is available for students and practitioners of this modality who would like to officially recognize their expertise in the field, although this is not a legal necessity for setting up an MBSR practice. To receive professional certification for MBSR, students enroll in a mindfulness-based stress reduction class or program (typically one to two weeks), experience a minimum of teaching four eight-week MBSR courses under the supervision of an MBSR instructor, exemplify a commitment to the integration of mindfulness in everyday life, and participate in a five- to ten-day silent, teacher-led mindfulness meditation retreat. The Teacher Certification Review, primarily run though the University of Massachusetts Medical School, may be of interest to the advanced practitioner because the requirements and standard of practice are higher than most other centers in the country.

RESOURCES

BOOKS

Mindfulness for Beginners by Jon Kabat-Zinn

Full Catastrophe Living: Using the Wisdom of Your Body and Mind to Face Stress, Pain, and Illness by Jon Kabat-Zinn

Mindfulness-Based Cognitive Therapy for Depression: A New Approach to Preventing Relapse by Zindel V. Segal, J. Mark G. Williams, and John D. Teasdale

Mindfulness Meditation: Cultivating the Wisdom of Your Body and Mind (audio book) by Jon Kabat-Zinn

ONLINE

Coping with Pain Mindfully

www.mindfullivingprograms.com/coping.php

An interesting and eloquent article by Steven Flowers, MFT, about living mindfully. Outlines the philosophy and world-view articulated by MBSR.

Mindfulness in Plain English

www.urbandharma.org/udharma4/mpe.html

A Buddhist slant to mindful living, written by the Venerable Henepola Gunaratana. This e-book is free of charge and acts both as a meditation guide and a well-articulated explanation of mindfulness.

Examples of research on the practice of mindfulness:

Staying Well: A Clinical Trial of Mindfulness-Based Stress Reduction and Education Groups for HIV

www.clinicaltrials.gov/ct/show/NCT00271856?order=4

A Mindfulness-Based Approach to HIV Treatment Side Effects

www.clinicaltrials.gov/ct/show/NCT00312936?order=5

Meditation-Based Stress Reduction in Rheumatoid Arthritis

www.clinicaltrials.gov/ct/show/NCT00071292?order=9

Mindfulness-Based Art Therapy for Cancer Patients

www.clinicaltrials.gov/ct/show/NCT00034970?order=12

Mindfulness-Based Stress Reduction for Hot Flashes

www.clinicaltrials.gov/ct/show/NCT00317304?order=1

ORGANIZATIONS

Center for Mindfulness at UMass Medical School

www.umassmed.edu/cfm

The parent organization for MBSR techniques. Contains lists of training programs, history of the discipline, and all the teacher certification requirements.

Omega Workshops

omega-inst.org/omega/workshops/
6dc781c075f5f828b2418b3a7ad18fa2

A list of holistic workshops related to MBSR. Its seven-day program is usually led by Jon Kabat-Zinn, PhD.

University of Iowa: Hospitals and Clinics

www.uihealthcare.com/depts/mindfulness/services.
html#mbsr

A MBSR and MBCT class by way of a medical university. Includes a twenty-three-hour instructional program for students beginning these practices.

Mindful Living Programs

www.mindfullivingprograms.com

A center for online programs about mindful living and MBSR. Publishes an online newsletter, lists retreats in the United States, and acts as a practitioner network for certified teachers and the public.

University of Minnesota: Center for Spirituality and Living

www.csh.umn.edu/csh/programs/MBSR_stress_
reduction_program/home.html

A MBSR training program for patients, students, and certified teachers.

Mindfulness-Based Cognitive Therapy for Relapse Prevention in Depression

mindfulness.ucsd.edu/mbct5day.htm

A five-day professional training seminar in MBCT.

Spirit Rock

www.spiritrock.org

A Buddhist meditation center that offers some classes and workshops.

TRAINING

Training in MBSR is mostly done on an independent practitioner basis through seminars and workshops. Though there are several programs in MBSR listed in this section, there are many institutionally independent, practitioner-run MBSR programs in the United States. Once trained via an institutional program I apprenticeship, students of MBSR may then receive their certification—but only after they have assembled a proper portfolio. For more on teacher certification, see www.umassmed.edu/Content. aspx?id=41322&linkidentifier=id&itemid=41322.

To search for MBSR practitioners/programs in your area, consult www.umassmed.edu/cfm/mbsr.

Awareness and Relaxation Training
www.mindfulnessprograms.com

A list of programs in MBSR, postgraduate education, and information on MBSR teacher training.

Valley Mindfulness
www.valleymindfulness.com

Stress reduction and wellness programs for groups and individuals. Based in Northampton, Massachusetts.

Steve Shealy, PhD
www.bemindful.org/mbsrhome.htm

MUSIC THERAPY

Music therapy uses music as a way of accessing emotions and experiences not easily accessible by way of conventional, verbal-based psychotherapies, also collectively known as "talk therapy." A music therapist often works with people who have trouble communicating verbally, such as the developmentally delayed, mentally challenged, and certain geriatric patients. However, almost every person has a strong enough reaction to hearing specially chosen music (and to singing or playing specific songs) to potentially make music therapy a potent transformer of acute and chronic physical, psychological, and spiritual states.

Five general aspects of music therapy are listed below:

1. Music therapy is prescribed by members of the client's treatment team. Members can include doctors, social workers, psychologists, teachers, caseworkers, or parents.

2. Music is the primary therapeutic tool. Using music to establish a trusting relationship, the music therapist then works to improve the client's physical and mental functioning through carefully structured activities. Examples can include singing, listening, playing instruments, composition, moving to music, and music and imagery exercises.

3. Music is administered by a trained music therapist. A music therapist's education and training is extensive. Musical interventions are developed and used by the therapist based on his or her knowledge of the music's effect on behavior, the client's strengths and weaknesses, and the therapeutic goals.

4. Music therapy is received by a client, and it targets a wide range of clinical populations and client ages.

5. Music therapy works toward specific therapeutic goals and objectives. Goal areas include communicative, academic, motor, emotional, and social skills. It is important to be aware that while clients may develop their musical skills during treatment, these skills are not the primary concern of the therapist. Rather it is the effect such musical development might have on the client's physical, psychological, and socioeconomical functioning.

There are two professional organizations for music therapists. The first, the American Association for Music Therapy (AAMT), is a spin-off of the second, the National Association of Music Therapy (NAMT). The separation between the two represents different philosophies regarding the practice of music therapy: NAMT focuses on entry-level BA programs, whereas AAMT focuses on graduate MA programs. NAMT awards the title of MTR (registered music therapist); AAMT awards the tide MTC (certified music therapist). According to some professionals in the field, NAMT's listing of approved schools is curriculum-based, whereas AAMT's listing is competency-based—that is, based on the degree of practical experience already acquired in any classroom or nonclassroom environment.

A certification board administers a standardized test for both groups, which enables practitioners to add BC (board certified) to their title. This helps the profession garner recognition and societal legitimacy while providing another step toward state licensure. Because it was one of the first creative arts therapies to possess an independent certification board ("psychodrama" also has one), other therapists look toward music therapy as an indicator of where the established field of creative and expressive arts may be moving at this time.

RESOURCES

BOOKS

The New Music Therapist's Handbook by Suzanne B. Hanser

Musicophilia: Tales of Music and the Brain by Oliver Sacks

Case Studies in Music Therapy by Kenneth E. Bruscia

Music Therapy: Another Path to Learning and Communication for Children in the Autism Spectrum by Betsey King

An Introduction to Music Therapy: Theory and Practice by William B. Davis, Michael H. Thaut, and Kate E. Gfeller

A Comprehensive Guide to Music Therapy: Theory, Clinical Practice, Research and Training by Tony Wigram, Inge Nygaard Pedersen, and Lars Ole Bonde

Receptive Methods in Music Therapy: Techniques and Clinical Applications for Music Therapy Clinicians, Educators, and Students by Denise E. Grocke, Tony Wigram, and Cheryl Dileo

Defining Music Therapy by Kenneth E. Bruscia

PERIODICALS

International Journal of Arts Medicine
www.barcelonapublishers.
com/international_journal_of_mt.htm

Nordic Journal of Music Therapy
www.njmt.no

A peer-reviewed journal published biannually and based out of Scandinavia

Music Therapy Journal
www.musictherapyjournal.com

A peer-reviewed academic "voice" of music therapy

Contributions to Music Education
homepage.mac.com/wbauer/cme

A refereed journal published by the members of the Ohio Music Education Association in recognition of the importance of research in guiding music education practice

Journal of Research in Music Education
www.jstor.org/journals/00224294.html

A quarterly publication of music education research studies published by the Society for Research in Music Education

Medical Problems of Performing Artists
www.sciandmed.com/mppa

The first clinical peer-reviewed journal dedicated to the diagnosis of medical, including psychological, disorders related to the performing arts

Music Therapy Perspectives
journalseek.net/cgi-bin/journalseek/journalsearch.
cgi?field=issn&query=0734-6875

Appeals to professional and nonprofessional music therapy interests

Psychology of Music
pom.sagepub.com/archive

Archive of journal articles via Sage Journals online

Psychomusicology
www.jstor.org/sici?sici=0148-9267(198423)8%3A3%3
C80%3AP%3E2.0.CO%3B2-8

First two issues of peer-reviewed journal

The Arts in Psychotherapy
www.elsevier.com/wps/find/journaleditorialboard.
cws_home/833/editorialboard?navopenmenu=1

General peer-reviewed journal centered on dance, drama, art, music, and poetry therapy

ONLINE

Music Therapy
http://en.wikipedia.org/wiki/Music_therapy

Music Therapy Info Link
http://members.aol.com/kathysl

General information on music therapy by Katherine A. Lindberg, MT-BC

Worldwide Internet Resource: Music Therapy

http://library.music.indiana.edu/music_resources/
mtherapy.html

A list of Internet projects related to music therapy

ORGANIZATIONS

American Association for Music Therapy

www.musictherapy.org

The AAMT provides the MTC (certified music therapist) credential. Contact the association for a listing of approved graduate programs. The group publishes a journal and sponsors conferences.

Certification Board for Music Therapists

www.cbmt.org

The CBMT oversees the certification process for both the AAMT and the NAMT.

Society for Music Perception and Cognition

www.musicperception.org

The Society for Music Perception and Cognition is a not-for-profit organization for researchers and others interested in how we sense, and react to, music. Includes links, membership, scientific network, and related academic journals.

Society for Research in Music Education

www.menc.org/research.html

Arts in Therapy Network

www.artsintherapy.com

The AT Network is a nonprofit organization dedicated to providing an online community for creative arts therapists and those who are interested in the healing arts.

Expressive Therapy Concepts

www.expressivetherapy.org

A group dedicated to the art and culture of expressive therapies

Association for Creativity in Counseling

www.aca-acc.org

The ACC was established in 2004 as a forum for counselors, counselor educators, and counseling students interested in creative, diverse, and relational approaches to counseling.

Association for Music and Imagery

www.ami-bonnymethod.org

All the members of AMI have been trained in the Bonny Method of Guided Imagery and Music. The organization was created to maintain and uphold the integrity of the Bonny Method and to nurture and support its members. It offers information on training programs in this method of psychotherapy, which combines music therapy with guided imagery.

National Board for Certified Counselors, Inc.

www.nbcc.org

National Coalition of Creative Arts Therapies Associations

www.nccata.org

TRAINING

Bonny Foundation: An Institute for Music-Centered Therapies

www.bonnyfoundation.org

The Bonny Foundation, founded by Helen Bonny in 1988, is a nonprofit organization that provides resources and training in the therapeutic use of the arts for professional therapists. It offers complete training and credentialing in the Bonny Method of Guided Imagery and Music.

Institute for Music, Health and Education

www.educationhq.org/college-422905.php

The IMHE was established in 1988 by Don Campbell to provide cutting-edge programs for those with an interest in the therapeutic and educational uses of sound, including music. It offers independent and yearlong training programs.

PILATES

The Pilates method is a physical fitness system that was developed in the 1920s by Joseph Pilates. Joseph Pilates moved to England in 1912, earning a living as a boxer, circus performer, and self-defense trainer. During World War I, the British interned him with other German citizens in a camp on the Isle of Man, where he trained other inmates in fitness and exercises. Here the beginnings of the Pilates method began to take shape. Around 1925, Joseph Pilates migrated to the United States. On the ship to America he met his future wife Clara. The couple founded a studio in New York City and taught and supervised their students well into the 1960s. Joseph and Clara Pilates soon established a devout following in the local dance and the performing arts community of New York. Well-known dancers such as George Balanchine and Martha Graham (both European immigrants, too) became devotees and regularly sent their students to the Pilates studio for training and rehabilitation.

Since then the technique has grown in popularity, reaching its way into television commercials and fitness fads. A consumer report study done by the *New York Times* in late 2005 revealed that there were more than 11 million people practicing Pilates (predominately women) and over 14,000 certified Pilates instructors in the United States.

Joseph Pilates originally called his method Contrology, because he thought that his method allowed a practitioner's mind to control his or her muscles. Since the 1920s, our scientific understanding of the human body has changed, yet "mind over matter" continues to be the prevailing adage in current Pilates practice. The Pilates program targets the postural muscles (at the core of the body), providing balance for the spine while strengthening the body from the inside out. Pilates exercises teach patients to constantly be aware of the breath, the alignment of their spine, and the relative strength or weakness in their torso muscles. In this way, it is a postmodern, secular version of Hatha Yoga, which also encourages practitioners to always be aware of their breath and spinal alignment—both when doing Yoga postures and when performing general daily activities as a constant moving meditation.

There was a cloud of controversy in the Pilates community in 2000. Prompted by a federal intellectual property lawsuit, the U.S. courts ruled that the term "Pilates" is generic and "free for unrestricted use." As a result, any untrained or under-qualified Pilates practitioner may call himself or herself an instructor without going through any of the training originally considered necessary for a Pilates pro. *The Wall Street Journal* investigated "phony" Pilates instructors in a 2005 exposé. Though the controversy was a damaging blow to the Pilates community, Pilates is still a method that—if done properly and under the supervision of a professionally certified practitioner—can help patients get into shape, sculpt their posture, increase their immune system's strength, elevate their overall well-being, and decrease blood pressure and other responses to stress. It offers all the benefits that any well-rounded exercise routine can.

Unlike other forms of exercise, training is one-on-one. This is similar to being personally trained at a gym, except that Pilates work is performed within a series of wood and metal framed machines that look different than normal gym equipment. The instructor stands nearby and gives instructions and encouragement throughout the hour-long session, focusing on torso muscles, breath, and spine. Small group classes are also available, which is important to many due to the high price of individual sessions. Pilates teachers tend to avoid large group classes, however, so that individual adjustments can be performed as needed.

Joseph Pilates claimed his method has a philosophical and theoretical foundation. He insisted that Pilates was not merely a collection of exercises but a method developed and refined over more than eighty years of use and observation. One interpretation of Pilates principles is listed below:

Mind over Matter

According to practitioners, the central aim of Pilates is to create a fusion of mind and body, so that without thinking about it, the body will move with economy, grace, and balance. The end goal is to produce an attention-free union of mind and body. Practitioners believe in using one's body to the greatest advantage, making the most of its strengths, counteracting its weaknesses, and correcting its imbalances. The method requires that one constantly pay attention to one's body while doing the movements.

Breathing

Joseph Pilates believed in circulating the blood so that it could awaken all the cells in the body and carry away the wastes related to fatigue. For the blood to do its work properly, it has to be charged with oxygen and purged of waste gases through proper breathing. Full and thorough inhalation and exhalation are part of every Pilates exercise. Joseph Pilates saw forced exhalation as the key to full inhalation. "Squeeze out the lungs as you would wring a wet towel dry," he is reputed to have said. Breathing, too, should be done with concentration, control, and precision. Breathing not only oxygenates the muscles, but proper breathing reduces tension in the upper neck and shoulders. Pilates breathing is a posterior lateral breathing, meaning when inhaling you breathe deep into the back and sides of your rib cage. At the same time as you exhale, you feel the engagement of your deep abdominal and pelvic floor muscles and maintain this engagement as you inhale. Each exercise is accompanied by breathing instructions.

Centering

Joseph Pilates called the large group of muscles in the center of the body—encompassing the abdomen, lower back, hips, and buttocks—the "powerhouse." All energy for Pilates exercises begins from the powerhouse and flows outward to the extremities. Physical energy exerted from the center coordinates one's movements. Pilates' founder believed that it was important to build a strong powerhouse in order to rely on it in daily living. Modern instructors call the powerhouse the "core."

Concentration

Pilates demands intense focus. Beginners learn to pay careful attention to their bodies, building on small, delicate fundamental movements and controlled breathing. In 2006, at the Parkinson Center of the Oregon Health and Science University in Portland, Oregon, the concentration factor of Pilates was being studied in providing relief from the degenerative symptoms of Parkinson's disease.

Control

Joseph Pilates built his method on the idea of muscle control. That meant no sloppy, uncontrolled movements. Every Pilates exercise must be performed with the utmost control, including all body parts, to avoid injury and produce positive results. Pilates emphasizes not intensity or multiple repetitions of a movement, but proper form for safe, effective results.

Precision

Every movement in the Pilates method has a purpose. Every instruction is vitally important to the success of the whole. To leave out any detail is to forsake the intrinsic value of the exercise. The focus is on doing one precise and perfect movement, rather than many halfhearted ones. Eventually, this precision becomes second nature and carries over into everyday life as grace and economy of movement.

Flow or Efficiency of Movement

Movement is kept continuous between exercises through the use of appropriate transitions. Once precision has been achieved, exercises flow within and into each other in order to build strength and stamina.

Pilates training seminars are available in many places all over the country. Because it is an unlicensed health modality, there are no standard requirements between different education programs. Most respectable Pilates programs have two different levels of training. The first level of training is a basic practitioner course—usually a weekend retreat—in which students are introduced to a host of different Pilates repertories, the history behind the art, and techniques for leading Pilates sessions. In the second-level, more in-depth courses, students learn how to be leaders during Pilates sessions. There is no formal accreditation agency for Pilates, but the programs in this book have been included because of their reputation within the Pilates community.

RESOURCES

BOOKS

Modern Pilates: The Step-by-Step, At-Home Guide to a Stronger Body by Penelope Latey

Pilates by Rael Isacowitz

A Pilates' Primer: The Millennium Edition by Joseph Pilates and Judd Robbins

Pilates: Body in Motion by Alycea Ungaro

Pilates' Return to Life Through Contrology by Joseph H. Pilates and William Miller

ONLINE

Pilates Insight

www.pilatesinsight.com

An independent consumer-targeted resource for nonbiased information on the methods and concepts used in Pilates

CVS Caremark

http://healthresources.caremark.com/topic/pilates

General consumer information on getting started with Pilates

ORGANIZATIONS

Balanced Body Pilates

www.pilates.com

This leader in Pilates equipment and education is a great resource for navigating the online Pilates community.

Body Arts and Science International

www.basipilates.com

A professional certification group that informally accredits various Pilates education programs around the world. Designed and developed by Rael Isacowitz, this organization is one of many striving to raise the standard of practice for Pilates instructors and practitioners.

Pilates Method Alliance

www.pilatesmethodalliance.org

The PMA made history in 2005 by launching the first industry-wide certification exam for the Pilates method in the United States. It has established recommended industry performance parameters guiding the practice of all PMA-certified and noncertified Pilates teachers. The alliance has established these standards to further bring professionalism to Pilates.

United States Pilates Association

www.pilates-studio.com

The mission of USPA is to preserve and continue to promote the highest standards in Pilates and professional training for future generations. It lists training centers on its Web site. The association intends to extend its resources and mission into the areas of teacher training and certification and continuing education through the New York Pilates Studio Teacher Certification Program.

Balanced Body University

http://bbu.pilates.com

Partnered with pilates.com, BBU has been certifying Pilates instructors for more than thirty years. BBU is the most regarded Pilates program in the United States.

Pilates Certification Center

www.pilatescertificationcenter.com

Based out of Raleigh, North Carolina, the Pilates Certification Center is an independently run institution that hosts training seminars for students of Pilates.

POETRY THERAPY

The focus of poetry for healing is self-expression and personal growth for the individual, whereas the focus of poetry as art is the poem itself. Both use the same tools and techniques: language, rhythm, metaphor, sound, and image, to name a few. Word therapy, after all, comes from the Greek word, *therapeia,* meaning to nurse or cure through dance, song, poem, and drama, which is another way of saying the expressive arts. The ancient Greeks tell us that Asclepius, the god of healing, was the son of Apollo, god of poetry, medicine, and the arts. Thus poetry therapy is a psychotherapy that can be traced back to primitive humankind.

At the dawn of civilization, we used poetic chants and rituals to promote the well-being of the tribe or for the benefit of an individual patient. Ritual rites, incorporated by tribal Shaman, have been documented as far back as the fourth millennium in ancient Egypt. Archaeologists have discovered words and symbols written on papyrus, which patients would ingest after it was dissolved in a liquid solution.

The first hospital in the United States, Pennsylvania Hospital (founded by Benjamin Franklin in 1751), employed literary treatments for psychiatric patients, including reading, writing, and even publishing. The so-called "Father of American Psychiatry," Dr. Benjamin Rush, introduced music and literature as effective complementary treatments to conventional psychotherapy in the beginning of the nineteenth century.

In 1928, Eli Greifer, an inspired poet, pharmacist, and lawyer, sought to prove that a poem's didactic messages had therapeutic healing power. His student, Dr. Jack Leedy, continued Griefer's dream and created the Association for Poetry Therapy in the early 1970s. Around the same time, scholarly literary circles began using the term "bibliotherapy" to refer to the therapeutic value of literature, which included poetry, prose, and nonfiction. By 1980, the American psychological community had accepted poetry as a legitimate style of complementary psychotherapy. The field was represented by different institutions creating their own private certification programs, using different techniques and psychological approaches. To gain solidarity and representation in the larger psychotherapeutic community, the various institutions and enthusiasts merged their interests, creating the National Association for Poetry Therapy. This group has now taken over the function of credentialing poetry therapists with designations as certified poetry therapist or registered poetry therapist. As our knowledge of the human psyche continues to grow, so do the methods and techniques of poetry therapy.

Practicing therapists are usually nationally certified in a larger modality of healing, such as psychotherapy, counseling, psychology, social work, psychiatry, nursing, massage therapy, or spiritual/pastoral direction. Because the discipline is diverse and unlicensed, sessions may take the form of either reading or writing poetry. Patients are encouraged to reflect on what they have written and/or heard, and incorporate literary themes and ethics into their own personal lives. The therapy is tailored to the patient's individual needs. Skilled therapists need to be attentive and receptive to their patients' ever-changing mental states. Poetry therapy is usually incorporated in conjunction with larger therapeutic approaches, depending mostly on the practitioner's area of expertise and training.

In the words of one poetry therapist: "One of the benefits of poetry reading and writing is not only does it help to define a patient's sense of self, but also strengthens it. This is necessary if we are to be a healthy part of this world. The poetry process attaches us to the greater part of ourselves, to all that is whole and good and beautiful. And when we feel ourselves as not alone in the world, but a part of and integrated with all that exists, self-esteem grows. The good news is we discover we are the same heroes and heroines of the old mythology, and in writing poetry ourselves, we extend it into the present, and forward, creating new stories to mark us."

RESOURCES

BOOKS

Poetry Therapy: Theory and Practice by Nicholas Mazza

Poetic Medicine: The Healing Art of Poem-Making by John Fox

Poetry, Therapy and Emotional Life by Diana Hedges and Gillie Bolton

Creative Arts Therapies Manual: A Guide to the History, Theoretical Approaches, Assessment, and Work with Special Populations of Art, Play, Dance, Music, Drama, and Poetry Therapies by Stephanie L. Brooke

Verse Therapy by Anna M. Vincent

Con-Versing With God: Poetry for Pastoral Counseling and Spiritual Direction by Cynthia Blomquist Gustavson

Biblio/Poetry Therapy: The Interactive Process, A Handbook by Arleen McCarty Hynes (1994)

Biblio/Poetry Therapy: The Interactive Process: A Handbook by Arleen McCarty Hynes and Mary Hynes-Berry (1986)

PERIODICALS

Journal of Poetry Therapy
http://springerlink.metapress.com/content/105729

Peer-reviewed research and writing in the field of behavioral science, psychology, and clinical psychology with an emphasis on the therapeutic value of poetry

The Arts in Psychotherapy
www.elsevier.com/wps/find/journaleditorialboard.cws_home/833/editorialboard?navopenmenu=1

General peer-reviewed journal about dance, drama, art, music, and poetry therapy

The Museletter
www.poetrytherapy.org/publications.htm

The Museletter is the official newsletter of the National Association for Poetry Therapy.

ONLINE

Poets House

www.poetshouse.org

An archive of amateur poetry

Poets and Writers

www.pw.org

Poet's Lane

www.poetslane.com

ORGANIZATIONS

The National Association for Poetry Therapy

www.poetrytherapy.org

The main resource for information on training, legislation, publication, research, and trends in poetry therapy, this is the largest nonprofit advocacy group in the United States. For a large list of independent poetry therapy practitioners' home pages, consult www.poetrytherapy.org/members.sites.html.

The Institute for Poetic Medicine

http://poeticmedicine.org

A general advocacy and training resource led by poet and author John Fox

Creative "Righting" Center

http://users.erols.com/sreiter

Provides training, treatment, and information on Dr. Sherry Reiter's approach to poetic therapy

Center for Journal Therapy

www.journaltherapy.com

Kathleen Adams explores the healing power of keeping a journal

National Coalition of Creative Arts Therapies Associations

www.nccata.org

Integrates different forms of creative and expressive psychotherapy into a general advocacy group. The coalition hosts integrative conferences several times a year.

POLARITY THERAPY

Polarity therapy is a synthesis of ancient Eastern health care ideas centered around energy work. Developed in the mid-1940s by osteopath, chiropractor, and naturopathic doctor Randolph Stone, polarity therapy seeks to balance and restore the flow of subtle energy that is believed to flow into all human bodies. Stone agreed with the Yoga/Vedanta tradition in that this energy is said to come from God the Universe and enter bodies through the invisible energy centers, called chakras, along the human spine. This life force, called "the breath of life" by Stone, is then distributed from the chakras throughout the human nervous system in order to animate and maintain life.

Stone was an aficionado of mysticism early in life, then a lifelong practitioner of an Indian Raja Yoga spiritual path from his fifties onward. He freely used the jargon from a multitude of spiritual systems, including Yoga, Taoism, Buddhism, Sufism (mystical Islam), Kabbalah (mystical Judaism), and mystical Christianity, for describing his polarity work. Prana and chi, from the spiritualized medical systems of Yogic ayurveda and Taoist Chinese medicine, were synonyms for the polarized life force he claimed was the key to health. Stone also believed that when this life force is naturally polarized into a negative and positive charge by God at the beginning of creation, it is the same as the Taoist "yin and yang" concept. When it is further polarized into positive, neutral, and negative charges, it is the same as the Yogic forces named, "sattva, rajas, and tamas."

Blockages in the flow of this vitalistic force are claimed to lead to pain and disease, or be experienced as stuck emotions and lack of vitality. The result of restoring balanced energy flow is a heightened sense of awareness, improved health, and general well-being on all levels. Polarity therapy has four distinct areas of technique by which proponents believe life force energy can be influenced and vitality enhanced: polarity bodywork, specific polarity Yoga exercises, counseling/positive thinking, and nutritional recommendations. Polarity bodywork is similar to old school osteopathy and chiropractic, as well as craniosacral therapy. Polarity therapists claim expertise in "energetic anatomy" and may also work with these energetic body patterns in a manner similar to acupressure along acupuncture meridians. Various esoteric energetic patterns inherent in the body, such as the five-pointed star and six-pointed star referred to in Yoga, Kabbalah, and other traditions, may be traced upon a patient's body.

Most polarity therapists are licensed or certified in another base discipline. They can be found working in private practice and counseling centers, as well as with physicians and chiropractors. There are two certification levels: associate practitioner of polarity, which allows professionals in other fields to use polarity as a complementary technique, and the registered practitioner of polarity, a more advanced form of certification enabling practitioners to use polarity as a primary technique. Both certificates require coursework and hands-on experience.

Many hybrids and other systems of polarity therapy have evolved out of the initial work of Stone, so consistency among schools and treatments can be different. The original polarity therapy, as well as Randolph Stone himself, became famous in the 1960s during the holistic counterculture movement. At age eighty-four, Stone moved in with his spiritual community in northern India, teaching free Yoga and polarity classes to many thousands of fellow Yogis until his physical demise seven years later. Polarity therapy can thus be viewed as Stone's attempt to Westernize Yoga, ayurveda, and other relatively unknown spiritual-medical systems of his time, so that Americans could reap the many benefits of Eastern philosophy and medicine. In this manner, Stone was a health pioneer, bringing Indian medicine to the United States decades before ayurveda awareness arose again with the arrival of Deepak Chopra.

RESOURCES

BOOKS

Polarity Therapy: Healing with Life Energy by Alan Siegel and Phil Young

Polarity Therapy: The Complete Collected Works, Volume I by Randolph Stone

The Polarity Process: Energy as a Healing Art by Franklyn Sills

Polarity Therapy: The Power That Heals by Alan Siegel

Foot Polarity Therapy by Wilfried Teschler

The Art of Polarity Therapy: A Practitioner's Perspective by Phil Young

Gale Encyclopedia of Medicine: Polarity Therapy by Gloria Cooksey

ONLINE

Natural Healers
www.naturalhealers.com/qa/polarity.shtml

A consumer-targeted FAQ about practicing polarity therapy professionally

What Is Polarity?
http://users.erols.com/rosediana/wipol.html

Rose Khalsa, a registered and advanced polarity practitioner, discusses and explains the various theories on polarity within the body

ORGANIZATIONS

The American Polarity Therapy Association
www.polaritytherapy.org

The APTA is the largest advocacy group for polarity therapy in the United States. For all inquiries into practice, education, and legislation, consult its Web site.

PSYCHODRAMA AND DRAMA THERAPY

Psychodrama is a form of communication founded around 1925 by Jacob Moreno, MD. It is often, but not exclusively, used as a form of psychotherapy. A student of Sigmund Freud, Moreno departed from his professor's psychoanalytical techniques before he had even graduated from medical school. Moreno claimed that as a student he once challenged his elder in this way: "Well, Dr. Freud, I start where you leave off. You meet people in the artificial setting of your office. I meet them on the street and in their homes, in their natural surroundings. You analyze their dreams. I give them the courage to dream again. You analyze and tear them apart. I let them act out their conflicting roles and help them to put the parts back together again."

Part of what may have given Moreno such confidence was that he was developing, in his mind, the therapeutic potential of group therapy. He made his initial claim to fame in 1932, when for the first time, he announced the concepts of group therapy and psychodrama to the American Psychiatric Association. For the next forty years, he developed and shared his "Theory of Interpersonal Relations," as well as a variety of tools useful in the social sciences. Moreno's most notable tool within his field of psychodrama is called "sociometry," or the measurement of predictable interpersonal dynamics within a group. To assist with sociometry Moreno also created the "sociogram," a fluid pictorial representation of sociometry using a systematic method for graphically representing individuals as nodes and the relationships between them as arcs. In his monograph, *The Future of Man's World*, Moreno describes how he developed his work in order to counteract "the economic materialism of Marx, the psychological materialism of Freud, and the technological materialism" of our modern industrial age. Moreno was a rare vitalistic MD, unafraid to stand by his spiritual and humanistic beliefs as most of his colleagues embraced the opposing forces celebrating modern technologies over nature.

Moreno's autobiography describes his life teaching as threefold:

1. Spontaneity and creativity are the propelling forces in human progress.

2. Love and mutual sharing are powerful, indispensable working principles in group life. It is imperative that we have faith in our fellow man's intentions, a faith that transcends mere obedience arising from physical or legalistic coercion.

3. A "superdynamic" community based on these principles can be brought to realization through new techniques.

In these principles, Moreno heralds the encounter groups, love-ins, and communes of the counterculture 1960s, although Moreno would also have predicted the failure of most communes due to their lack of effective group therapy performed within. That specific form of group therapy he named psychodrama utilizes dramatic enactment and reenactment, primarily of real-life events and issues but also including role play, role reversals, mimicry, mirrors, soliloquy, sociometry, and improvisation. More recently, the offshoot field of drama therapy now includes theater games, storytelling, puppetry, and performance.

Psychodrama tends to focus on one person in a group at a time. Therapists encourage clients to reenact events, especially traumas and unresolved issues from their past. Psychodrama attempts to create an internal restructuring of individuals' dysfunctional mind-sets, especially regarding other people. It challenges participants to discover new answers to unsolved situations and to become more spontaneous and independent by choice. Unlike the other creative and expressive arts, psychodrama is available only to students who have already completed a master's degree in a related field (such as counseling or social work); therefore, training in psychodrama is primarily conducted through private training centers and by individual trainers who conduct workshops. Certification is available through the American Society of Group Psychotherapy and Psychodrama.

Drama Therapy

Drama therapy is a modern branch of psychodrama defined by the National Association for Drama Therapy as the systematic and intentional use of drama and theater processes to achieve psychological change and emotional growth. Drama therapists use a wide variety of techniques, including reenactment of real-life events. Drama therapy, an expressive therapy modality, is used in a wide variety of settings, including hospitals, schools, mental health centers, prisons, and businesses. Drama therapy exists in many forms and can be applicable to individuals, couples, families, and various groups.

Although the use of dramatic process and theater as a therapeutic intervention began with Moreno's psychodrama, the field has expanded to allow many more creative forms of theatrical interventions as therapy. Drama therapy capitalizes on the healing properties of play and pretending, and tends to utilize the fictional mode as much as the more direct confrontational modes typical of psychodrama. Scenes enacted in drama therapy become personal and highly emotional over time, but the focus is generally on group process and group interaction. Drama therapy is extremely varied in its use, based on the practitioner, the setting, and the client. From full-fledged performances to empty chair role-play, sessions may involve as many variables as exists in human group dynamics. Aside from their therapeutic training, drama therapists have a background in theater and in psychotherapy. Completion of an approved master's program plus 1,500 hours of paid work experience as a drama therapists leads to recognition as a registered drama therapist.

Renee Emunzh, the director of the drama therapy program at the California Institute for Integral Studies, contributed to this introduction.

RESOURCES

BOOKS

The Living Stage: A Step-by-Step Guide to Psychodrama, Sociometry and Group Psychotherapy by Tian Dayton and Zerka Moreno

Psychodrama: A Beginner's Guide by Zoran Djuric, Jasna Veljkovic, Miomir Tomic, and Zoran Uric

The Drama Within: Psychodrama and Experiential Therapy by Tian Dayton

Psychodrama Since Moreno: Innovations in Theory and Practice by Paul Holmes

Psychodrama: Resolving Emotional Problems Through Role-Playing by Lewis Yablonsky

A Clinician's Guide to Psychodrama: Third Edition by Eva Leveton

Psychodrama/Foundations Psychotherapy Volume II by J.L. Moreno

The Handbook of Psychodrama by Marcia Karp

PERIODICALS

Journal of Group Psychotherapy Psychodrama and Sociometry
www.heldref.org/ijam.php

Features articles on the theory and application of action methods in the fields of psychotherapy, counseling, education, management, and organizational development. Its articles bridge research and practice appropriate to clinical and educational simulations, behavior rehearsal, skill training, and role-playing within group settings. The focus is on action interventions, psychodrama, and sociometry.

International Journal of Arts Medicine
www.barcelonapublishers.
com/international_journal_of_mt.htm

This publication is the official journal of the International Arts Medicine Association and the International Society for Music in Medicine.

ONLINE

Psychodrama FAQ
www.blatner.com/adam/pdntbk/Psychodrama-FAQ.
html

A well-written FAQ by Dr. Adam Blatner on some of the misconceptions about psychodrama

Lesley University
www.lesley.edu/faculty/estrella/psychodrama.html

General information on academic studies done in expressive therapies

ORGANIZATIONS

National Association for Drama Therapy
www.nadt.org

Incorporated in 1979, this nonprofit upholds professional competence and ethics among drama therapists, develops criteria for training and registration, sponsors publications and conferences, and promotes the profession of drama therapy through information and advocacy.

American Society of Group Psychotherapy and Psychodrama
www.asgpp.org

The ASGPP is a membership and advocacy organization that grants the titles: certified practitioner and trainer, educator, and practitioner by way of the American Board of Examiners in Psychodrama, Group Psychotherapy and Sociometry. This organization also provides a list of nationwide trainers and institutes offering workshops in these areas of study.

American Occupational Therapy Association, Inc.

www.aota.org

Although occupational therapy tends to work with physical rehabilitation more than it does the expressive arts, some occupational therapists use art and music therapy to augment their practices. Most occupational therapists are licensed.

Association of Schools of Allied Health Professions

www.asahp.org

The ASAHP is a membership and advocacy organization composed of various health professions. The increasing use of expressive and creative arts therapists has pushed an integrative approach to psychotherapy into the mainstream health professional networks.

Creative and Expressive Arts Therapies Exchange

www.ciis.edu/academics/exa.html

Established in 1989, CREATE is a membership organization open to therapists, educators, artists, and others interested in psychotherapy and the arts. The association is a network of individuals who are working or have an interest in the creative and expressive arts therapies. CREATE embodies all creative and expressive therapies— multi model, art, music, drama, psychodrama, dance/movement, and poetry. Participation allows members to share resources and find strength through a sense of common purpose. Membership is open to all who are interested in the use of the expressive arts in therapy. The organization publishes a journal and holds an annual conference.

The International Network for the Dances of Universal Peace

www.dancesofuniversalpeace.org

This network, a nonprofit membership organization founded by Samuel Lewis, links the many worldwide dance circles via a registry of meetings and leaders, newsletters, archives and publications, and trainings. Although sometimes called Sufi dancing, the Dances of Universal Peace use sacred phrases, chants, music, and movements from many traditions around the globe for the promotion of peace and integration. Contact the network for a listing of regional groups.

Arts in Therapy Network

www.artsintherapy.com

An online community for creative art therapists

Expressive Therapy Concepts

www.expressivetherapy.org

A group dedicated to the art and culture of expressive therapies

Association for Creativity in Counseling

www.aca-acc.org

A forum for counselors, counselor educators, and counseling students interested in creative, diverse, and relational approaches to counseling

National Board for Certified Counselors, Inc.

www.nbcc.org

National Coalition of Creative Arts Therapies Associations

www.nccata.org

United States Association for Body Psychotherapy

www.usabp.org

Dedicated to developing and advancing the art, science, and practice of body psychotherapies

TRAINING

National Psychodrama Training Center

www.nationalpsychodramatrainingcenter.com

The mission of the center is to teach and train others in the methods, theories, and philosophy of J.L. Moreno, MD, founder of psychodrama, sociometry, role training, and sociodrama.

Psychodrama Training Associates

Locations include Miami, Princeton, Tampa, and West Palm Beach.

www.psychodramatraining.com

Training at Lifestage

www.lifestage.org/training.html

Seminars and training sessions can be organized across the country.

KELLEY-RADIX WORK

Kelley-radix (or radix for short) is a psychotherapeutic methodology developed by psychologist Charles Kelley, PhD. Kelley studied with Wilhelm Reich toward the end of his life and devoted the remainder of his life to clarifying Reich's concepts and trying to improve upon Reich's system of orgonomy, the groundbreaking vitalistic, body-centered psychotherapy developed in the 1930s. Being an expert in physiology as well as psychology, Kelley contributed valuable data that is used to this day in the area of dispersing neurotic muscular "armoring" around the eyes. Thirteen years after Reich's tragic death in prison, Kelley split from his fellow orgonomists and developed an offshoot that he called radix.

Whereas Reich had labeled the vital force of life "orgone," Kelley renamed it "radix" (meaning "root" or "cause") in order to set his teachings apart from Reich. He founded Radix Education in 1970 to further develop Reich's system of therapeutics, which he believed was being ignored within the field of psychotherapeutics. Kelley had applied himself to Reich's physical, atmospheric, and laboratory experiments before focusing on the phenomenon of "muscular armoring," which appears as chronic muscular contractions, an inherent part of the human condition. Reich believed that these contractions restrict the free and balanced flow of human life force. This comprehensive, prescient theory, called "character analysis," was developed during Reich's days of study under Sigmund Freud.

Unlike Reich, Kelly believed that even though the negative effects of a patient's armoring restrict his or her experience of general well-being, it enables the patient's positive application of self-direction in everyday life. In his later years, Kelley's training programs evolved from teaching Reichian, "express your feelings" work to more focus on "feeling with purpose." This more recent attention of Kelley upon the importance of the interplay between feeling impulses, as well as upon volitional self-control of these feeling impulses, is known as Kelley-radix.

One of Reich's nicknames was "Fury on Earth," due to his constant, free-flowing expression of both positive and negative emotions at all times. Kelly's updating of orgonomy to include discriminative self-expression is perhaps more appropriate to our twenty-first century times, or perhaps a therapeutic cop-out regarding Reich's ideal of childlike fluidity of emotion regardless of circumstances. Given the strong connection between Reich's orgonomy and Kelly's radix, it should not be surprising that they share large overlap regarding therapeutic techniques.

This quote from the Kelley-Radix.org Web site could have come directly from an orgonomist: "Individual sessions are the heart of Kelley-radix work. The core of the Kelley-radix experience is learning to recognize and contact the chronic muscular tensions that hold back long-repressed emotions. Learning to surrender to these emotions, having the encouragement and opportunity to safely express fear, pain, rage, and their counterparts of trust, pleasure, and love while staying present in full eye-to-eye (reality) contact with the practitioner as the emotions are released is a powerful experience. The individual session gives the client an opportunity to delve deeply into his or her personal process while having the full attention of the practitioner. It provides the added time and space to work through whatever issues and emotions are in the day-to-day life of the client. Kelley-radix work uses a rich diversity of verbal and nonverbal techniques based upon the needs of each client. Physical exercises, breathwork, body awareness, energetic practices, and other nonverbal and verbal techniques are combined in order to discover purpose and authentic self-direction; awaken a greater sense of aliveness; enhance the capacity for love, trust, and joy; strengthen self-acceptance, self-confidence, and self-esteem; integrate body, mind, feelings, and behavior; release anxiety and negative or "stuck" feelings; and free chronic physical tensions."

The primary difference in radix seems to be that Kelley-radix patients (called "radix persons" since Kelley did not like to "pathologize" his clients) learn to control their emotions while learning to surrender to emotions only when it is "safe, appropriate, and desirable." This balance between control and expression leads to much improved relationships in both the personal and professional arenas. Gaining the ability to achieve meaningful longer-term life objectives, and to be able to enjoy them once attained, is to have earned a degree of satisfaction and happiness unavailable to those limited by excessive armoring or by the lack of sufficient containment of feeling.

Postmodern psychotherapies frequently rely upon verbal dialogue as the main vehicle for creating emotional release and transformation within a patient. Reich, Kelley, and most other body-centered therapists agree that the relative health or ill health of the body-mind is much deeper than mere verbiage.

Instead, it is contained and reflected in our cells and musculature, as well as in our emotional and sexual expression, all other actions, thoughts, and, finally, words. Whereas a clever patient can talk circles around an unsuspecting talk therapist, it is difficult for a patient to hide his or her issues from a body-centered therapist. This is because humans learn to control their words much better than their bodies, and also because many emotional traumas are held in one's musculature before the ability to verbalize has even appeared in a child. A skilled and observant body-centered psychotherapist is thus able to assess pathological armoring, in which the patient only perceives his or her "normal" way of moving and expressing emotions. Learning to use, or to dissolve, this armoring at will is one of the definitions of well-being within the radix system. If you are ready for intensive therapy and self-examination, which will make you a better healer, consider trying body-centered psychotherapy for yourself (also see also bioenergetics and core energetics).

It is important to note that while many radix therapists are also massage therapists, radix is not a form of massage. Practitioner training is available in the United States at either the Kelley-Radix Center or the Radix Institute. Radix is not a widely practiced form of psychotherapy, so its therapeutic community is small.

RESOURCES

ORGANIZATIONS

The Radix Institute
www.radix.org

The Radix Institute is a nonprofit organization that trains and certifies people to do radix work. The institute also provides continuing education and other professional services for certified radix practitioners.

The Kelley-Radix Center
www.kelley-radix.org

The Kelly-Radix Center is dedicated to extending and exploring the work of Charles R. "Chuck" Kelley, the founder of radix psychotherapy.

The Institute for Individual and Group Psychotherapy
www.iigp.org/default2.asp.html

The Institute for Individual and Group Psychotherapy, formerly the Bar-Levav Educational Association, is a radix-friendly institute specializing in long-term intensive psychotherapy with a bodywork component.

Marie Schils
www.marieetmarie.be/marieschils.htm

A Belgian site featuring the work of Marie Schils, a body-psychotherapist and certified radix teacher in Liège, Belgium.

United States Association for Body Psychotherapy
www.usabp.org

A nonprofit membership association dedicated to developing and advancing the art, science, and practice of body-centered psychotherapy.

ROLFING (STRUCTURAL INTEGRATION)

Structural integration is based on a premise which, when applied skillfully, healthfully aligns the human body with the Earth's gravitational field. Its practitioners attempt to alleviate tension by way of "unlocking" the myofascia, web-like connective tissue that surrounds every muscle of the body. This is done via a series of about ten sessions using manipulative techniques to regulate muscle position and function. Largely based on the work of Ida Rolf (hence *rolfing*), structural integration is focused on rebalancing and aligning the body physically, biochemically, and kinesiologically. This interdisciplinary modality attempts not to change a patient's internal structure, but to restore balance by focusing on manipulating the aforesaid myofascia into appropriate anatomical position. Ultimately, this allows practitioners to indirectly target entire body segments, shifting them into their natural, optimal positions. Structural integration corrects misalignment of fascia and "waits" for the body's response to the change. Once the therapist has a good assessment regarding his or her patient's physiological responses, the practitioner can cater the therapy to patients' individual needs, massaging specific tissue zones more rigorously than others.

In medical literature, the term myofascial was

used by Janet Travell, MD, in the 1940s referring to musculoskeletal pain syndromes and "trigger points"—small areas of muscle tenderness that when pressed cause distant pain somewhere else. Some current medical practitioners use the term "myofascial therapy" or "myofascial trigger point therapy" for their fascia-oriented work, especially naturopaths, physical therapists, and chiropractors. In rolfing and other similar nonmedical arts, however, the term myofascial release refers to soft tissue manipulation techniques. There are also two main schools of myofascial release: the direct and indirect methods, with rolfing being an example of the direct approach.

Rolf hypotheorized that "bound up" myofascia often restricts opposing muscles from functioning independently from one another. Her practice aimed to separate adhered fascia by deeply separating the fibers manually so as to loosen them up and allow effective movement patterns. Rolf believed that an adequate knowledge of living human anatomy and hands-on training were required in order for practitioners to safely negotiate the appropriate manipulations and depths necessary to free the bound-up fascia in their clients.

Rolfers usually prescribe an initial patient sequence of ten, ninety-minute sessions to gradually "unlock" the whole body, usually beginning with the muscles that regulate and facilitate breathing. During a rolfing session, a client generally lies down and is guided through specific postures. During this time, a rolfer manipulates a patient's fascia until it is believed to have returned to its anatomically correct position. There are also advanced rolfing sessions that incorporate patient movement as well as static bodywork positions.

Ida Rolf's methods were solidified in the 1950s, with the goal of organizing the human structure in relation to gravity. Her work evolved synergistically out of osteopathy, Hatha Yoga, Alexander Technique, and Feldenkrais Technique. Many patients report that some of the methods can be painful, yet the technique has evolved to be more gentle than in its early days. Rolf asserted that her bodywork modality was a life philosophy, though she was a woman of few words: "Put the tissue where it should be, and then ask for a moment."

Recent research has demonstrated that rolfing al-

lows for a more efficient use of the musculoskeletal system, channeling the body to conserve energy and allocate resources more economically. The refined patterns of patients' movements, which are encouraged after rolfing sessions, can significantly reduce chronic stress and degenerative changes in anatomical structure. Studies have also indicated that rolfing significantly reduces spinal curvature in subjects with lordosis (excessive curvature of the lower spine). Current research is testing the hypothesized "enhanced neurological functioning," a proposed yet unsubstantiated positive side effect of rolfing.

There are several certifications that rolfers/structural integrators can attain, yet there are few states in the country that have standards for licensure. There is one organization in particular—the International Association of Structural Integrators—that is lobbying the federal government to institute a national certification for rolfers. According to the IASI, its mission is to "to be structural integration's leading organization for the creation of standards of practice, review, and certification of practitioners and the advancement of structural integration as a cornerstone to human health and well-being through education, community, and communication." National certification usually means more income, more practitioners, more research, and more legitimacy for a modality. Needless to say, this organization envisions a bright and optimistic future for structural integration.

RESOURCES

BOOKS

Rolfing: Reestablishing the Natural Alignment and Structural Integration of the Human Body for Vitality and Well-Being by Ida P. Rolf

Rolfing Structural Integration: What It Achieves, How It Works and Whom It Helps by Hans Georg Brecklinghaus

Rolfing and Physical Reality by Ida P. Rolf

Rolfing in Motion: A Guide to Balancing Your Body by Mary Bond

Balancing Your Body: A Self-Help Approach to Rolfing Movement by Mary Bond

Rolfing by Dr. Ida P. Rolf

The Rolfing Experience: Integration in the Gravity Field by Betsy Sise

Equine Structural Integration: Myofascial Release Manual by James Vincent Pascucci, Nicholas David Pascucci, and Carol J. Walker

PERIODICALS

Medline
www.unboundmedicine.com/medline/ebm/research/Rolfing

Articles in various peer-reviewed journals related to rolfing

Journal of Bodywork and Movement Therapies
www.sciencedirect.com/science/journal/13608592

A general body-oriented holistically minded medical journal

ONLINE

Crystalinks
www.crystalinks.com/rolfing.html

General information about the techniques and poses used in typical rolfing sessions

The Rolf Method of Structural Information
www.rolfmethod.com

General consumer information about rolfing and structural integration

Aetna IntelliHealth
http://intelihealth.com/IH/ihtIH/WSIHW000/8513/34968/362156.html?d=dmtContent

A consumer resource for the relationship of rolfing with health insurance plans

ORGANIZATIONS

The Rolf Institute
www.rolf.org

The leading institution, endorsed by founder Ida Rolf, for structural integration. It provides information on recommended education programs and a network for practitioners.

The International Association of Structural Integrators
www.theiasi.org

A general advocacy group lobbying for national rolfing certification and licensure

The Guild for Structural Integration
www.rolfguild.org

An advocacy, educational, and membership group that raises public awareness regarding the efficacy and benefits of structural integration. It maintains a massive archive of practitioner links on the Web

European Rolfing Association
www.rolfing.org

Dedicated to spreading the work of Ida Rolf throughout Europe

The International Schools of Structural Integration
ww.theissi.org

An educational institution committed to increasing standards of practice in the structural integration community

TRAINING

Body Therapy Center
Palo Alto, California
www.bodytherapycenter.com

International Professional School of Bodywork
San Diego, California
www.ipsb.edu

Florida School of Massage
Alachua and Gainesville, Florida
www.floridaschoolofmassage.com

The Core Institute
Phoenix, Arizona
www.thecoreinstitue.com

School of Integrative Therapies
Holmdel, New Jersey
www.thesoit.com

Scherer Institute of Natural Healing
Santa Fe, New Mexico
www.schererinstitute.com

Body Therapy Institute
Siler City, North Carolina
www.massage.net

Cortiva Institute—Brian Utting School of Massage
Seattle, Washington
www.cortiva.com/locations/busm/

Institute of Structural Medicine
Twisp, Washington
www.structuralmedicine.com

RUBENFELD SYNERGY METHOD

The Rubenfeld Synergy Method (RSM) is a body-centered therapy that emphasizes the use of gentle touch, verbal expression, and directed movement. It combines techniques used in the Alexander Technique and Gestalt therapy as well as those of the Feldenkrais Method and Ericksonian hypnotherapy. Like other similar therapies, RSM helps to open a patient's gateways to contacting, expressing, and understanding past memories and feelings. It is based on the belief that blocked emotional expression in the past has resulted in "dis-ease" somewhere within the patient's present-day body-mind.

The premise in RSM is that skillful touch combined with talk therapy can release repressed and suppressed emotions and help to heal body-mind pain. The method was founded by Ilana Rubenfeld, and though it is only forty years old, it has established a small foothold within the holistic medicine community. In the 1950s, Rubenfeld was seeking relief from partial paralysis of her arm muscles that were about to truncate her successful career as an orchestra conductor. She decided to study the F.M. Alexander Technique, a body awareness training especially used by performers to rid themselves of body movements that are inefficient and fatiguing. She also began participating in psychotherapy. Once she learned to listen to her body in a greater way, emphasizing awareness, her physical pain and paralysis ceased. Intrigued with this approach, she became an "Alexander teacher," where her reputation grew as a facilitator of both domains: the physical and the emotional. In the 1970s, at a fortuitous meeting with Buckminster Fuller, he suggested the name "Rubenfeld Synergy" for her slightly unique integration of touch and talk.

The eighteen principles and theoretical foundations of RSM are listed below. They are not exclusive to RSM, as this is by definition a synergistic therapy. Most body-centered, humanistic, and transpersonal psychologies adhere to a similar list, although this version has its own unique flavor:

1. **Each individual is unique.** Rubenfeld synergists approach clients and their sessions with this principle of honoring their uniqueness.

2. **The body, mind, emotions, and spirit are dynamically interrelated.** Each time a change is introduced at one level, it has a ripple effect throughout the entire system.

3. **Awareness is the first key to change.** By bringing the unconscious into awareness, clients have the opportunity to explore alternate choices and to develop possibilities for emotional, physical, and psychophysical change.

4. **Change occurs in the present moment.** Clients may experience memories of the past and fantasize about the future, but change itself can occur only in the present.

5. **The ultimate responsibility for change rests with the client.** Rubenfeld synergists can support clients to recognize dysfunctional behavior and guide them to try new ones. They cannot force clients to change.

6. **Clients have the natural capacity for self-healing and self-regulation.** Innate healing ability already exists in clients, waiting to be actualized. Rubenfeld synergists do not "cure" or "correct" but rather facilitate clients' healing.

7. **The body's energy field and life force exist and can be sensed.** Rubenfeld synergists use gentle touch to sense energy, its pulsations and movement. When tight holding patterns in the body-mind are released, there is a marked change in the energetic quality.

8. **Touch is a viable system of communication.** Rubenfeld synergists develop "listening hands" to dialogue with clients, thus opening new gateways to their unconscious mind.

9. **The body is a metaphor.** Clients' postural positions and movements may represent emotional issues in their lives.

10. **The body tells the truth.** Often what clients communicate verbally is not congruent with their body's story. Rubenfeld synergists guide their clients to listen to their body's message.

11. **The body is the sanctuary of the soul.** Rubenfeld synergy sessions may progress toward a spiritual dimension when clients deal with their "soul" issues—questioning their life values in relationships, families, communities, and the world.

12. **Pleasure needs to be supported to balance pain.** Rubenfeld synergists help clients contact their strengths and joy so that they can experience pleasure to balance pain.

13. **Humor can lighten and heal.** Appropriate humor, not sarcasm, interrupts habitual, painful patterns. Laughing invites deeper breathing, releases tense muscles, and can heal pain.

14. **Reflecting clients' verbal expressions validates their experience.** When clients hear what they have said, they often use this opportunity to reflect on their initial statements and take them to a deeper level.

15. **Confusion facilitates change.** Confusion usually interrupts habit patterns, creating a window of opportunity in which the client can experiment with new and nonhabitual behavior.

16. **Altered states of consciousness can enhance healing.** Altered states are pathways to the unconscious mind. They facilitate heightened awareness and enable clients to access physical and emotional memories that still inhabit their bodies.

17. **Integration is necessary for lasting results.** Many physical problems change when their associated emotional material is processed. Unless clients integrate their new insights and behaviors into their daily lives, they may revert back to their previous problems.

18. **Self-care is the first step to client care.** Rubenfeld synergists are trained to take care of themselves and prevent burnout by maintaining personal boundaries, paying attention to their physical environments, and listening to their bodies, minds, and emotions.

RSM training has evolved over three decades regarding structure, length of each study module, and location of study, but its goals remain the same: to teach the integration of a gentle listening touch with verbal tools; to help clients gain self-awareness, self-esteem, a relief of emotional wounds, and the encouragement to be true to their own "music"; and to build a loving, supportive community of healers.

Professional certification and postgraduate training is available through several institutions below. Because the practitioner community is relatively small, most institutions retain a strong connection to the original method as taught by Ilana Rubenfeld.

RESOURCES

BOOKS

The Listening Hand: Self-Healing Through the Rubenfeld Synergy Method of Talk and Touch by Ilana Rubenfeld and Joan Borysenko

Healing Journeys: The Power of Rubenfeld Synergy by Vicki Mechner

Gale Encyclopedia of Alternative Medicine: Rubenfeld Synergy by David Helwig

ONLINE

American Cancer Society
www.cancer.org/docroot/ETO/content/ETO_5_3X_Rubenfeld_Synergy_Method.asp?sitearea=ETO
A research study on the efficacy of the Rubenfeld synergy approach in cancer patient therapy

Answers.com
www.answers.com/topic/rubenfeld-synergy?cat=health
General consumer information on the practice and method of Rubenfeld synergy

ORGANIZATIONS

Rubenfeld Synergy Method

www.rubenfeldsynergy.com

A membership group that certifies and trains practitioners

Ilana Rubenfeld

www.ilanarubenfeld.com

The students of Ilana Rubenfeld's method created an organization to educate the public about the benefits of the method and train practitioners through semiannual workshops.

SOMATIC MOVEMENT THERAPY

Somatic movement therapy training (SMTT) is a course of study originally founded by Martha Eddy in 1991. In her therapy, Eddy synthesized a deep understanding of somatic education, movement science, and human communication into a single modality of body-oriented therapy. The therapy stems from Eddy's experience and practice of Laban movement analysis (LMA), Barteniff fundamentals, and body-mind centering. She claims that by paying close attention to the internal body, one's "deepest and healthiest intensions" can be made clear and effect change. Using LMA to give a precise vocabulary to the sometimes elusive signs of the body's movements, reflective practices help patients connect to and proceed with meaningful parts of their lives. Somatic movement therapy employs powerful body-based skills that are taught as a safe response for the ever-growing stress in our often overly stimulating world.

Advanced professional training in SMTT is available through SOMAction Institute, with various locations around the United States. It is broken down into four phases. The first starts with basic courses on SMTT theory, postures, and techniques. The second phase is an interim independent study period with assignments specially designed by Eddy to bring one to a deeper understanding of one's own body. The third phase is a six-week intensive retreat (held biennially) where practitioners new and old can discuss their progress with the technique. The fourth and final phase of training might be thought of as continuing education, which requires practicing somatic therapists to attend integrative seminars.

RESOURCES

BOOKS

Somatics: Reawakening the Mind's Control of Movement, Flexibility, and Health by Thomas Hanna

Authentic Movement by Mary Starks Whitehouse, Janet Adler, Joan Chodokow, and Patrizia Pallaro

Somatic Practices, Movement Arts, and Dance Medicine by Gale Reference Team

ORGANIZATIONS

SOMAction: Moving on Center

www.movingoncenter.org

The largest somatic therapy institution on the Web, it includes training locations, certification requirements, membership boards, links, and much more.

The Center for Kinesthetic Education

www.wellnesscke.net/pt.htm

Co-founded by Martha Eddy, the center offers information on professional certification in somatic therapies.

Tamalpa Institute

Kentfield, California

www.tamalpa.org

A movement-based expressive arts training center that offers training programs and workshops in the Halprin Process, a healing arts approach that integrates movement/ dance, visual arts, performance techniques, and therapeutic practices.

YOGA THERAPY

Unlike ayurveda and Chinese medicine, which are therapeutic systems bolstered by the religious philosophies of Yoga/Vedanta/Hinduism and Taoism /Buddhism, respectively, Yoga therapy is the only medical system directly plucked from a religious practice, desecularized, and reintroduced to the public as a mainstream health and fitness aid for all. Unbeknownst to many "gymrats," Yoga is one of the world's oldest religions, originating on the India subcontinent approximately 7,000 years ago, according to data derived from modern archeological sites.

Yoga literally means "union" or the process of fully remembering our inherent soul union ("Yoga") with the sole substance, God. It is the art of consciously choosing to leave the delusive "matrix" of the external universe behind, at times and then permanently, so that glimpses of our true relationship with creation can be felt and so that eventually our actual godly nature can be experienced at will. Omniscience, omnipresence, omnipotence, and ever-changing contentment and bliss are the promised results for successful Yoga practitioners, perhaps over many lifetimes, as are the desire and ability to teach others to accomplish this same type of final freedom from the matrix (called "maya" in Yoga philosophy).

If the similarities between this story of Yoga and the story of Neo, Morpheus, and *The Matrix* movie series seems suspiciously similar, that is because the Matrix story takes a nod from the philosophy of Yoga. It spread to Greece before the fourth century B.C.E. and appeared again in Plato's famous recounting of Socrates' short story, "The Cave." Soon afterwards, Alexander the Great travelled to India and brought from there his guru, the Yogi Kalyana, illustrating further the ancient India-Greece spiritual connection. In Socrates' version of "The Cave," humans firmly chained in a deep cave can only see shadows of themselves and others that appear on a nearby wall due to a fire shining behind them. These cave dwellers spend their whole lives believing that their shadowy world is the real one. When one of the prisoners is unchained and dragged toward first the fire and then the outdoor sunshine, the prisoner's experience is at first disorienting and overwhelming. Gradually, the newly freed one acclimates to the new lights and sights, and understands that his old shadowy world was the merest fraction of the much more thrilling truth of existence.

When he descends to teach his old prison mates the good news, they jeer him, accuse him of madness, and threaten to kill him. Ignorance is bliss? Well, to metaphorical cave dwellers, ignorance is comfortable; waking up is a hassle; and there's probably nothing better to wake up to anyway. But Yogis from pre-history through Socrates (considered a Yoga master by contemporary Yogis) and on to postmodernity have always claimed that it is ultimately soul knowledge, not ignorance, that brings bliss. In Yoga, human ignorance is synonymous with our craving for maya's flickering pleasure and aversion to its shadowy pain. This can be at the very least unsatisfying, and at the worst chronically miserable. But since that's the only life of which most of us are aware, cravings and aversions continue for millions of lifetimes until one by one individuals realize that they've been duped. Waking up from their delusive cave dream, though challenging, becomes the only game worth playing.

In the Hollywood version, the maya-matrix is a sinister delusion perpetuated by intelligent machines that extract their fuel from cave-imprisoned, barely living humans. These billions of humans are plugged into a virtual reality system that convinces them they are living an amusing human life outside the machines' cave, when in fact they are only viewing virtual reality shadows and missing out on the thrilling and fulfilling knowledge that awaits them if they could only discover maya's deception; be willing to escape it; and then be instructed how to actually make happen the step-by-step escape to truth. Enter Morpheus, who has already received help, gradually freed himself, and now devotes his life to awakening others. This is a direct mirroring of the traditional Yogic guru-disciple relationship. Neo follows Morpheus's lead, trains hard, and eventually attains even greater mastery over the matrix than Morpheus (just as ego-free Yoga gurus delight if their disciples surpass them in spiritual attainment). Neo is now a "satguru" in Yoga jargon, one with a vast public mission such as Krishna or Moses or Jesus, and is karmically chosen to free masses of humans from their delusive existence in maya's cave.

In Yoga philosophy, however, the matrix is much less sinister. In fact, it is more a lark, a game, a divine play or hobby of God not to be taken seriously—even if at times it feels scarier than the Devil incarnate, also known as maya personified. This is the case no matter how much delusive pain or pleasure you are feeling. The inherently deluding five senses can only report back on maya's virtual cave reality. Yoga cosmology says that one day God was somehow a bit bored and lonely in the pre-creation unitary consciousness-existence-bliss mode that described God's effortless enjoyment. This was before the first thought, feeling, or body was even conceived of by the eventual creator. And then: BIG BANG BOOM!

A sphere of vibration emanated due to the desireless desire for companionship from the nonexistent point of bliss we sometimes call God, and the rest is history. From that massive vibration, reverberating now and forever like a huge roaring ocean of om (that sacred sound turned temporarily into a cliché in the 1960s) has come all of time, space, atomic forces, and the relatively quaint Earth dramas that so beguile terrestrial cave dwellers. God is still always blissed out and no longer even slightly bored and lonely since a small part of God, a tip of the divine iceberg, is now teeming in trillions of entities living out entertaining lives on billions of physical, astral (light), and causal (thought) worlds. Meanwhile, the metaphorical cave dwellers (namely you and me) experience the opposites of heat and cold, pleasure and pain, likes and dislikes, as alternately smile- or frown-inducing; and sometimes just plain boring.

If all of us awakened from our cave delusion too soon, so the story behind Yoga goes, then God's jig would be up, and there would be no more game of creation to eternally entertain God as us. Eventually, we each earn our own inevitable enlightenment, or awakening, from the maya-matrix. But so many impediments have been placed in our way—one of which is instinctively thinking that the shadow cave is the only real game in town and another of which is our tendency to ignore or despise those who try to come to our aid with both news of the sunnier world of individual enlightenment as well as a variety of routes out of the cave.

The good news of Yoga is that eventually every deluded "prodigal son" wakes up and gets to feast forever with the rest of God on the "fatted calf" of blissful wisdom. The bad news is that, as long you don't wake up, you'll suffer unnecessarily for eons with your fellow cave dwellers. To Yogis, this is unnecessary, when all you have to do is work hard to hike out of the cave with your helpful friends and revel in your omnipresent playground for as long as you choose. But make no mistake: the trail that exits the cave is steep and challenging for even the hardiest souls. An easy stroll it is not.

The varieties of escape routes from the maya-matrix have been called by a variety of names: the eightfold paths of both Yoga/Hinduism and Buddhism, Taoism, Kabbalah (mystical Judaism), Sufism (mystical Islam), mystical Christianity (so *uncommonly* practiced at present that it no longer has a separate name). You name the religion—it shares an escape route suspiciously similar to the generic escape route promoted by the deep meditators of all faiths: unplug from obsession with the external world; tune in with one's internal, core, divine nature; and compassionately help the blind once you've regained your own more accurate spiritual sight.

Yoga was the original matrix-dissolving religion, as far as historians of religion know, just as ayurveda was the original holistic medicine system. Of course, the original does not necessary mean better. But let us give credit where credit is due, and not buy into the modern tendency to believe that everything new (Neo) will always surpass everything old. Yoga cosmology is cyclic, with long periods of advancing awareness following long periods of declining awareness in an endless, ever-changing, kaleidoscopic loop. In Yoga, our job is simply to find the appropriate escape route for ourselves and to find freedom as quickly as we can for everyone's sake (except for the rest of God, who's totally amused and ecstatic no matter what happens).

The history of Yoga as a comprehensive, matrix-healing therapy could be detailed from Yogi-to-Yogi and doctrine-to-doctrine leading up to the present year. That exercise would be boring for everyone, however, and completely out of tune with the spirit of Yoga itself. What is more important to understand is that, as far as modern historians know, Yoga remained an all-consuming lifestyle and religion for millennia until the modern age.

Five doctrinal texts, memorized via the oral tradition for millennia before being written down, stand out from all the others regarding the philosophy and practice of Yoga:

- "The Vedas" or "The Truths" are the oldest known religious doctrines and the source of ayurveda medical knowledge.

- The Upanishads are placed at the end of the Vedas and therefore known as "Vedanta," the name given by Indians to the source of Yoga philosophic.

- The *Mahabharata* or "Great Battle" metaphorically explains Yoga philosophy as an amusing war (remember, this is a game!).

- The *Bhagavad Gita* or "Song of God" occurs within the story of the Great Battle and records the Yoga conversations between liberated Krishna (Morpheus) and "cave-dwelling" but freedom yearning warrior, Arjuna (Neo).

- The "Yoga Sutras" come to us from Patanjali, the maya-liberated author who opted to help free others by, among other things, succinctly writing down the essentials of Yoga philosophy and practice so that everyone could understand it.

The last of these texts was written around 200 B.C. at the latest. The British overthrow of India in 1858 resulted in a great meeting of worlds.

The British named the Indians "Hindus" because many of them lived by the "Indus" River, and for the first time in 2000 years, Yogic philosophy was unleashed upon Europe and North America. Soon intellectuals picked out the most inspiring threads (including Patanjali's Yoga Sutras, literally "Threads on Divine Union") and began to include them in their books and lectures. Leo Tolstoy and Ralph Waldo Emerson are two of the most famous initial converts from the nineteenth century, but the trickle turned into a flood. Swami Vivekananda wowed his audience with a short speech affirming the unity of all religious paths at the World Parliament of Religions in Chicago on another profound 9/11—this one in 1893. In that same year, Paramahansa Yogananda was born in India. An earnest Yogi from around the age of six, Yogananda was trained to become Yoga teacher to the West. Between the ages of seventeen to twenty-seven, he played Neo to the Morpheus training of Swami Sri Yukteswar, a rigid disciplinarian and strong supporter of Western logic, efficiency, and ingenuity. Arriving in the U.S. in 1920, Yogananda spoke to overflow auditorium crowds for years before settling in to play Morpheus himself for hundreds of devoted Neos in America. The first Yogi to spend the majority of his life in the U.S., Yogananda is credited with being one of the founding fathers of American Yoga. Yet it took another "great battle" before Yoga become popular enough to inhabit gyms and certification programs nationwide: the war between the gray flannel suits and the counterculture in the psychedelic '60s.

One reason Yoga recrested in the '60s is that the very criticism leveled at the mainstream culture of the times (cave dweller-like rigidity regarding sex roles, dress, music, economic institutions, heaven-and-hell Christianity, U.S. hegemony) were some of the very areas answered by the always tolerant, ever fluid, kaleidoscopic, reincarnational, it's-all-a-game, lighten up, be creative, "we're all gonna be enlightened someday" message emanating from Asia in general and Yoga/Buddhism/Taoism in specific.

The mass counterculture's desire to break new boundaries resulted in millions of folk experimenting with psychedelics that had been known about for decades, including LSD, psilocybin mushrooms, and mescaline cacti. Lo and behold, the psychedelic experience shared by many experimenters seemed suspiciously similar to the out-of-the-matrix reports that had been recorded by Vedanta/Taoist/Buddhist Yogis for millennia. Some Yogis even reported that their ancestral comrades had used psychedelic plants for millennia in order to afford them encouraging glimpses of the overwhelmingly engrossing enlightenment that lay ahead. Modern day quantum physics and the quest for a grand unified, as in integrated, theory of the universe are at the heart of mysticism. Stephen Hawkings of Oxford and other contemporary pioneers are pondering such far out things as string theory, time and space, anti-matter, and the likelihood of other dimensions. Finally, the great institutions of science and technology meet the wisdom of the heart. And not a moment too soon.

Many of the sixties' youngest members picked up a daily meditation habit or Hatha Yoga practice and copied the colorful draping dress of the Hindus, as well as other lifestyle practices from just about any culture that had maintained beliefs different from the materiality obsessions of the West. Of course, the majority of the population in Europe and the U.S. stuck to their philosophical guns, and eventually, the counterculture fads of the 1960s passed away. Psychedelics were made illegal; most users hadn't wanted the hassle of Yoga practice anyway and switched to the unenlightening replacements of cocaine and amphetamines. Soon disco led to Reaganomics, and maya easily repositioned the matrix veil of external materiality over our sleepy, cave-dwelling eyes.

But the dogmas of the East were here to stay, gradually infiltrating themselves into popular slang (karma, guru, yin/yang, the dharma bums, the fifth dimension, and so on); political speeches; and especially health care. Acupuncture had been in the American colonies since the 1700s due to immigrating French doctors' previous exposure to the native medicine of Indochina. However, Chinese medicine took off in the U.S. only when a journalist accompanying the Nixon administration's convoy to China fell ill and reported back his favorable impressions of acupuncture and Chinese herbal medicine to his *New York Times* readers.

Ayurvedic medicine made its popular reappearance in the 1980s when Deepak Chopra, an Indian MD, met "the Beatles' guru," Maharishi Mahesh Yogi. Chopra had become disillusioned with allopathy over a decade of work in U.S. hospitals, so he was receptive when the Maharishi ("Great Yogi") requested that Chopra become the prophet of ayurveda for the Western world. Soon Chopra was selling millions of books based on Vedanta and ayurveda, especially following a 1991 appearance on *Oprah*. And although ayurveda has not approached the level of popularity that the (secularized) version of Chinese medicine has in America, without Chopra's ascent, it is possible that Yoga would not have reached its own peak interest of late.

Another alternative health figure who paved the way for mass Yoga is Andrew Weil, MD, a Harvard-trained doctor from the (surprise) late 1960s. Probably the most recognizable doctor in the U.S. today, Weil teaches deep Yogic breathing to many of his clients and claims that proper breathing is the one treatment he would use for all patients if he could only choose one—strong words from an allopath, holistic or not.

Evolution of Yoga Therapy

Yoga therapy as a medical modality has traditionally been a subset of ayurveda, practitioners of which usually prefer treatment plans based on diet and herbs. They know that most patients wouldn't be disciplined enough to practice daily Yogic exercises anyway. Until the fifteenth century, the contorting postures most Westerners think of as Yoga (asana, meaning "immobile" in Sanskrit) were merely a small but important third step along the eight-step Yogic path. The cultivated ability to remain immobile is designed to aid in keeping the Yogi's body healthy, supple, and strong.

This is done not so that the Yogi's delusive matrix body could be kept well as an end in itself, but so that the Yogi could withstand long hours of meditation without moving a muscle or being distracted by the pain of disease or inflexibility.

In the fifteenth century, sage Swami Svatmarama removed asana from its important but minor role, and expanded its importance into a new style of Yoga he called "hatha" or "sun-moon." This referred to the Yogi's gentle but firm manipulation of energy currents along the spine, currents that were usually ignored but were also potentially enlightening. Since these two main currents have opposing polarities, Yogis refer to them as hatha, which also has a secondary meaning of "forceful." Swami Svatmarama labeled Hatha Yoga not as a replacement for the religion of Yoga but instead as a "stairway to the heights" of Raja (meditation- and enlightenment-focused) Yoga. The hatha Yogi simply spent more time on asana than the norm and, presumably, less time on meditation. Over the centuries, however, strands of Hatha Yoga began to appear that distanced asana from the traditional end goal of enlightenment. Instead Hatha Yoga was sometimes used as an effective route to retain or regain one's body-mind health. This was an effective use for Yoga but far from its original lofty intent.

Many Hatha Yoga teachers have been born and buried since Swami Svatmarama. Some have been traditionalists who encourage students to free themselves from maya's matrix, some have positioned themselves as little more than physical education instructors, and many have inhabited the vast gray areas in between. When ayurveda and Yoga therapy re-emerged in the West during the 1980s, however, there was little question as to which form would take precedence. There was no way that a heavily Christian-based culture, approximately 40 percent of whom have recently been evangelicals believing in a 6000-year-old universe, were going to embrace Yoga therapy as the religious practice it once was—and still is.

Hatha Yoga

Today there are two streams in the West. The first branch is the Hatha Yoga that most Americans simply know of as "Yoga," with practitioners not knowing that Yoga is an ancient religion. Even Hatha Yoga teachers will sometimes claim that Yoga is not a religion, but rather a philosophy or lifestyle similar to what the religion of Buddhism has become in some Asian countries. But millions of religious zealots in India practice daily Yoga meditation, while sitting in an immobile asana as their chosen route out of God's playful, though often painful, matrix called maya. Modern Yoga teachers sometimes even change the meaning of the word "Yoga" from "uniting, or yoking, the soul with God" to "uniting the mind with the body." In original Yoga, the mind and body are both part of maya's matrix, so uniting them together gets you little more than more enjoyable matrix software to enjoy within your prison cave.

Our recent Hatha Yoga fad, fueled by celebrity Yogis like Madonna and fitness chains, has brought more Americans in contact with Yoga than ever before. Improved relaxation, flexibility, and health in general is a welcome cultural side effect, so as a whole, there is nothing to deride about this process. What is unfortunate, perhaps, is that the Yoga "baby" of all-around body-mind-spirit development has been thrown out with the "bathwater" of nonessential religious dogma so uncomfortable to Westerners. Yet as far back as the 1920s, teachers such as Paramahansa Yogananda were already Westernizing Yoga practice while still retaining its original spiritual goal of God union (ironically, Yogananda removed most of the asana practice from his Kriya Yoga system, aware that Americans were already far too obsessed with their physical bodies). So it was not a given that Hatha Yoga would be secularized beyond recognition in our postmodern times, just a strong likelihood without a twenty-first-century nationwide Yoga representative as influential as a Vivekananda or a Yogananda.

The influential teacher representing spiritual Yoga has not yet arrived in our new millennium. Chopra and Maharishi mixed Yoga and ayurveda with a high-margin business model that rarely mentioned practical day-to-day spiritual practice. Bikram Choudury brought Yogananda-style asana to the West and become Hollywood's "Yoga Teacher to the Stars," while removing any trace of spiritual focus from his boot camp-like asana sessions. And the current celebrity-driven Hatha Yoga fad has become little more than "yog-ercise" for those bored with previous aerobics classes.

Yoga in the West

Yoga therapy as a specialized health modality is sometimes attributed to Swami Sivananda from Rishikesh, India. Sivananda founded the Divine Life Society on the banks of the Ganges and taught many Yoga disciples using the traditional and spiritual eightfold path. This included the young Krishnamurti, who later went on to teach "guru-less" Yoga in the U.S.; Swami Satchidananda, the guru who spoke to Woodstock crowds and trained Peter Max, John Coltrane, Alan Ginsberg, and many others in the U.S. during the promotion of his version of traditional, religious, "Integral Yoga"; and Swami Satyananda Saraswati, who founded the Bihar School of Yoga a year after his guru's passing. Satyananda's school combined an applied scientific approach to Yoga with the spiritual obsession typical of any Yoga school in India. Although Sivananda himself was a traditionalist, he was also an MD who helped modern Yogis see and experience the worldly practicality that has always come along with the spiritual practice of Yoga.

A similar combination of spiritual depth and mundane practicality has filled the lives of other Yogis believed to have contributed to, if not founded, modern Yoga therapy: Tirumalai (T.) Krishnamacharya, an ayurvedic doctor, and his disciples B.K.S. Iyengar, K. Pattabhi Jois, Indira Devi, and son T.K.V. Desikachar. All have had a significant impact on the popularization of Hatha Yoga practice in America. These Yogis devoted their lives to spiritual evolution, believing that encouraging Hatha Yoga in the West was at least fostering some degree of spiritual practice. So the question remains: who "desacralized" Hatha Yoga in the West?

In yet more cosmic irony, the most likely candidate is the most famous student of Bishnu Ghosh, youngest brother to Paramahansa Yogananda. Yogananda was the Yogi who, from 1920–52, made the biggest initial impact on traditional God-, guru-, and meditation-focused Yoga practice in the United States. His brother Bishnu, however, preferred what was then called "physical culture" and what is now called bodybuilding, gymnastics, and public performance combined. Bishnu trained Bikram Choudury (Choo-dree), the current "Bad Boy of Yoga," according to *Yoga Journal*. Choudury become a Hatha Yoga champion starting when he was around five years old.

Yet there is no such thing as a "Hatha Yoga champion" within the religion of Yoga.

In fact, such a classification would normally have been pegged by gurus as egotistical, and thus anti-Yoga, in the first place. Regardless, Choudury won the National India [Hatha] Yoga Contest three years in a row before retiring as champ, becoming an "Olympic quality" bodybuilder, suffering a weight-lifting knee injury, and returning to guru Bishnu, who helped him regain his health via Hatha Yoga therapy. After founding Hatha Yoga schools in India and Japan, in 1974 Choudury followed Yogananda's lead and made his way to Los Angeles. There he set up shop in Beverly Hills and became a "Yoga Teacher to the Stars," including the then popular Michael Jackson, Raquel Welch, and Tom Smothers. Choudury's unusually braggadocio-like personality insists to this day that only his version of twenty-six postures—practiced only in a specific order and only in a room heated to a specific temperature—is the true Hatha Yoga. This would include, apparently, all the asana recommendations prescribed by Yoga teachers for thousands of years, as well as all of the Hatha Yoga training from the days of Hatha Yoga founder Swami Svatmarama to the present time. Choudury has, in fact, called these teachers, "circus clowns."

From the 1970s on, Choudury's Hatha Yoga has possibly had the greatest numerical influence on Hatha Yoga practice across America. This is probably due to the franchising of Bikram's Yoga schools, versus the more pedestrian spread of spiritualized Hatha Yoga schools promoting Iyengar, Integral, Ananda, and Sivananda styles.

Yoga as a healing art and fitness method has become acceptable to Americans as long as it works on their fat cells, aches, and pains. And Yoga therapy, the use of Hatha Yoga postures to act as preventive and curative medicine for healing the body-mind, can now be learned through certification programs nationwide. This is both a wonderful thing for our culture and a missed opportunity to help Americans relax and rejuvenate to a much greater degree.

Yoga Therapy Definition

In January 2007, the International Association of Yoga Therapists (IAYT) defined Yoga therapy as "the process of empowering individuals to progress toward improved health and well-being through the application of the philosophy and practice of Yoga." This definition could scarcely be a broader umbrella, and, as the IAYT authors agree, it does little to distinguish Yoga therapy from the practice of Yoga without a trained therapist present. Seemingly content with working unhurriedly within the infinite cycles of Hindu cosmology, the IAYT has decided to wait at least a year before releasing its definition of "Yoga therapist." Until that time, Yoga therapy is what you make it, as there are no other standards that define Yoga protocols leading to certification as a Yoga therapist.

Another unofficial definition of a Yoga therapist might be: the instruction of Yogic practices and principles, from a trained practitioner to a client, for the promotion of greater client well-being as well as toward prevention and treatment of all potential and actual pathologies. This definition is also broad enough to cover all Yoga therapies but replaces the unnecessarily vague verb, "empower," with a specific verb, "instruct," and also includes treatment of disease by a practitioner.

If Yoga therapists hope to see their system spread nationwide, they will likely have to embrace both sides of the political-medical system and agree that they are making money by responding to clients' desires to treat pathology as much or more than they are responding to clients' desires to proceed from health toward super-health via an empowerment process. They will probably also have to clarify that what they do is instruct clients toward greater health via their own increasing expertise in Yoga postures, breathwork, and meditation. These Yoga practices are learned in a step-by-step approach that also may include Yoga spiritual philosophy. The extent that this philosophy will be included in any Yoga therapy session lies on a spectrum from traditional God-obsessed to postmodern secular, depending on the individual practitioner.

At this stage, Yoga therapy by this name is so new that any person who teaches, or "empowers" another with Yoga, be it at a gym, a meditation hall, or a doctor's office, can include themselves in the mix as long as they hold a certification in Yoga therapy.

Hatha Yoga teachers are found in studios across the country, from bare bones YMCAs to the most elite and glitzily mirrored clubs. These teachers sometimes come from lineages and Hatha Yoga schools developed around the teachings of particular Yoga gurus mentioned earlier, such as Krishnamacharya and Sivananda. And sometimes they come from offshoots far removed from these teachers but evolutionarily beholden to them still, such as many generic "Power Yoga" trainings. In general, Yoga teacher trainings focus heavily on asana and minimally on pranayama and meditation. Although the training itself may include plenty of Yoga cosmology and philosophy, it is understood that this can be used for purely academic purposes or for a student's chosen spiritual path. Students may learn one set of Yoga postures to be taught always in the same order, or they may learn hundreds of postures that can be presented to the public at random.

Coursework is extremely varied in depth and content by who's doing the teaching. What teaching certifications have in common is to help students provide the health-bestowing effects of Hatha Yoga practice to all comers.

The Yoga teacher or Yoga therapist may teach any aspect of Yoga, and it might be useful to understand the steps of the traditional eightfold Yogic path and the different forms Yoga can take.

1. **Yama (the five "restraints"):** *ahimsa*—no harm to others in word, thought, or deed; *satya*—tell the truth without being insensitive; practice no deceit in word, thought, or deed; *asteya*—no stealing; simply don't take or "borrow" what isn't yours, and give back what you've agreed to return; *bramacharya*—chastity or non-lusting; ideally be celibate if single and sexually moderate if coupled, keeping at least some control over this powerful force for good and ill; *aparigraha*—non-greediness; live simply within your means and celebrate the successes of others.

2. **Niyama (the five "observances"):** *shauca* (SAH-sha)—purity of body and mind via healthful habits; *santosh*—contentment, to be practiced as sincerely as possible no matter what the circumstances; tapas—discipline; delayed sensory gratification in exchange for later spiritual reward; *svadhyaya* (svahd-YA-ya)—study

and introspect; absorb wisdom from scripture, wise folk, and self-analysis; *ishvara-pranidhana*—"God-devotion"; think and feel God as much as possible.

3. **Asana ("immobile"):** following your teacher's instructions, learn to keep your body strong and supple enough to sit for extended periods, in immobile meditation position. This is the isolated form most Westerns are familiar with.

4. **Pranayama ("life force control"):** because this often involves using specific breathing patterns, it is usually assumed that pranayama means "breathing exercises"; there are other Yogic methods for life force control, however, including using visualization or nonbreath-oriented meditation techniques.

5. **Pratyahara ("withdrawal from the senses"):** the state reached upon the "successful" practice of step four; this goal is to be kept in mind during pranayama practice, as once freed from the senses' distractions, the rest of the steps begin to flow more effortlessly. Easier said than done.

6. **Dharana ("concentrating on one thing"):** this can be concentration upon anything: a worldly thing, a spiritual thing; concentration is the sole key in step six, and here the Yogi is oblivious to anything other than his or her object of concentration.

7. **Dhyana ("meditation (upon God)"):** here the attention is riveted upon God in whatever version is being manifest—Light, Sound (Om and its tributaries), Peace, Love, Joy, Wisdom, Compassion. The Yogi is now both oblivious to the outside world and entering temporary spiritual rapture.

8. **Samadhi ("merging"):** the first stage of step eight is "sabikalpa" samadhi, or samadhi "with difference." Here the Yogi is completed merged with God's ever-new bliss, and knows it. However, the Yogi must remain immobile or his or her felt divine connection fades. The second stage of "nirbikalpa," or samadhi "without difference," is when the Yogi can retain

God-communion even when moving freely about in the world. Even this isn't really the last step of Yoga, as things only keep improving spiritually from here on out. But once you're at the nirbikalpa samadhi stage, there's believed to be no backsliding possible. So, for all practical purposes, this is the Yogic endgame.

Removing one step from this ancient process and calling it "Yoga" is perhaps similar to handing out edible wafers to a roomful of people and calling it "Catholicism." Nonetheless, step three (asana) also has many benefits for the participants who incorrectly believe that by practicing it they are automatically practicing the "Yoga" of God-union. The thousands of asana postures that have been developed over millennia are extremely beneficial for those wanting to maintain or regain all-round body flexibility at the joints, tendons, and ligaments. These postures also assist in the healing processes for many musculoskeletal injuries by improving circulation to and from structures. This is especially important for structures, such as joint cartilage, that take a longer time to heal due to inherent poor circulation. An increase in circulation toward a body tissue brings nutrients to that area. Return circulation carries away naturally occurring cellular toxins created during the healing process or simply during normal "wear and tear."

Hatha Yoga postures also result in a unique "massaging" of internal organs due to the mild to wild contortions that are part of the posture requirements. No Western science has been done to affirm whether this organ massage is healthful or not. But we do know that the stimulation organs receive from jogging, for example, helps them to function optimally. Hatha Yoga is also a moderately effective muscle strengthener and cardiovascular workout aid, depending on the Yoga style performed. Ananda Yoga, for example, gives mild benefits regarding increasing muscle strength and aerobic capacity, while "flow" yogas such as Ashtanga Yoga offer excellent benefits toward increased strength and cardiovascular health because of their rigorous pace and frequent lifting of the body off the ground.

On a psychological basis, regular Hatha Yoga practice is believed to lessen depression and anxiety, two sides of the same illness coin that is near epidemic in America. So does exercise in general, however. While every ailment of the body-mind might hypothetically improve with Hatha Yoga practice, what is needed is for Western scientific institutions to begin rigorous research on claims made for "treatment" postures regarding specific disease states. If hatha Yogis are making the claim, for example, that a certain neck-stretching "cobra" pose is helpful for many thyroid ailments because it places therapeutic pressure on the thyroid gland due to the nature of the stretch, it is time to verify these claims. The same is true if headstands are claimed to improve memory or mental illness. Without such proof, it is probably better to let Hatha Yoga remain a fitness aid; whereas, with such proof, we will have begun to categorize an effective, drug-free and side-effect free system of healing not unlike that classified by Western osteopaths.

Because of these likely medical benefits, combining healing and fitness, both Yoga teachers and Yoga therapists will have an increasing client base into the foreseeable future. As for how Yoga evolves in America, the jury is still out.

Techniques

There have literally been thousands of Hatha Yoga postures invented over the centuries. Yoga teachers and trainers use their own favorite combinations for instructing students or helping clients heal. However, there are certain core asanas that one will routinely experience in most classes and clinics.

Core and none-core postures are used within different schools of Hatha Yoga. Although the postures may be the same in each one, the different styles are important to understand since the experience feels as different as dancing jazz versus salsa versus ballet. Regardless of the specific style, Hatha Yoga postures are to be done slowly, fluidly, gracefully, and never brought past the point of pain. Slow, deep, diaphragmatic, "Yogic" belly breathing is usually recommended throughout, as is *vijayi* ("victory") breathing, which is a belly breath breathed in such a way as to sound like Darth Vader during both inhalation and exhalation. The mind is to be kept as calm as possible by focusing on the breath, the body movements, a spiritually inspiring thought. To assist this process, the eyes are kept soft yet firmly focused at one point. If the eyes are open, the focus is usually on an unmoving spot within your environment. If the eyes are closed, focusing at the heart area or point between the eyebrows are common traditional spiritual instructions. The stiller the eyes, the stiller the rest of the body-mind.

Since Yoga is not a competition, the relative skill of nearby Yogis is best ignored. Mental encouragement of yourself and others is far more helpful for everyone involved. Consciously cultivate a feeling of vitality and exuberance, especially during difficult poses. Channel emotional and physical discomfort into the felt sense of improving discipline, will power, flexibility, healing, and spiritual connectivity. Have fun! Remember, Yoga to union to bliss.

Ananda Yoga

Paramahansa Yogananda has left his mark on two of the most common Hatha Yoga systems available today, even though he preferred to de-emphasize the importance of Yoga postures. For Yogananda, asana meant simply to be able to keep the back straight and body relaxed during long hours of meditation. Although he taught Yoga postures as part of his comprehensive Raja ("royal," or comprehensive) Yoga training for disciples, he also felt that practicing too many postures took time away from the more important Yogic techniques of pranayama and meditation. Yogananda also noticed that Americans tended to already be too concerned with their bodies and external displays of superior appearance. He counseled his youngest brother, Bishnu Ghosh, to no avail regarding this same obsession. Ghosh went on to become a star as a traveling "physical culturist" and in the process also trained Bikram Choudury. This is the same expert hatha Yogi who secularized Yoga as he brought his series of postures to southern California in the late '60s. One of Yogananda's direct disciples, however, began teaching the postures he'd learned in Yogananda's Self-Realization Fellowship (SRF) ashrams. This disciple is Swami Kriyananda (J. Donald Walters), who founded the yogically traditional Ananda organization in the late 1960s just as Choudury was arriving in California. Nearly identical to the posture series advanced by Choudury, the Ananda version is soothing, relaxed, and highly spiritualized. Meditations are led several times throughout Ananda Ha-

tha Yoga classes, and spiritual affirmations are said in unison during the holding of the postures themselves. The postures are not rigorous, and there is little felt competition compared with many other Hatha Yoga classes.

Ashtanga Yoga

In this form of Hatha Yoga, the student learns a series of flowingly connected Yoga poses linked with specific breathwork. The entire series of poses is called a "vinyasa." Students move in smooth fashion from one pose to the next, from standing to backbends to balancing and twisting poses. Once they've mastered a series, they move on to a more difficult one. Controlled breathing is important in Ashtanga Yoga. Sometimes the room is heated to help muscles become relaxed and flexible. Because students don't stop or pause between poses, this is one of the best Hatha Yoga styles to practice for cardiovascular benefits. If the flow of postures is performed correctly (one can "cheat" and make them easier), this is also one of the best hatha yogas for strengthening muscles. Classes tend to have a competitive feel due to the rigorous nature of the exercise, so this style is not the first choice for those wanting a calming, spiritual environment. The Ashtanga posture series is said to have been discovered written on palm leaves in a Calcutta library by Hatha Yoga expert, T. Krishnamacharya, and his student, K. Pattabhi Jois, in the 1930s. Jois still teaches Ashtanga classes in his Indian homeland to this day.

Bikram Yoga

This type of Yoga involves a series of twenty-six poses practiced in a heated room. This is often not the best beginner's Yoga as it requires an already good fitness level and is psychologically challenging from the get-go. Bikram Yoga is an excellent way to stretch muscles, ligaments, and tendons; improve your cardiac capacity; and strengthen your will power. Be prepared for assertive, sometimes critical, instructors copying the style of founder Bikram Choudury. There are no flowing transitions between postures as in Ashtanga Yoga. Instead, the instructor commands to "Change!" postures, each of which is practiced two times in succession. Although there are several more series of postures beyond the initial twenty-six, few students are given permission to move past step one due to perceived skill imperfections.

Integral Yoga

Trademarked by Swami Satchidananda, and not to be confused with Sri Aurobindo's (non-hatha) Yoga of the same name. Satchitananda's Integral Yoga is very much based on the traditional eight-step Yogic path to enlightenment. But most people experience it via the Integral Hatha Yoga classes offered in cities across America. These classes blend asanas, pranayama, and meditation in a calming manner that feels more spiritualized compared with many other Hatha Yoga styles today.

Hatha Yoga

Started in the fifteenth century as a slight variation on the traditional eight-step Yoga spiritual path, Hatha Yoga has now come to mean only step three—asana. Whereas founder Swami Svatmarama wanted students to merely increase their emphasis on asana as they made their way toward step-by-step enlightenment, current practitioners do little else other than asana. All the other Yoga styles mentioned in this list are currently considered Hatha Yoga styles, regardless of whether or not they also were originally designed to offer training in the entire eight-step Yogic path.

Kundalini Yoga

Like Integral Yoga, Kundalini Yoga is actually a type of Raja Yoga—the inclusive style of religious Yoga that focuses most importance on meditation and devotion to God. It has been commercialized, however, into a specialized form of vigorous Hatha Yoga combined with breathwork, expressive utterances, visualizations, and meditations. These practices are designed to permanently raise the Yogi's energy from the lower spine to the brain stem and top of the head. Since Yogis believe this same process occurs spontaneously with other styles of Yoga, Kundalini Yogis simply put most of their focus on accomplishing this specific spiritually enlightening task. Expect more Indian philosophy and esoteric practices in Kundalini Yoga classes compared with other styles listed here.

Kripalu Yoga

Also a type of religious Raja Yoga, this Yoga was named in 1972 by founder, Amrit Desai, in honor of his guru, Swami Kripalu. Hatha Yoga within this style is heavily focused on pranayama via breathwork, as well as on the cultivation of "Witness Consciousness." This is a nonjudgmental observation of all one's thoughts, feelings, sensations, and spiritual experiences, more commonly known as "mindfulness" within Buddhist terminology. Mastering physical poses is secondary in importance to spiritual work, and poses tend toward the gentler, more relaxing side of the Hatha Yoga spectrum.

Iyengar Yoga

B.K.S. Iyengar is one of the nephews and students of T. Krishnamacharya, founder/discoverer of Ashtanga Yoga. After forming a successful school of his own in India, Iyengar began teaching classes in England and the rest of Europe from 1961–76 via elite connections with violinist Yehudi Menuhin. His 1966 book, *Light on Yoga,* became the most influential book on Hatha Yoga to date, and his status as one of the founding fathers of Hatha Yoga in both the East and West continues to grow with each passing year.

Iyengar Yoga focuses on anatomical detail and precise body alignment. Poses are held for a longer number of minutes compared with other types of Hatha Yoga. Iyengar Yoga is most recognizable by its heavy reliance upon props such as cushions, benches, wood blocks, straps, and sand bags, all of which are used to help students maintain proper form. Although firmly based in traditional eight-step Yoga, typical Iyengar-style classes mention mostly Yoga postures versus pranayama and meditation. Iyengar is also one of the founding fathers of Yoga therapy as physical therapy. His Ramamani Iyengar Memorial Yoga Institute is dedicated to treating ailments with Yogic medicine alone and is especially known for using specific asanas for specific ailments.

Power Yoga

This secularized Hatha Yoga is similar to Ashtanga, but no special sequences are followed. Instead, teachers are free to improvise in order to create vigorous workouts. Sometimes Power Yoga is done in a heated room, which helps muscles maintain flexibility and prevents injury. It is designed for people who want to feel stimulation and rigor when they practice Yoga.

Madonna, one of the central Hatha Yoga harbingers of our generation, is a Power Yoga advocate.

Application

Both Hatha Yoga instructors and Yoga therapists use a variety of postures within a variety of styles. A Hatha Yoga instructor will normally lead a class of from three to one hundred persons, with the teacher facing the rest of the class and a full-length series of mirrors behind the teacher. The mirrors allow the students to compare where they think their body parts are with where the more objective mirrors tell them they are. The teacher can also occasionally face the mirror while leading the class, giving students the perspective of an anatomically correct Yoga posture from behind. Frequently, the instructor will lead the class in a simple pranayama ("life force control") exercise, usually instructing the class to breathe in a precise pattern.

One classic example of pranayama is to breath in through the nose at two beats per second while beginning a traditional Yogic belly breath. Count the number of breaths it takes to perform a full inhalation through the nose, letting the inhalation begin with the belly fully expanding. This allows the lungs to fully expand as well. Hold the breath for the same count that it took to inhale, then exhale for the same number of counts. Repeat six times or so. If this practice is done with the body immobile, the eyes closed, and the concentration at one particular point in the body (the heart area or point between the eyebrows are two common traditional spots), the mind usually begins to quickly calm down. It is now better prepared for concentrating on anything, including performing Yoga postures.

Chosen postures usually include a variety of forward bends, backward bends, side bends, standing postures, twisting postures, lying down postures, and sometimes inverted postures with the feet over the head in some way. A Yoga posture series normally lasts anywhere from thirty to ninety minutes, after which the supine "corpse pose" is usually done for final relaxation purposes. At this time, the instructor often leads the class in a group visualization exercise, which can then lead into a more traditional silent meditation. Rarely is there any mention of Yoga dogma, such as the importance placed on chanting Sanskrit-based hymns, or listening to nonphysical sounds (such as "Om"), or revolving life force around the chakras lining the nonphysical spine in order to speed spiritual evolution. Instead, students are generally encouraged to feel more peaceful, loving, compassionate, and forgiving.

Most modern classes leave out the preliminary pranayama exercises and final visualizations and meditations. (Since most Hatha Yoga instructors are in business at some level, they usually alter their class offerings to meet the desires of their clients.) With most Americans doing Yoga for the physical benefits, it is understandable that Yoga postures will dominate almost any Hatha Yoga class in America. With that said, there is a growing trend of Yoga studios offering a more Integral Yoga class.

Yoga therapists differ in their approach compared with Yoga instructors in that they are often meeting with a client on a one-on-one basis. This allows Yoga therapists to impart more of their personal Yoga philosophy to individual clients, and it is easier for therapists to sense the receptivity of an individual client to esoteric Yogic information and tailor their approach accordingly. Clients normally come to Yoga therapists due to chronic musculoskeletal difficulties, similar to the reason why clients visit chiropractors or physical therapists. Because each Hatha Yoga asana has been classified as to which muscles it stretches, which organs it massages or stimulates, and which nerves or other tissues are delivered more life force, any physical complaint can be offered treatment. A client will be led through specific postures during his or her appointment with a therapist, and then instructed on how, and how often, to perform the same or similar postures at home.

Yoga therapists can also treat psycho-spiritual ailments, since regular Hatha Yoga practice can also aid in calming the pathologically restless, uncontrolled, obsessive, compulsive, neurotic, egotistical mental state that most people quickly acknowledge is present when they attempt to practice asanas—especially if these asanas precede an attempt at concentration and meditation practice. At present, however, it is the minority of individuals who seek treatment for their neuroses. Those who seek assistance rarely move beyond pharmaceutical drug treatment and talk therapy. So Yoga therapists will likely find their psycho-spiritual assistance to clients is only as much a part of their treatment plan as they believe their client will comply with. Mostly they will offer support for the physical complaints the client has presented to them and provide on-the-side encouragement regarding ideal Yogic breathing, emotional control, focused thought, prayer, and devotion. This can be secularized as "life coach."

Careers and Trends

Today Yoga is a lucrative and growing business across the entire country and much of the planet. About 16.5 million Americans now spend nearly $3 billion annually on Yoga classes and products, a February 2005 poll by Harris Interactive and *Yoga Journal* magazine revealed. And it is currently estimated that around 30 million Americans and 5 million Europeans regularly practice some form of Hatha Yoga.

One opinion concerning the globalization of Yoga is that it is co-opting an ancient spiritual philosophy and lifestyle. Because Yoga invokes ideals of harmony, health, and balance, it fits well as a potentially therapeutic balancing agent within the frenetic postmodern environment. So, on one hand, the acculturation of Yoga in America and Europe might be viewed as a welcome celebration of multiculturalism, promoting more open and tolerant cultural dispositions. On the other hand, the processes of Yogic commercialization may be considered to have diluted the sacredness of Yoga practice beyond recognition.

Yoga as exercise or physical therapy has morphed into numerous subdivisions and variations, moving farther and farther from the original sources within ancient Indian culture. Naked Yoga, chair Yoga, acro Yoga, and hip-hop Yoga are just some of the more creative variations emerging for consumers, who ultimately will decide the shape of Yoga in the West.

Regardless of what occurs concerning the re-spiritualization of Yoga, or lack thereof, it seems that we have not yet seen the peak of interest in Hatha Yoga practice in the West. Hatha Yoga classes will probably only become more and more Americanized, and thus more attractive to the U.S. mainstream consumer base. And Yoga therapy is only now emerging as a subspecialty of physical therapy within the holistic allopathic medical movement. However, this doesn't yet mean that receiving certification in either Yoga teaching or Yoga therapy will result in a lucrative individual practice. Similar to other CAM certifications, financial success will largely hinge on personal business skills and charisma. There won't be much of an existing system of career hierarchy to fit into after receiving your certification, as there would be, for example, if you gained a physical therapy degree. Instead, you will likely need to make your own business connections, start your own practice with other medical practitioners or alternative therapists, and in general find your personal Yoga niche that sets you apart from your peers.

Upon certification as a Yoga teacher, your income will vary greatly depending on the hours worked and the type of classes taught. For a class taught in a community center, the teacher may receive $5 to $10 per student, while private instruction may be $50 or higher per hour. Certification as a Yoga therapist will normally also result in marketing yourself as a self-employed practitioner, although more and more clinics and hospitals are responding to patient demand and carrying a Yoga therapist on staff. Per hour rates are a bit higher for Yoga therapists than for Yoga teachers, averaging from $50 to $100 per hour.

This debate will no doubt continue to simmer, but the prospective student can take heart that Yoga has finally been made acceptable enough to the global mainstream that it is possible to make a living via the practice and instruction of asana alone. If you are a Western Yoga practitioner of any sort, this news should be of great comfort, since it has never been true before and is a clear sign of increasing multicultural open-mindedness in America. And if you simply enjoy the Yoga postures but have no interest in practicing the philosophy and lifestyle that has until recently always been fused with the postures, you can also take heart that you can offer this unique form of healing to your future clients without joining any Eastern-style "cult" or religion of any sort. Neither teaching Hatha Yoga, nor offering it as therapy, are likely to bring huge financial rewards at the present time, but working with calmness- and flexibility-inducing Yoga movements as your career path will bring many other obvious, lifelong advantages.

RESOURCES

BOOKS

Note: There are hundreds of books written about Yoga. Below is a sampling geared toward future practitioners of Yoga.

Yoga Anatomy by Leslie Kaminoff, Amy Matthews, and Sharon Ellis

Light on Yoga: The Bible of Modern Yoga by B.K.S. Iyengar and Yehudi Menuhin

Yoga as Medicine: The Yogic Prescription for Health and Healing by *Yoga Journal* and Timothy McCall

The Heart of Yoga: Developing a Personal Practice by T.K.V. Desikachar

Anatomy of Hatha Yoga: A Manual for Students, Teachers, and Practitioners by H. David Coulter

Hatha Yoga Illustrated by Martin Kirk, Brooke Boon, and Daniel Di'Turo

The Yoga Sutras of Patanjali: Commentary on the Raja Yoga Sutras by Sri Swami Satchidananda

The Language of Yoga: Complete A to Y Guide to Asana Names, Sanskrit Terms, and Chants by Nicolai Bachman

PEER-REVIEWED PERIODICALS

Yoga Journal
www.yogajournal.com

A peer-reviewed publication for practitioners in the United States

International Journal of Yoga
www.ijoy.org.in

A multidisciplinary quarterly scientific Yoga journal, dedicated to Yoga research and applications. The journal is an official publication of the Swami Vivekananda Yoga Anusandhana Samsthana.

International Association of Yoga Therapists' Publications Overview
www.iayt.org/publications_Vx2

A free online archive of several Yoga journals

ONLINE

Yoga Directory
www.yogadirectory.com

A directory of Web sites for all types of Yoga enthusiasts

HolisticMed.com
www.holisticmed.com/www/Yoga.html

A comprehensive list of Yoga Web links for practitioners and the public

Anusara
http://anusara.com

A general consumer and practitioner resource for information on the growth and practice of Anusara Yoga

Yoga to Health
www.yogatohealth.com.au

Based on the philosophy that YOGA stands for Your Opening to Growth and Awareness. This group, which is dedicated to the body-mind connections in Yoga practice, publishes a newsletter and hosts several workshops and classes.

International Association for Yoga Therapists
www.iayt.org

A group dedicated to disseminating information on Yoga therapy; mostly a resource for current Yoga practitioners

Satyananda Yoga
www.satyananda.net

Information on Satyananda Yoga and retreats in this modality

ORGANIZATIONS

The American Yoga Association
www.americanyogaassociation.org

A nonprofit educational organization that serves the public to provide the highest quality Yoga instruction and education resources to anyone interested in Yoga. The AYA is one of the largest comprehensive Yoga advocacy and membership groups in the United States, incorporating many types of Yogic practice and philosophy.

International Yoga Teachers' Association

www.iyta.org.au

IYTA is an international organization founded in Australia in 1967. The association has branches in four countries, contacts in another ten, and members in twelve countries. It is dedicated to promoting the growth and understanding of Yoga principles throughout the world.

International Yoga Association

www.holisticbenefits.com/ima/international-Yoga-association.html

Insurance and liability plans for Yoga practitioners

Iyengar Yoga Links

www.iyengar-Yoga.com/Associations/United_States

Catalogue of different Iyengar Yoga sites

National Iyengar Yoga Association

www.iynaus.org

A membership and advocacy group for Iyengar Yoga

Yoga Alliance

www.yogaalliance.com

Registers individual Yoga teachers and Yoga training programs in a network of practitioners, consumer, and institutions. Registered schools, accredited by Yoga Alliance, are well-regarded in the Yoga community.

Yoga Research and Education Foundation

www.yrec.org

The YREF conducts and promotes research in any aspect of Yoga practice and efficacy.

Yoga Research Society

www.yogaresearchsociety.com

Hosts professional seminars and workshops for advanced Yoga practitioners. Subjects usually include new research and developments in the field of Yoga and holistic medicine.

Yoga for Health and Educations Trust

www.Yoga-health-education.org.uk

A nonprofit U.K. group dedicated to developing a unique teacher-training scheme for advanced Yoga practitioners

EDUCATIONAL RESOURCES

A note on Yoga schools: As Yoga is both increasing in popularity and diversifying in the United States, there are hundreds of individual practitioner training programs. Because there is no standard for what makes a Yoga practitioner, different programs will vary in tuition, instructional hours, and requirements. The list below is hardly comprehensive.

International Yogalayam

www.discover-Yoga-online.com

An online school of Yoga-related instructional resources

Kripalu Center

www.kripalu.org

One of the leading Yoga institutions and training schools in the United States

Yoga Works

www.yogaworks.com/teacher_training

An organization that has teacher training in several different locations around the United States

YogaFit

www.yogafit.com

A similar network of Yoga practitioners and instructional programs

YogaSite

www.yogasite.com/teachertraining.html

A great list of different Yoga training programs in every state

Yoga Network

www.yoganetwork.org/school_search.cfm

Search for accredited Yoga schools in your area. A great resource for finding top-notch practitioner training programs

Yogafinder

www.yogafinder.com/Yoga.cfm?yogateachertraining=y

Search for Yoga training centers by geography

Chakra Yoga

www.chakrayoga.com

International Yoga training seminars and retreats

Yandara Yoga Institute
www.yandara.com
An esteemed Yoga training seminar-type program

American Viniyoga Institute
www.viniyoga.com/index.
php?cn=what_training_teacher
Special one hundred-hour program based in California

ZERO BALANCING

Zero balancing is a hands-on bodywork system developed by Fritz Smith, MD, osteopath, licensed acupuncturist, and mystic. During the 1960s and 1970s, Smith went in pursuit of a deeper understanding of illness and health, becoming a student of rolfing, Raja Yoga (including asana and meditation), and other Eastern philosophies. Already a DO and MD since 1961, he became a licensed acupuncturist in 1972 and later studied with noted "five-element" instructor, J.R. Worsley, of the Chinese College of Acupuncture in England. It was during this time that he also experienced personal revelations under the teaching of Swami Muktananda. These latter two experiences became the catalysts for zero balancing in 1975.

Zero balancing integrates Western anatomical conceptions with Eastern concepts of a separate, invisible, near identical body of energy that acts as a functional template for physical life. By fusing a practical with a spiritual model, zero balancing teaches practitioners to use energy as a working tool in relation to body structure.

The fundamental principles of zero balancing are centered on one's interpretation of the mind's energy within the context of the body's structure. This type of therapy seeks to solidify the body-mind connection by balancing emotional energy in the physically densest tissues of the body—the skeletal system. The results of a zero balancing session are said to be manifold: it may help to reduce present stress while enhancing the body's ability to cope with future stress, as well as promote a general sense of metaphysical wholeness, happiness, and well-being. Just like the dual-part model for zero balancing, the benefits of this therapy are both psycho-spiritual and physical.

The specific touch used in zero balancing is described as having "characteristic clarity," and attempts to engage in a harmonious relationship between body and energy. Pressure is applied to focus points around the bones and joints, rather than tissues. Some somatic techniques rely upon deliberate stillness, as opposed to constant movement. A typical session, which lasts around thirty minutes, begins with a brief consultation about the patient's lifestyle and specific complaints. Sessions begin in a seated position, moving from there to a comfortable reclining position on your back. Using touch, the zone balancing practitioner evaluates your energy fields and energy flow in these two positions and balances the structures as needed. He or she may focus on body, mind, spirit, or all three, depending on where the fields are disturbed or the energy is blocked. Throughout the zero balancing session, attention is given to the skeleton in particular because it contains the deepest and strongest currents. This fully clothed bodywork begins with the lower back, legs, and feet, and eventually moves to the upper body and the head. Hereafter, the therapist will revisit the feet before finishing whatever other bodywork is to be performed that session. The touch is gentle and distinct and should not be painful. This modality uses specific stretching forms, including "dorsal hinge fulcrums," hip evaluations, and "half-moon vectors." The stretches infer a cooperative relationship between the therapist and the patient, so the style and efficacy of the treatment varies depending upon the chemistry of the pair. A zone balancing session is designed to promote maximum relaxation and well-being. It is supposed to be pleasant for both the zone balancing practitioner to give and the client to receive. Some people describe experiencing "expanded awareness," others that it's like "feeling balanced to zero," which sounds pretty good.

RESOURCES

BOOKS

Zero Balancing by John Hamwee

Zero Balancing: Touching the Energy of Bone by John Hamwee

The Alchemy of Touch: Moving Towards Mastery Through the Lens of Zero Balancing by Fritz Frederick Smith

ORGANIZATIONS

Zero Balancing Association

www.zerobalancing.com

The main advocacy and membership Web site for zero balancing. It includes information on training, certification, philosophy, and helpful Web links to other somatic therapies.

TRAINING

There is no formal accreditation for this nondegree training. There are many programs in the United States. Listed here are only a few.

American College of Traditional Chinese Medicine

San Francisco, California
www.actcm.edu

Connecticut Center for Massage Therapy

Groton, Newington, and Westport, Connecticut
www.ccmt.edu

Helma Institute of Massage Therapy

Saddle Brook, New Jersey
www.helma.com

Baltimore School of Massage

Linthicum, Maryland
www.bsom.com

The Lauterstein-Conway Massage School

Austin, Texas
www.tlcschool.com

Section III

PRACTITIONER RESOURCES

CONTINUING EDUCATION, RETREAT AND CONFERENCE CENTERS

These resources are general in nature and are relevant to all health care providers. For consideration in the next edition, please e-mail: updates@thehunterpress.com

Breitenbush Hot Springs
Willamette National Forest, Oregon
www.breitenbush.com

Breitenbush offers workshops as well as individual retreats and is well known as being a common meeting center for various holistic conferences.

Canyon Ranch Spa
www.canyonranch.com

With three locations in Tucson, Arizona; Lenox, Massachusetts; and Miami Beach, Florida, Canyon Ranch was one of the first holistic spas and has since become one of the largest integrative spa programs in the United States. Emphasizing preventative, holistically minded health, Canyon Ranch hosts retreats, conferences, and large events several times a year.

Center for Spiritual Awareness
Lakemont, Georgia
www.csa-davis.org

The center offers meditation retreats in the northeast Georgia mountains from May to September. Its spiritual director, Roy Eugene Davis, is a direct disciple of Paramahansa Yogananda.

Chinook Conference Center and Retreat Facility of the Whidbey Institute
Clinton, Washington
http://www.whidbeyinstitute.org

Chinook was founded in 1972 as a contemplative learning center. As a nonprofit educational organization committed to creating a sustainable future for the planet, Chinook shares and stewards its resources in a way that demonstrates and teaches the sacred interconnection of Earth, spirit, and all living things. Chinook offers individual retreats, work retreats, and internship programs.

Claymont Society
Charles Town, West Virginia
www.claymont.org

The society was founded in 1975 as a community and school to promote the principles of continuous education and integrated human development. In 1985, Claymont Court Seminars, sponsored by the society, was established to host and facilitate retreats, workshops, and seminars.

Esalen Institute
Big Sur, California
www.esalen.org

Esalen was founded in 1962 as a nonprofit education center and soon after found itself a pioneering representative of the human potential movement. Esalen offers seminars, workshops, and invitational conferences in the area of personal and social transformation. It also offers certification courses in Esalen's massage method and a month-long certification course in hypnotherapy.

Feathered Pipe Ranch
Helena, Montana
www.featheredpipe.com

Feathered Pipe offers retreat-style workshops on topics such as astrology, Yoga, women's wisdom, and Shamanism. It has received notable publicity from various vacation and retreat magazines.

Fellowship Renewing Experience, Strength and Hope Renewal Center
Augusta, Missouri
www.freshrenewal.org

FRESH Renewal Center, founded in 1990, is dedicated to a spiritual renewal process in which individuals recovering from addictions and their families can find sanctuary, support, and personal growth. The center follows the Twelve-Step recovery program.

Heartwood Institute

Garberville, California

www.heartwoodinstitute.com

Heartwood provides resources for attaining higher physical, psychological, and spiritual well-being. Besides offering an array of somatic nondegree training programs (such as massage, polarity, and shiatsu), Heartwood conducts various personal growth retreats, often within an educational framework.

Holistic Networker's Guide to Holistic Conferences Expos and Events

www.holisticnetworker.

com/directory/Holistic-EventsExpos/82-0.html

A general guide to the various conferences and seminars in holistic medicine that are going on all over the United States. Holistic Networker includes many smaller conferences that are not explicitly listed in this book.

The Himalayan Institute

Honesdale, Pennsylvania

www.himalayaninstitute.org

A leader in the field of Yoga, meditation, spirituality, and holistic health, the Himalayan Institute was founded by Swami Rama of the Himalayas. The mission of the Himalayan Institute is to discover and embrace the link between East and West, spirituality and science, and ancient wisdom and modern technology. It hosts several programs, retreats, and seminars in various holistic modalities.

Insight Meditation Society

Barre, Massachusetts

http://dharma.org

Founded in 1975 by Jack Kornfield, PhD, Joseph Goldstein, and Sharon Salzburg, the society is a nonprofit retreat center whose purpose is to foster the practice of vipassana (insight) meditation and to preserve the essential teachings of Theravada Buddhism. IMS offers a year-round program of intensive meditation retreats and various opportunities for volunteer service.

Joseph Campbell Foundation

New York, New York

www.jcf.org

Joseph Campbell was a famous professor of mythology; Bill Moyers featured him in a PBS series called *The Power of Myth*. Founded in 1990, the foundation explores "a mythopoetic response to contemporary literalism and cultural retrenchment." The foundation preserves, protects, and perpetuates Campbell's work by publishing his books and cataloging his papers and recorded lectures; promotes mythological education; and sponsors conferences, workshops, and seminars.

Kalani Honua Conference and Retreat Center

Pahoa, Hawaii

www.kalani.com

Kalani Honua was founded in 1980 as an intercultural conference center devoted to supporting physical, spiritual, and emotional healing; the arts; and traditional Hawaiian culture. The center is a multicultural, shared living community that presents a spectrum of educational events including workshops, conferences, and retreats.

Kripalu Center for Yoga and Health

Lenox, Massachusetts

www.kripalu.org

Kripalu Center is a nonprofit, volunteer organization founded in 1972. Staff live and work full time at the center, practicing the spiritual teachings of Yoga as modeled and taught by Yogi Amrit Desai, the center's founder. Dedicated to promoting personal and spiritual growth, the center provides humanitarian service and education based on the Yogic principle that harmony of the body and mind are central to inner growth. The center offers programs in Yoga, self-discovery, spiritual attunement and meditation, bodywork, and health and wellness.

Mount Madonna Center

Watsonville, California

www.mountmadonna.org

Mount Madonna Center for the Creative Arts and Sciences is a community designed to nurture the creative arts and the health sciences within a context of spiritual growth. The center is inspired by Baba Hari Dass and is sponsored by the Hanuman Fellowship, a group whose talents and interests are unified by the common practice of Yoga. Personal and group retreats as well as weekend programs are available. The center also maintains a work-study program.

Mountain Light Retreat Center

Crozet, Virginia

www.findthedivine.com/retreatcenter/ml/wedding.html

The center offers services in holistically inspired non-religious celebrations in the Blue Ridge Mountains of Virginia.

New York Open Center
New York, New York
www.opencenter.org

The New York Open Center is a nonprofit holistic learning center that was founded in 1984 by Walter Beebe and Ralph White. Located in Soho downtown Manhattan, the center offers a broad array of programs in all aspects of the emerging spiritual, holistic, and ecological worldview, including a three-year program in integrative therapy for those seeking training in alternative approaches to counseling. Program formats include weekend workshops, ongoing courses, and evening lectures. As a prototype of the urban holistic learning center, the NYOC also offers workshops on how groups can start holistic centers in their own towns or cities.

The North East Directory of Holistic Retreats
www.neholistic.com/Dretreats.htm

This comprehensive guide includes information on retreat centers that are not listed in this book.

Ojai Foundation
Ojai, California
www.ojaifoundation.org

Founded by Joan Halifax, PhD, Ojai offers weekend workshops, group retreats, educational programs, and ceremonies.

The Omega Institute
Rhinebeck, New York
http://eomega.org

The Omega Institute for holistic studies was founded by the Sufi Order of the West 1977 with a handful of participants and a few weekend classes. In 1982, the institute purchased a former summer camp in the rural woodlands of the Hudson Valley, ninety miles outside of New York City. Programs at Omega are varied and include new ideas in health, psychology, family and relationships, the creative arts, sports, spiritual understanding, and global studies. It also sponsors an annual conference.

Pangaia
Hawaii
www.pangaia.cc

This rejuvenating green retreat center is situated on the eastern edge of the volcanic rift zone of Hawaii.

Resources for Ecumenical Spirituality
Mankato, Minnesota
http://resecum.org

Founded in 1987, RES is a Minnesota-based nonprofit organization that fosters mutual understanding among religious faiths through shared spiritual practice and dialogue. It sponsors retreats, colloquia, publications, and other projects related to spiritual practice and study.

Rest of Your Life Retreat
La Vernia, Texas
http://roylretreat.com

Nestled on a crystal clear lake, ROYL provides a peaceful, restful, relaxing, and rejuvenating health center.

The Rim Institute
Phoenix, Arizona
www.well.com/user/dpd/rim.html

The Rim Institute is a research and retreat center specializing in the field of altered consciousness. The center offers retreats, seminars, and workshops in the field.

Rowe Camp and Conference Center
Rowe, Massachusetts
www.rowecenter.com

Rowe was founded in 1973 in the Berkshires of western Massachusetts. It is committed to creating a space where the sacred enters into the everyday, and where personal, social, and spiritual transformation is encouraged and experienced. Most of Rowe's various programs are in the form of weekend workshops.

Satchidananda Ashram-Yogaville
Buckingham, Virginia
www.yogaville.org

Founded in 1979, this spiritual center located in the foothills of the Blue Ridge Mountains in central Virginia sponsors programs, including workshops and retreats, in Hatha Yoga, Raja Yoga, meditation, and vegetarian cooking—all based on the Integral Yoga teachings of Sri Swami Satchidananda, the founder of the Integral Yoga Institute.

Sedona Retreats
Prescott, Flagstaff, and Phoenix, Arizona
www.sedona.net

Sedona offers referrals to hundreds of luxury retreats and spas in the southwestern United States. It also offers restaurant guides, maps, and art galleries for the holistic traveler.

Sevenoaks Pathwork Center

Phoenicia, New York

www.sevenoakspathwork.org

Pathwork is a spiritual path of purification and transformation concerned with self-responsibility, self-knowledge, and self-acceptance. The practice is based on 258 lectures given over twenty years by a spirit entity known as the Guide and transmitted through Eva Pierrakos. The Sevenoaks Center, formerly the Phoenicia Center, is the largest of a number of Pathwork communities around the world.

Southern Dharma Retreat Center

Hot Springs, North Carolina

www.southerndharma.org

Southern Dharma Retreat Center, founded in 1978, is a nonprofit foundation whose purpose is to offer silent group meditation retreats led by teachers from a variety of spiritual paths. The center is located in the North Carolina mountains about an hour from Asheville.

Spirit Rock Center

Woodacre, California

www.spiritrock.org

Spirit Rock Center offers insight meditation retreats that are designed for both beginning and experienced mediators. The center is nonsectarian, although the ethics and traditions of Buddhist psychology offer guidance. Advisors include the Venerable Thich Nhat Hanh, Ram Dass, and Stanislav and Christina Grof.

Tai Sophia Wellness School

Laurel, Massachusetts

www.tai.edu

From a small healing arts clinic founded in 1975, Tai Sophia Institute has grown to become a preeminent academic institution for wellness-based education, clinical care, research, and public policy discourse.

Taos Institute

Taos, New Mexico

www.taosinstitute.net

The Taos Institute is a center for dialogue, inquiry, and consultation aimed at achieving more humane and ecologically viable forms of relationship: from the level of daily intimacies, to local communities and organizations, and onward to the global community. The institute offers conferences, consulting, and workshops.

Temenos at Broad Run Conference and Retreat Center

West Chester, Pennsylvania

www.temenosretreat.org

Established in 1986, Temenos is a service of the Swedenborgian Church. Temenos sponsors programs for psychological and spiritual growth directed toward integration of body, mind, and spirit. Regular offerings include healing arts, dream sharing, family relationships and communication, couples retreats, creative expression, inner child work, holotropic breathwork, world community, creation spirituality, universal peace dances, and Swedenborgian spiritual perspectives.

Tree of Life Rejuvenation Center

Center Patagonia, Arizona

www.treeoflife.nu

This beautiful retreat center in the Arizona mountains occupies 166 acres south of Tucson. Organic gardens contribute to the gourmet, organic, kosher, vegetarian, live-food cuisine created and prepared by its innovative chefs. It also offers several self-healing courses and retreats, which empower participants to take responsibility for their healing and awakened living.

Vallecitos Mountain Refuge

Santa Fe, New Mexico

www.vallecitos.org

Vallecitos, established by Grove T. Burnett and Linda M. Verlarde, is dedicated to awakening and cultivating the spiritual dimension of environmental and social activism. Applicants must have at least ten years of experience as an activist and the endorsement of the organization that employs them or with which they work closely. Accepted applicants are awarded full fellowships. Vallecitos has held an annual mediation retreat for environmental leaders since 1994.

GENERAL AND INTERNATIONAL RESOURCES

This chapter is also dedicated to general and international holistic organizations that do not belong to a specific practice. For consideration in the next edition, please e-mail: updates@ thehunterpress.com

ORGANIZATIONS

American Academy of Environmental Medicine
www.aaemonline.org

The AAEM was founded in 1965 and is an international association of physicians and other professionals interested in expanding our understanding of individuals and their environment.

The American Anthropological Association
www.aaanet.org

The AAA is an interdisciplinary organization concerned with cross-cultural experimental, experiential, and theoretical approaches to the study of consciousness. The primary areas of interest include: states of consciousness, religion, possession, trance, and dissociative states; ethnographic studies of shamanistic, mediumistic, mystical, and related traditions; indigenous healing practices; linguistic, philosophical, social, and symbolic studies of consciousness phenomena; and psychic (psi) phenomena, including their roles in traditional cultural practices and applications such as in psychic archaeology. It publishes the newsletter *Anthropology of Consciousness.*

American Association of Integrative Medicine
www.aaimedicine.com

The AAIM was founded to establish a network of related integrative health care providers to disseminate information. Its membership group is a vast network of holistic practitioners from many different systems of healing. It facilitates diplomat programs, continuing education, conferences, newsletters, and general resources links.

American Board of Integrative Holistic Medicine
www.holisticboard.org

The ABIHM, founded in 1996, seeks to establish and maintain the highest standards of medical care, ignite and sustain the joy and passion of physicians in their work, establish the role of unconditional love as the basis of healing and support, and recognize the importance of the health of the planet as integral to human health. The intention of this process is the transformation of medical systems toward holism, by combining science and compassion.

The American College for the Advancement of Holistic Medicine
www.acamnet.org

The ACAM is a not-for-profit association dedicated to educating physicians and other health care professionals on the latest researching findings and methods in complementary medicine. While the ACAM has specific programs for holistic MDs and nurses, it is an excellent resource the holistic practitioner. It represents more than 1,000 physicians in thirty countries.

The American Holistic Health Association
Anaheim, California
http://ahha.org

Formed in 1989, the AHHA was the amalgamation of two national holistic medical associations. It encourages practitioners to incorporate holistic health care into their practices. Besides being an active membership organization and offering useful articles about the benefits of self-help, the AHHA is a networking organization for geographically specified holistic member associations.

American Humanist Association
www.americanhumanist.org

The AHA promotes naturalistic humanism, a philosophy which holds that human beings determine the moral principles by which they live. The AHA publishes *The Humanist*, a bimonthly magazine of critical inquiry and social commentary, and *Free Mind*, the association membership magazine.

The Association for Integrity in Medicine
www.integrityinmedicine.org

As a 501c6 nonprofit lobby organization, AIM advocates on behalf of integrative health services and medicine through greater accountability, standards, professionalism, and education.

Bioneers

www.bioneers.org

Formerly the Collective Heritage Institute, Bioneers were founded in 1990. It represents a union of scientists and social innovators who have demonstrated visionary and practical models for restoring the Earth through environmental restoration and social work. It holds a large consumer-oriented conference.

The Bravewell Collaborative

www.bravewell.org

The Bravewell Collaborative organizes community philanthropists dedicated to advancing integrative medicine. It supports several holistic boards and associations. The Bravewell clinical network includes eight members: the Scripps Center for Integrative Medicine, the Continuum Center for Health and Healing, the Duke Center for Integrative Medicine at Duke University, the Jefferson-Myrna Brind Center for Integrative Medicine at Thomas Jefferson Medical College, the Center for Integrative Medicine at the University of Maryland School of Medicine, the Osher Center for Integrative Medicine at the University of California, the Alliance Institute for Integrative Medicine, and the Institute for Health and Healing at Abbott Northwestern Hospital.

California Pacific Medical Center

www.cpmc.org

As affiliate of Sutter Health, CPMC is one of the most progressive integrative clinics in California and the United States.

The Center for Mind-Body Medicine

www.cmbm.org

The CMBM is a nonprofit educational organization dedicated to reviving the spirit of medicine. The center is working to create a more effective, comprehensive, and compassionate model of health care and health education. Its model combines the precision of modern science with the wisdom of the world's healing traditions to help health professionals heal themselves, their patients and clients, and their communities. The center offers professional training and certification in several different healing modalities.

Cochrane CAM Field

www.compmed.umm.edu/cochrane.asp

A division of the University of Maryland School Of Medicine, Cochraine CAM Field was founded in 1996 and is an international group of individuals dedicated to facilitating the production of systematic reviews of clinical trials in holistic arts such as: acupuncture, massage, chiropractic, herbal medicine, homeopathy, and body-mind therapy. It is an entity of a larger network, the Cochrane Collaboration.

Consortium of Academic Health Centers for Integrative Medicine

www.imconsortium.org

The Consortium of Academic Health Centers for Integrative Medicine is supported by membership dues and grants from philanthropic partners including the Bravewell Collaborative for Integrative Medicine. Its membership currently includes forty-one highly esteemed academic medical centers. Many of the consortium's academic medical centers also offer clinical services.

The Continuum Center for Health and Healing

www.healthandhealingny.org

An initiative of Beth Israel Medical Center, the center offers an expanded practice of health care and educational offerings in the areas of wellness and prevention.

Cuyamungue Institute

www.cuyamungueinstitute.com/

Cuyamungue offers certification courses in dance and movement therapy, among other integrative topics.

The Eagle Connection

www.theeagleconnection.com

The Eagle Connection is an alliance of organizations and individuals working for personal, communal, and global transformation through a cross-cultural and spiritual exploration. Founding co-directors Jo Imlay and John Broomfield, PhD, disseminate information about individuals and groups developing imaginative holistic solutions to critical educational, social, economic, health, and environmental problems. They also teach workshops on these topics throughout North America. Membership is by subscription to its bimonthly newsletter *Eagle Connector*.

The EarthSpirit Community

www.earthspirit.com

The ESC is a Boston-based collective that coordinates a nationwide network of people following earth-centered spiritual paths. Members' spiritual practices are rooted in the ancient traditions of pagan, pre-Christian Europe that have at their core a respectful awareness of the sacredness of our planet.

Elsevier Journals

www.us.elsevierhealth.com/index.jsp

Elsevier is a leading publisher of health and science books and journals. Titles are available in print or online through its Web site.

Environmental Health News

www.environmentalhealthnews.org

This news archive is published daily by Environmental Health Sciences, a not-for-profit organization founded in 2002 to help increase public understanding of emerging scientific links between environmental exposures and human health.

The Federation of Therapeutic Massage, Bodywork, and Somatic Practice Organizations

Since 1991, this nonprofit membership organization has been a primary networking tool for professionals in the areas of massage, bodywork, and somatic practice. It recognizes the vast differences between the professions and emphasizes open communication between practitioners of different holistic therapies.

Four Winds Institute

www.fourwindsinstitute.org

The purpose of the Four Winds Institute is to stimulate and encourage personal growth and transformation. The institute's four areas of study include creativity, balance, the feminine, and listening. It has no religious affiliation.

Georgetown University CAM Masters Program

http://camprogram.georgetown.edu

This newly introduced master's program through Georgetown University can be completed in one year.

Healthopedia

www.healthopedia.com

A consumer information center resource for information on mental and physical illness, medications, and various other health topics.

Hippocrates Health Institute

www.hippocratesinst.com

This school is credited by Spa Management Group as being a top-tier teaching center. For a half of a century, the institute has taught generations how to access inner resources to transform quality of life through various programs and workshops.

Institute for Complementary and Alternative Medicine Newsletter

www.umdnj.edu/icam/newsletter/index.htm

A newsletter published through the University of Medicine and Dentistry of New Jersey. Topics covered range from ancient ayurveda techniques to current research in integrative therapy.

Interspecies Communication

www.interspecies.com

IC was founded in 1978 to promote human communication with animals (especially dolphins and whales) through music, art, and ceremony. Its methods consist of integrating the arts and the sciences with a strong emphasis on environmental preservation. It publishes a newsletter.

The John E. Mack Institute

www.johnemackinstitute.org

The institute, formerly the Center for Psychology and Social Change, works with community and corporate leaders, parents, educators, social planners, and journalists to promote a new consciousness as a means of changing human behavior and to define a new psychology for sustainability. It is interested in exploring the role human consciousness plays in building a sustainable world peace. The institute is affiliated with the Harvard Medical School at Cambridge Hospital and publishes the newsletter *CenterPiece*.

LifeSpan Medicine

www.lifespanmedicine.com

The LifeSpan program is a lifestyle, a "pathway to optimum health and function for the future." At this integrative clinic, a team of physicians analyzes your health and develops a custom, integrative treatment program.

The Lindisfarne Association

www.williamirwinthompson.org/lindisfarne.html

Lindisfarne is an association of individuals devoted to the study and realization of a new planetary culture. Lindisfarne brings together religious leaders, scientists, ecologists, architects, artists, and business people to enjoy the creative work of imagining and building a new world culture. Although its headquarters is located at the Episcopal Cathedral Church of St. John the Divine, the Lindisfarne Association is a nondenominational and independent, not-for-profit, educational corporation. The association offers conferences, concerts, lectures, exhibitions, poetry readings, and public workshops. It supports a publishing house (The Lindisfarne Press), a newsletter (*Annals of Earth*), and the Lindisfarne Mountain retreat center.

Menninger Clinic

www.menningerclinic.com

The Menninger Clinic is one of the most innovative international psychiatric and holistic treatment centers in the world.

The National Center for Complementary and Alternative Medicine

http://nccam.nih.gov

Funded by the U.S. Government and part of the National Institutes of Health, NCCAM offers grants to researchers and provides Congress and citizens with statistics on the most popular CAM modalities.

Natural Standard

www.naturalstandards.com

This organization was founded by clinicians and researchers to provide high-quality, evidence-based information about CAM therapies. This growing effort incorporates more than one hundred eminent academic institutions.

Our Ultimate Investment

www.children-ourinvestment.org

This nonprofit organization, founded in 1977 by Laura Huxley (spouse to Aldous Huxley), educates and informs the public about scientific research and humanistic ideals of human potential.

Physicians for Social Responsibility

www.psr.org

PSR is a group of physicians who lend their voice and authority to environmental issues such as global warming and toxic degradation of our environment.

Regenerate Design Institute

http://www.regenerativedesign.org

RDI is a nonprofit education organization with a vision that "people can live in a mutually enhancing relationship with the earth." It hosts several conferences, retreats, and seminars throughout the year on many different holistic techniques. The retreats usually emphasize green, sustainable living.

SaluGenectics Inc.

www.salugenecists.com

SaluGenecists create innovative, smart tools that assist individuals, practitioners, employers, and insurance companies to fundamentally change health care and break the vicious cycle of declining health and spiraling health care costs. Their tools provide personalized guidance to help target and reverse each individual's specific underlying causes of ill health and effectively promote wellness.

Science and Environmental Health Network

www.sehn.org

SEHN was founded in 1994 by a consortium of North American environmental organizations concerned about the misuse of science in ways that failed to protect the environment and human health. Granted not-for-profit status in 1999, SEHN operates as a virtual organization, currently with six staff and seven board members working from locations across the United States. Since 1998, SEHN has been the leading proponent of the Precautionary Principle as a new basis for environmental and public health policy.

Scripps Health

www.scripps.org

Scripps Health is a progressive, forward-thinking, not-for-profit, community-based health care delivery network that includes four acute-care hospitals on five campuses, more than 2,300 affiliated physicians, an extensive ambulatory care network, home health care, and associated support services. As a result of the July 2000 reaffiliation with Scripps Clinic, Scripps Health now has approximately 11,000 employees and also cares for patients at thirteen clinics throughout San Diego County.

Spa Trade Resources

http://www.spatrade.com/resources/index.phtml?act=associations

Spa Trade is a buyer's guide for spa owners and workers. Its resources section contains a directory of spa associations in the United States.

Teleosis Institute

www.teleosis.org

Teleosis is devoted to developing effective, sustainable health care provided by professionals who serve as environmental health stewards. It publishes a journal (*Symbiosis*) and has membership programs for green-minded practitioners to network with others.

Upledger Institute

www.upledger.com

The Upledger Institute is a holistic hospital and training center for an assortment of body-oriented healing modalities (such as craniosacral therapy and lymphatic drainage). This cutting-edge institution is at the forefront of integrative medicine. It employs more than 2,000 instructors.

The University of Arizona Program in Integrative Medicine

http://www.integrativemedicine.arizona.edu

Founded by the now famous Dr. Andrew Weil, the program is administered through the University of Arizona's School of Medicine. The mission of the program is to lead the transformation of the health care community by creating and supporting an active contingent of professionals who embody the practice of integrative medicine. Those interested in becoming an MD should look into this program and its resources before applying to medical school.

INTERNATIONAL RESOURCES

The Collaborative on Health and the Environment

www.healthandenvironment.org

The CHE is a diverse network of 2,900 individual and organizational partners in forty-five countries and forty-eight states who seek to address the link between human health and environmental factors.

Green Guide for Health Care

www.gghc.org

The Green Guide for Health Care is a best practice guide for healthy and sustainable building design, construction, and operations for the health care industry.

Health Care Without Harm

www.hcwh.org

HCWH is a global coalition of 473 organizations in more than fifty countries working to protect health by reducing pollution in the health care sector (i.e., mercury in hospital settings).

International Alliance of Healthcare Educators

www.iahe.com

Formed in 1996, IAHE is a coalition of health care instructors and curricula developers united to advance innovative therapies through high-quality continuing education programs. Each year it coordinates hundreds of workshops worldwide.

International Association for Near-Death Studies

www.iands.org

IANDS is the world's only organization devoted to scientifically grounded exploration of the "near-death experience." Representing five continents, its membership includes researchers and professionals interested in near-

death experience. It publishes the quarterly *Journal of Near-Death Studies* and sponsors a conference.

International Society for Scientific Exploration

www.scientificexploration.org

The ISSE is interested in the discussion and research of anomalous phenomena that lie outside the conventional disciplines of science. Most members are professional PhD and MD researchers in fields such as physics, astronomy, chemistry, biological sciences, engineering, and medicine. The society publishes the *Journal of Scientific Exploration*.

The International Spa Association

www.experienceispa.com/ISPA/

Created in 1991, ISPA is the leading professional voice of the institutional spa industry worldwide. It represents more than 3,000 health and wellness facilities and providers in seventy-five countries. It follows cutting-edge spas that are taking a more wellness, integrative approach.

Millennium Institute

www.millenniuminstitute.net

Formally called the Institute for 21st Century Studies, the Millennium Institute is a nonprofit organization founded in 1983 to promote long term integrated global thinking. Its programs construct frameworks for action by nourishing a worldwide network of individuals and organizations.

Practice Greenhealth

www.h2e-online.org

H2E is based on a vision of an environmentally aware and engaged health care community dedicated to the health of patients, workers, communities, and the global environment.

GEOGRAPHICAL INDEX

ALPHABETICAL INDEX

ACKNOWLEDGMENTS

Middlebury College senior Aaron Krivitzky was the backstop of this book, providing many first drafts, which were developed into chapters. He singlehandedly researched and authored the resource sections of the book. His performance suggests that he has taken a big step toward becoming the professional writer he aspires to become. Best of luck and thanks for your thoughtful, diligent efforts.

A handful of subject experts generously provided input when asked, notably Janet Kahn, PhD; Joseph Pizzorno, ND; and Karta Purkh Singh Khalsa.

Parts of this book were developed from the original *Common Boundary Graduate Education Guide,* which the author cowrote with publisher Charles Simpkinson, PhD, in Bethesda, Maryland, during the mid-1990s.

Finally, I would like to thank my many teachers, professors, and mentors over the years, who fueled my passion for learning and planted the seeds for an integral vision of my own.

ABOUT THE AUTHORS

DOUGLAS "LAS" WENGELL, MBA, has been an active participant in holistic health care for more than a decade, authoring a similar book while pursuing health psychology in his twenties. Growing up in Northern California, he embraced many aspects of the human potential movement, including exposure to East-West thinkers, humanistic psychology, integrative medicine, health and wellness, and the fine arts. He has been a practitioner of Raja Yoga since his teenage years. Las's expertise extends into the realms of ethics and environmental economics, philosophy, psychology, entrepreneurship, the Internet, and e-commerce. He studied rhetoric and philosophy at Rutgers (BA, *magna cum laude*), somatic and health psychology at San Francisco State, and entrepreneurship and finance at Emory (MBA).

He is the founder and CEO of Know Your Source, a distributor of transparent supplies to health care providers; the founder of the Association for Integrity in Medicine, a 501c6 nonprofit dedicated to integral health care reform; and the founder of The Hunter Press, devoted to a broad range of current affairs in the natural and social sciences.

NATHEN GABRIEL, ND, was trained as a naturopathic doctor at Bastyr University and consults on lifestyle and addiction in Southern California. He has extensive training in ayurveda, herbology, and positive psychology. He's been a practitioner of Raja Yoga for more than twenty five years. He also has a degree in holistic health education from John F. Kennedy University.

ADAM PERLMAN, MD, MPH, FACP, is the executive director for the Institute for Complementary and Alternative Medicine at the University of Medicine and Dentistry of New Jersey, where he is an assistant professor of medicine. In 2004, he was named the UMDNJ Endowed Professor in Complementary and Alternative Medicine.

His scholarly activities include numerous grants and publications. He was guest editor of the Complementary and Alternative Medicine volume of *Medical Clinics of North America,* as well as associate editor for the Complementary and Alternative Medicine section of the *Physician Information and Education Resource,* developed by the American College of Physicians and American Society for Internal Medicine.

Dr. Perlman received his BA from Tufts University and his MD from Boston University School of Medicine. He completed residencies in both internal medicine and preventive medicine at Boston Medical Center, as well as a general medicine research fellowship and master's of public health with a concentration in biostatistics and epidemiology from the Boston University School of Public Health. Dr. Perlman is the father of five children. He is a fifth-degree black belt and an instructor in martial arts, which he began practicing in 1982 and credits with spurring his interest in complementary medicine.

CONTINUE THE CONVERSATION ONLINE
JOIN THE KNOW YOUR SOURCE PRACTITIONER SOCIAL NETWORK!

knowyoursource

A mindful supplier to integrative health practitioners

COMMERCE • COMMUNITY • EDUCATION • ADVOCACY

knowyoursource.com

The Practitioner Social Network is FREE!

Here's what you can do on the Practitioner Social Network:

- Maintain your profile page, including your practice, philosophy, and personal blog
- Post your profile for prospective clients to view on knowyourhealer.net
- Review or post to the give-and-take community bulletin board
- Contact and network with complementary practitioners to your practice
- And more!

In addition, Know Your Source offers:

- Transparent, eco-oriented supplies for your practice
- Product reviews—read them and/or write your own
- Expert Ambassadors
- And more!

See you online. In good health.

Douglas "Las" Wengell, Founder/CEO
Know Your Source